RAPID
INTERPRETATION
OF
EKG's

... an interactive course

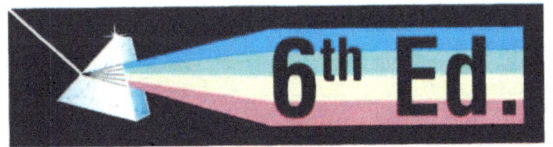

by
Dale Dubin, MD
Kiatoadec

Rapid Interpretation of EKG's

ISBN: 9798386910785   Paperback

1965 -1966 Hand-typed with freehand illustrations, unbound sheets as a course.

Initial Bound Ed. Copyright © 1967
numerous printings through 1968

First Edition Copyright © 1969
first printing, Janurary, 1969
second printing, May, 1970
third printing, July, 1970
fourth printing, October, 1970

Second Edition Copyright © 1971
fifth printing, February, 1971
sixth printing, May, 1971
seventh printing, July, 1971
eighth printing, November, 1971
ninth printing, March, 1972
tenth printing, May, 1972
eleventh printing, August, 1972
twelfth printing, November, 1972
thirteenth printing, April, 1973
fourteenth printing, December, 1973
fifteenth printing, June, 1974

Third Edition Copyright © 1974
sixteenth printing, October, 1974
seventeenth printing, February, 1975
eighteenth printing, August, 1975
nineteenth printing, April, 1976
twentieth printing, December, 1976
twenty-first printing, July, 1977
twenty-second printing, January, 1978
twenty-third printing, October, 1978
twenty-fourth printing, May, 1979
twenty-fifth printing, February, 1980
twenty-sixth printing, October, 1980
twenty-seventh printing, May, 1981
twenty-eighth printing, February, 1982
twenty-ninth printing, September, 1982
thirtieth printing, June, 1983
thirty-first printing, October, 1983
thirty-second printing, August, 1984
thirty-third printing, October, 1985
thirty-fourth printing, November, 1986
thirty-fifth printing, December, 1987
thirty-sixth printing, April, 1988
thirty-seventh printing, December, 1988

Fourth Edition Copyright © 1989
thirty-eighth printing, February, 1989

thirty-ninth printing, September, 1989
fortieth printing, March, 1990
forty-first printing, December, 1991
forty-second printing, July, 1993
forty-third printing, October, 1994

Fifth Edition Copyright © 1996
forty-fourth printing, February, 1996
forty-fifth printing, November, 1996
forty-sixth printing, March, 1997
forty-seventh printing, April, 1998
forty-eighth printing, October, 1999
forty-ninth printing, December, 1999

Sixth Edition Copyright © 2000
fiftieth printing, March, 2000
fifty-first printing, August, 2004
fifty-second printing, March, 2005
fifty-third printing, July, 2005
fifty-fourth printing, February, 2006
fifty-fifth printing, July, 2006
fifty-sixth printing, November, 2006
fifty-seventh printing, March, 2007
fifty-eighth printing, October, 2007
fifty-ninth printing, March, 2008
sixtieth printing, July, 2008
sixty-first printing, September, 2008
sixty-second printing, June, 2009
sixty-third printing, July, 2009
sixty-fourth printing, November, 2009
sixty-fifth printing, July, 2010
sixty-sixth printing, October, 2010
sixty-seventh printing, March, 2011
sixty-eighth printing, July, 2011
sixty-ninth printing, October, 2011
seventieth printing, June, 2012
seventy-first printing, August, 2013
seventy-second printing, October, 2013
seventy-third printing, May, 2014
seventy-fourth printing, July, 2014
seventy-fifth printing, December, 2014
seventy-sixth printing, April, 2015
seventy-seventh printing, August, 2015
seventy-eighth printing, May, 2016
seventy-ninth printing, December, 2016
eightieth printing, June, 2017
eighty-first printing, January, 2018
eighty-second printing, August, 2018
eighty-third printing, July, 2019
eighty-fourth printing, March, 2020

International Availability of *Rapid Interpretation of EKG's*

Rapid Interpretation of EKG's has been the international best seller for over fifty years. It is printed in 46 foreign language editions, which are available through publishers in most countries.

Our internet sites provide valuable, practical information on electrocardiography and cardiac monitors. Specific presentations are designed for each of three medical disciplines on the internet web sites.

The English edition of *Rapid Interpretation of EKG's*, now updated with each printing, is available internationally through the internet. Our three internet sites provide efficient book fulfillment to any location worldwide. Books can be ordered from any country with a major credit card. The internet sites provide foreign currency conversion information for instant value determination in all mediums of exchange.

Dedication

To those from whom I have learned:

Dr. George C. Griffith

Dr. Willard J. Zinn

Dr. Henry J. L. Marriott

Dr. Charles Fish

Dr. Suzanne Knoeble

Dr. William L. Martz

Dr. Nathan Marcus

Dr. Richard G. Connar

Dr. Jose Dominguez

Dr. Louis Cimino

Dr. David Baumann

Dr. Dale Dubin

Acknowledgments

With humility and gratitude, I acknowledge my indebtedness:

To God for the inspiration and for my persistent survival in spite of deadly warning shots. I do understand.

To all my mentors from whom I have learned principles of electrocardiography.

To all my family, living and deceased.

To my computer graphics guru Paul Heinrich, whose knowledge of computer science and graphic artistry made this 6th edition a beautiful reality.

And to my publisher, COVER Publishing Company, for their great understanding and cooperation. My association with the publisher represents the closest possible concert between author and publisher.

Some computer graphic illustrations utilize portions of *LifeART* clip art.

Table of Contents

Congratulations!

You are joining a coterie of knowledgeable medical professionals. *Rapid Interpretation of EKG's*, for over forty-five years the best seller in the US, has also educated millions of people around the world in 46 foreign languages.

Updated and refined with each of seventy printings, this classic text is now the most current and most referenced medical resource in the field.

But, for the understanding that is vital to your future, your personal success depends on certain subtle instructions in the book.

If advised to:

• "Review certain previous illustrations"… Do it! There's an important reason.

• "Place index tabs on certain pages"… This is necessary for your understanding.

• "Return to reread a specific page"… Respond willingly, without hesitation.

• "Study a chapter's summary *before* reading the chapter"… Preview it.

Your commitment to these details will reward you with **understanding** that ensures a lifetime of practical **knowledge**.

about sharing your knowledge…

My most sincere thanks to those persons, worldwide, who continue to send EKG tracings*. I am truly grateful. However, the number of people donating tracings has grown exponentially, making the publication of their names (as I've done previously) virtually impossible.

All of you will observe both classical and unusual tracings that should be preserved (use a copier, because EKG tracings tend to fade with time) for teaching purposes. Sharing this very special knowledge with others is a time-honored medical tradition.

This spirit of unselfish sharing of your knowledge continues to improve the level of care in this crucial medical discipline.

—DD

---

* I enthusiastically collect and study 12 lead EKG's, strips of classical and unusual tracings, and even those rolls of "code" tracings that are usually discarded. They may be sent to me via the publisher, COVER, Inc., P.O. Box 07037, Fort Myers, FL 33919. I regret that I cannot acknowledge all tracings. This rescued trash is an invaluable treasured resource; please know that it is appreciated!

"To make a great dream come true, the first requirement is a great capacity to dream; the second is persistence – a faith in the dream."

Hans Selye, MD

Most teachers are knowledgable.
Good teachers are intelligent.
Great teachers are patient.
Exceptional teachers are students themselves.
D.D.

Before you begin…

First, read the caption and associate it with the simplified illustration.

Master the concept. Your comprehension is important.

Then, carefully read the interactive text, filling in each blank as you go.

- If you need to return to the illustration, that's even better… because each time you review an illustration, the visual image becomes more indelibly impressed in your memory.

- Interactive (programmed) instruction assures UNDERSTANDING by employing visual imagery to explain and link important concepts. Understanding is the key to lasting knowledge…

… and it's enjoyable because it is entertaining audience participation. You are the audience, and I'm right here with you, highlighting your progress with helpful "Notes."

Let's have some fun!

"Lasting knowledge results from understanding."

Happy Learning,

Dale Dubin, MD

Chapter 1: Basic Principles

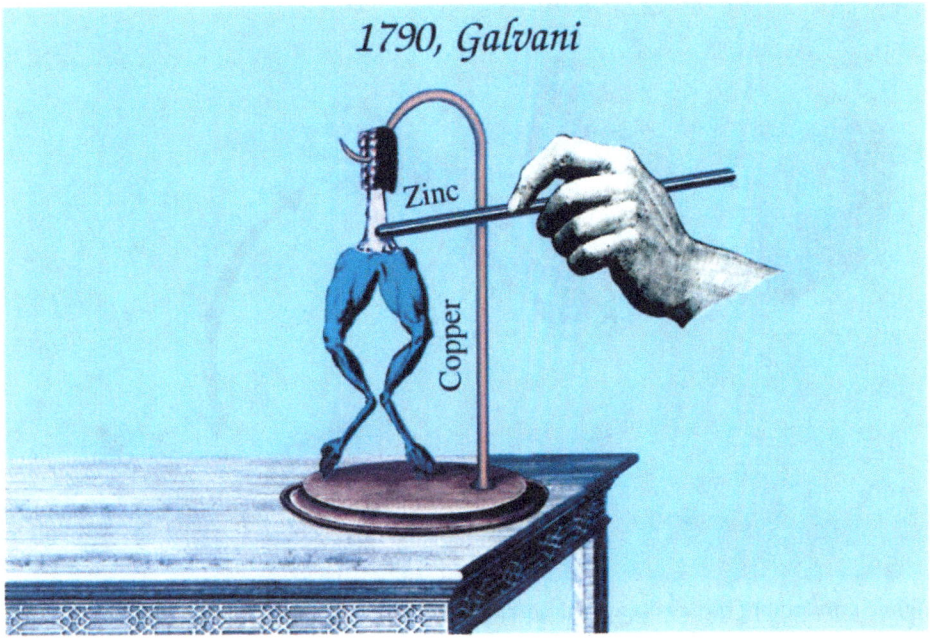

In 1790, an audience of usually sedate scientists gasped in disbelief as Luigi Galvani, with a flare of showmanship, made a dead frog's legs dance by electrical stimulation.

Galvani knew that completing a circuit connecting dissimilar metals to the legs of a recently deceased frog would create a stimulating _____ current.   electrical

The resulting electrical current would stimulate the frog's legs to jump, and with repeated stimuli he could make them _____.   dance

Note: But in those times, bringing a dead frog "back to life" was a shocking and ghastly "supernatural" feat. (And Galvani loved it!)*

* Get yourself a warm cup of coffee, relax and enjoy...
   the rest is just as easy and entertaining.

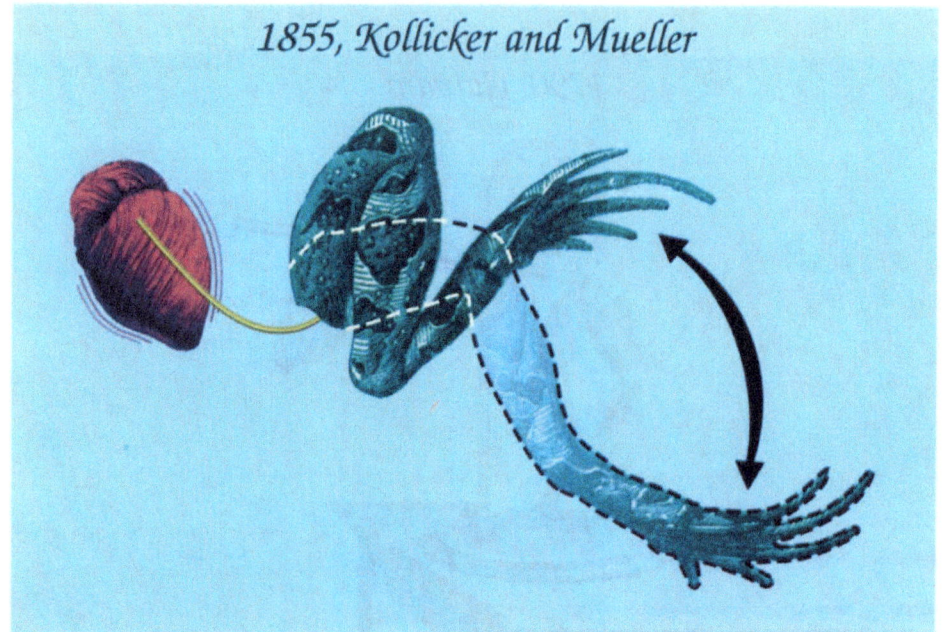

1855, Kollicker and Mueller

While conducting basic research around 1855, Kollicker and Mueller found that when a motor nerve to a frog's leg was laid over its isolated beating heart, the leg kicked with each heartbeat.

"Eureka!" they thought, "the same electrical stimulus that causes a frog's leg to kick must cause the heart to _____."   beat

So it was logical for them to assume that the beating of the heart must be due to a rhythmic discharge of _____ stimuli.   electrical

Note: And thus an association between the rhythmic pumping of the heart and electrical phenomena was scientifically established. Very basic and very important.

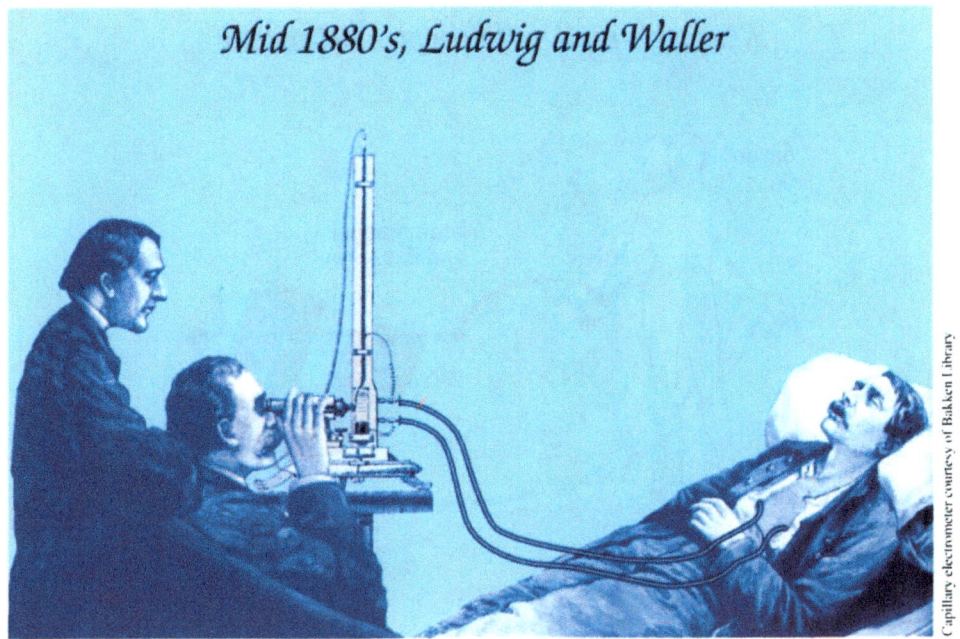

Mid 1880's, Ludwig and Waller

In the mid 1880's, while using a "capillary electrometer," Ludwig and Waller discovered that the heart's rhythmic electrical stimuli could be monitored from a person's skin.

This apparatus consisted of sensor electrodes that were placed on a man's _____ and connected to a Lippman capillary electrometer, which used a capillary tube in an electric field to detect faint electrical activity.

skin

The fluid level in the capillary tube moved with the rhythm of the subject's _____-beat… very interesting.

heart

This apparatus was a little too unsophisticated for clinical application, or even for economic exploitation, but it was _____ interesting.

very

Note: This momentous achievement opened the door for recording the heart's electrical activity from skin surfaces.

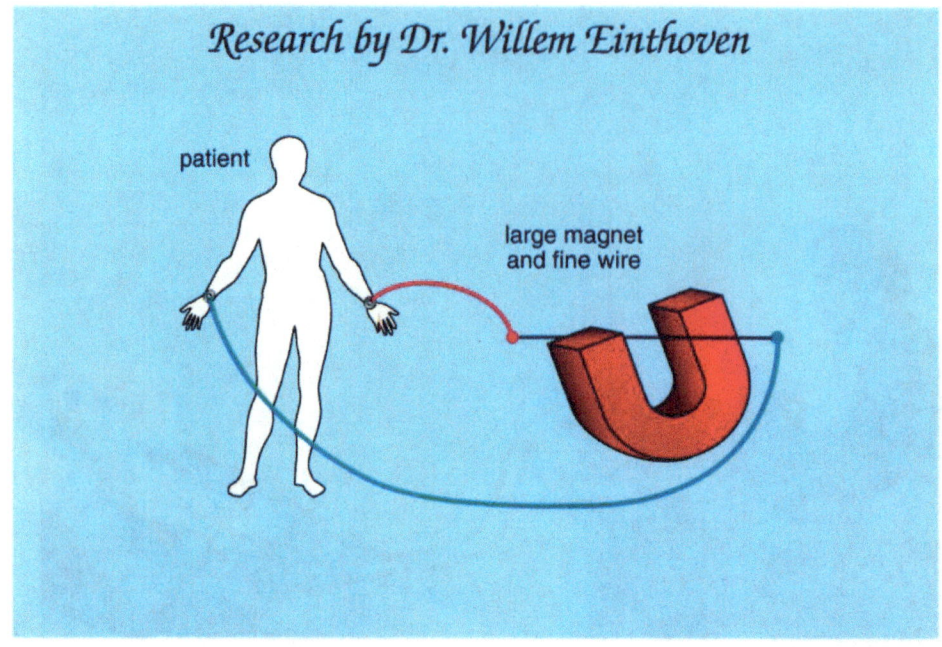

Enter Dr. Willem Einthoven, a brilliant scientist who suspended a silvered wire between the poles of a magnet.

Two skin sensors (electrodes) placed on a man were then connected to the ends of the silvered wire, which ran between the two poles of the _____.   magnet

The silvered _____ (in the magnetic field)   wire
twitched to the rhythm of the subject's heartbeat.

This was also very interesting, but _____   Einthoven
wanted a timed record.

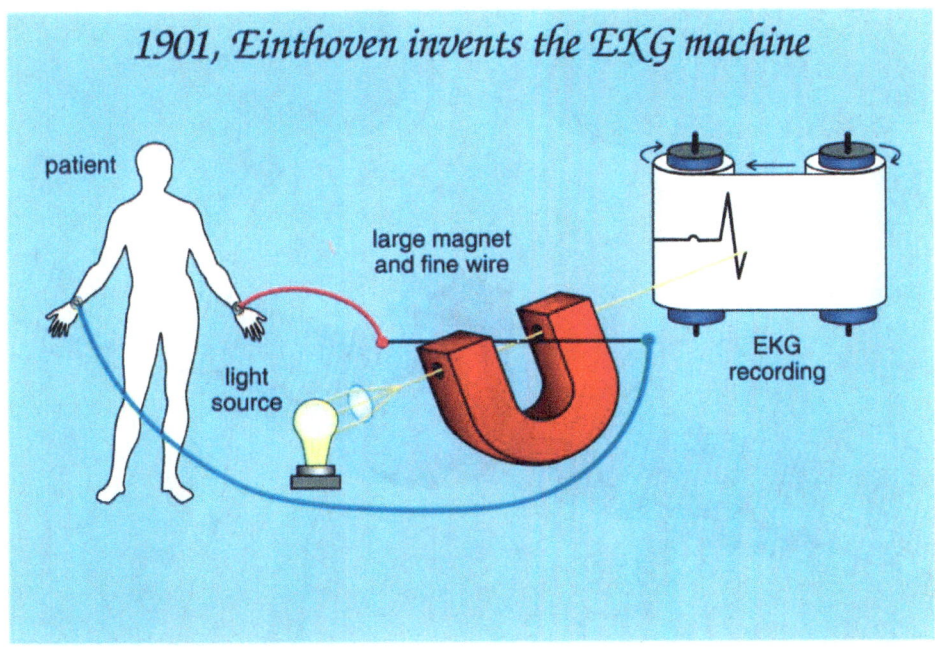

So Einthoven projected a tiny light beam through holes in the magnet's poles, across the twitching silvered wire. The wire's rhythmic movements were recorded as *waves* (that he named P, QRS, and T) on a moving scroll of photographic paper.

Very clever, that Einthoven! The _____ rhythmic movements of the wire (representing the heartbeat) created a bouncing shadow…

… that was recorded as a _____ series rhythmic of distinct waves in repeating cycles.

He named the waves of each cycle (alphabetically) P, QRS, and ____.   T

Note: "Now," thought the clever Einthoven, "we can record a heart's *abnormal* electrical activity… and compare it to the normal." And thus a great diagnostic tool, his "electrokardiogram" (Electro**K**ardioGram), evolved around 1901. Let's see how it works…

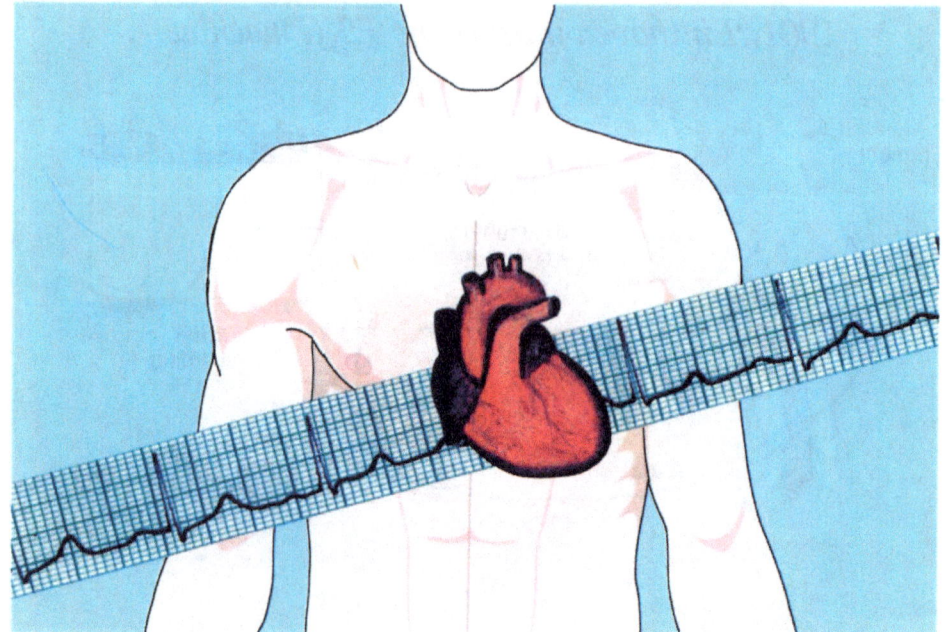

The **electrocardiogram** (EKG) records the electrical activity of the heart, providing a record of cardiac electrical activity, as well as valuable information about the heart's function and structure.

The electrocardiogram is known by the three letters _____;   EKG
it provides us with a record of cardiac electrical activity and
valuable information about the heart's function and structure.

Note: Since the time of Einthoven's "electrokardiogram," the medical
profession has used the letters EKG to represent the electrocardiogram.
Some say that "ECG" is more correct, and you may see it used in some
texts. However, Medicine honors tradition, and EKG has been used for
years. Also, ECG sounds like EEG (the brain wave recording), and this
can cause misunderstanding and confusion.

The EKG is inscribed on a ruled paper strip that gives
us a permanent _____ of cardiac activity and the   record
health status of the heart. Cardiac monitors and cardiac
telemetry provide the same information in real time.

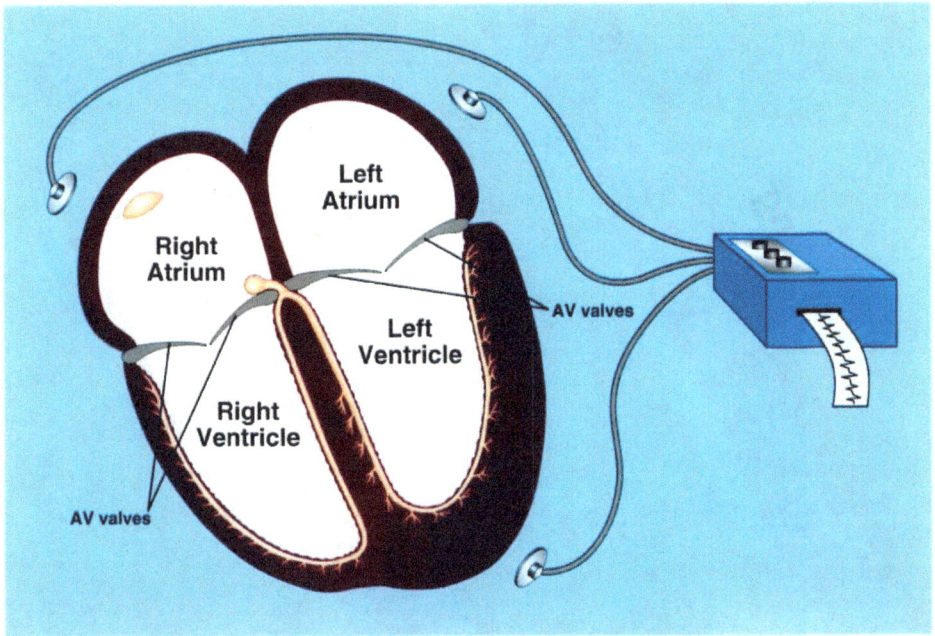

The EKG records the electrical activity of contraction of the heart muscle ("myocardium").

The information recorded on the EKG represents the heart's
_____ activity.   electrical

Most of the information on the EKG represents electrical
activity of _____ of the myocardium.   contraction

Note: The EKG also yields valuable information about the
heart's rate and rhythm.

When the myocardium (*cardium* = heart, *myo* = muscle)
is electrically stimulated, it _____.   contracts

Note: This illustration is intended to familiarize you with the
simplified cross-section of the heart and the (closed) AV valves.
The chambers are identified, and you should know them, for this
diagram will be used often.

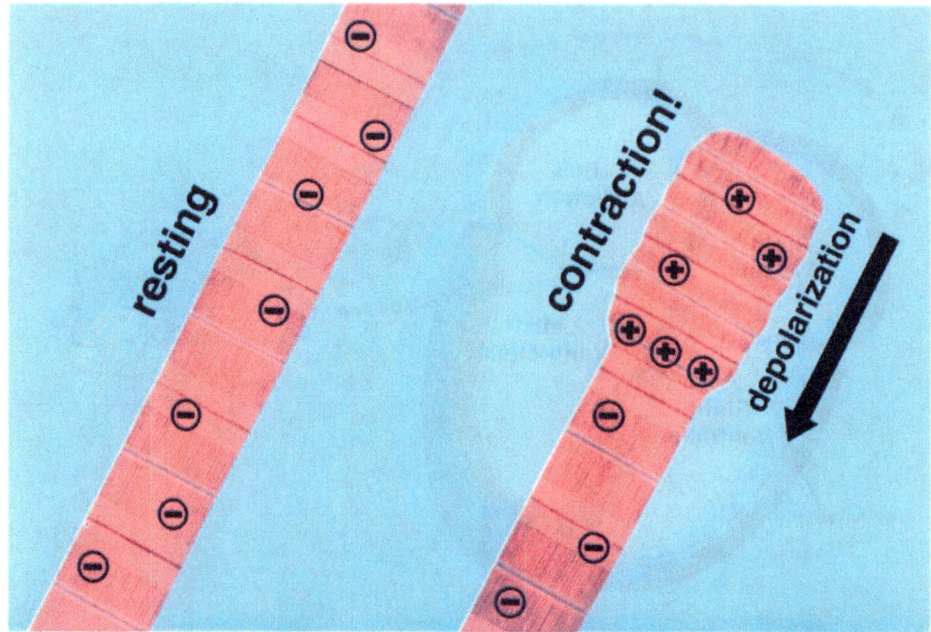

The interiors of heart muscle cells (myocytes*) are negative ("polarized") at rest, but when "depolarized" their interiors become positive and the myocytes contract.

While in the resting state, myocytes are *polarized*, the
interior of every cell being _____-ly charged.   negative

Note: In the strictest sense, a resting polarized cell has a
negatively charged interior and a positively charged outside surface, but
for simplicity we will consider only the negative interior.

The interiors of resting myocytes are negative, but
when these cells are *depolarized*, their interiors
become _____ and the cells contract.   positive

"Depolarization" moves as a wave through the myocardium.
As this wave of **depolarization** stimulates the heart's myocytes,
they become positive and _____.   contract

* Just as the heart muscle is called the *myocardium*, its cells are called "myocytes".

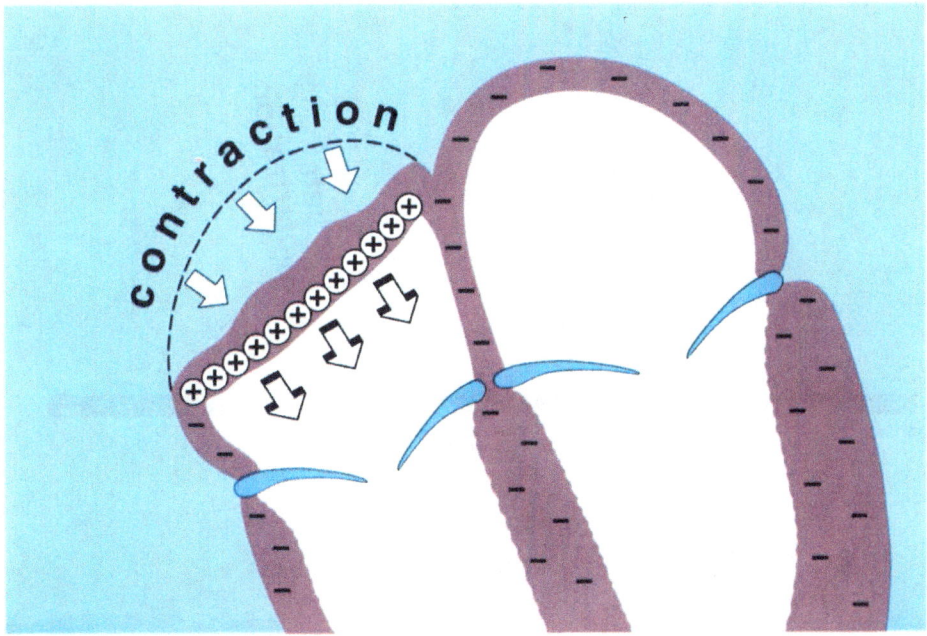

As a wave of depolarization progresses through the heart, it causes contraction of the myocardium. Depolarization begins in the right atrium and quickly spreads to the left atrium. The contracting atria force blood through the AV valves.

Depolarization may be considered an advancing wave
of _____ charges within the heart's myocytes.   positive

Note: The depolarization wave initiates contraction of the resting
myocytes as the charge within each cell changes to positive.

The advancing wave of depolarization causes progressive
contraction of the myocardium as this wave of _____ charges   positive
passes through the interiors of the myocytes.

Note: The cell-to-cell conduction of depolarization through
the myocardium is initiated by fast-moving sodium (Na^+) ions (the +'s
in the illustration above), within the myocytes.

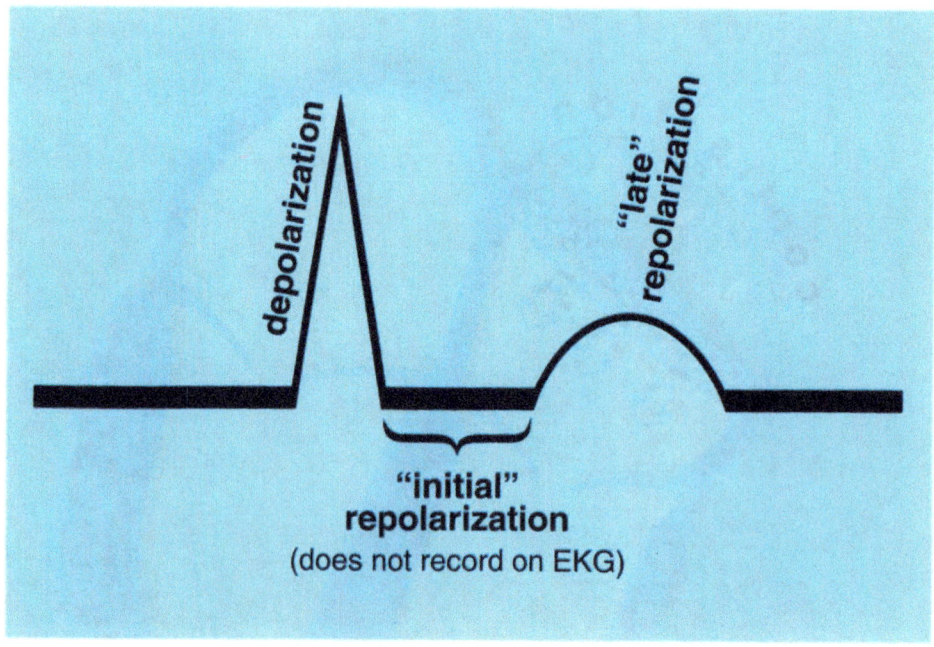

The depolarization wave (cell interiors become positive), and a phase of
repolarization (cell interiors return to negative) that follows, are recorded
on the EKG as shown.

This stimulating wave of depolarization makes the interiors
of the myocytes _____ and stimulates them   positive
to contract.

Then the myocyte interiors regain their resting negative
charge during the _____ phase that follows.   repolarization

Note: Repolarization is an electrical phenomenon that, in reality,
begins immediately after depolarization. The broad hump that
we see on EKG is the most active phase of repolarization.

Myocardial contraction is caused by _____ of   depolarization
the myocytes, which records on the EKG as shown above.
The recovery phase that follows depolarization is known
as _____ (see illustration).   repolarization

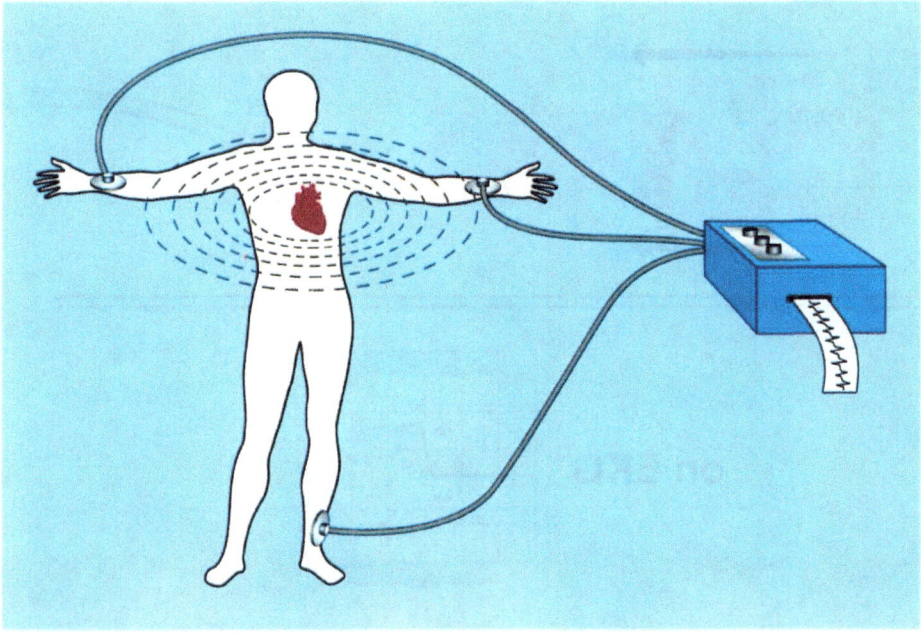

Sensors called "electrodes" are put on the skin to detect the heart's electrical activity. The EKG machine records this activity on moving paper as an electrocardiogram.

Both depolarization and repolarization of the myocardium are
_____ phenomena caused by the movement of ions.   electrical

The heart's electrical activity may be detected and recorded
from the _____ surface by sensitive monitoring equipment,   skin
including EKG machines, cardiac monitors, and
telemetry devices.

The EKG records the electrical activity of the heart
using skin sensors called _____.   electrodes

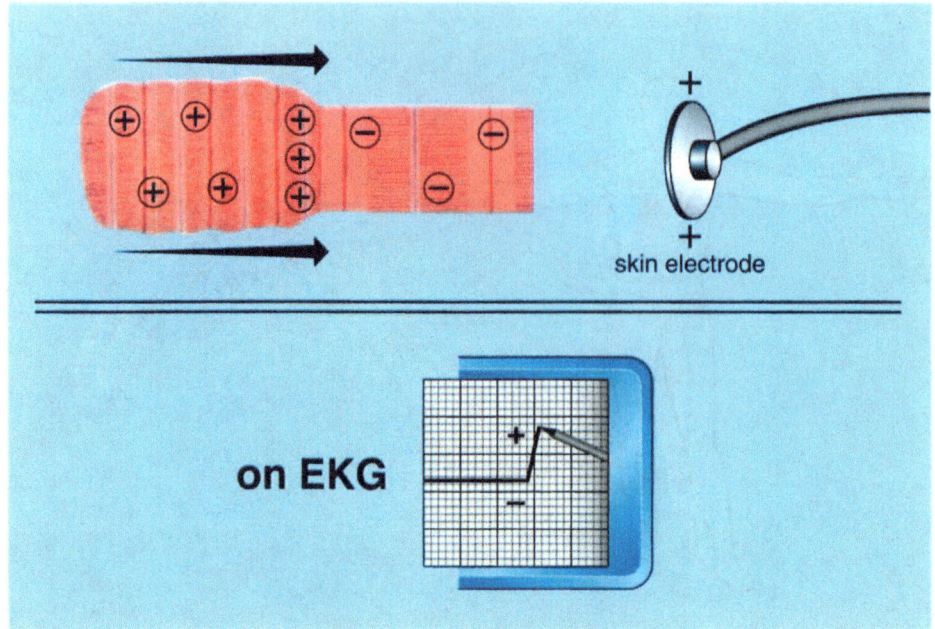

As the positive wave of depolarization within the myocytes flows toward a positive electrode, there is a positive (upward) deflection recorded on EKG.

Note: "Positive electrode," of course, refers to a positive electrode actively recording a patient's EKG.

A wave of depolarization advancing through the myocardium is a moving wave of _____ charges.   positive
(Here come the Na$^+$ ions!)

When this wave of positive charges (Na$^+$ ions) moves toward a positive electrode, there is a simultaneous upward deflection recorded on the _____.   EKG

In general, when you see an upward wave on EKG, you know that it represents a depolarization wave moving toward a _____ electrode.   positive

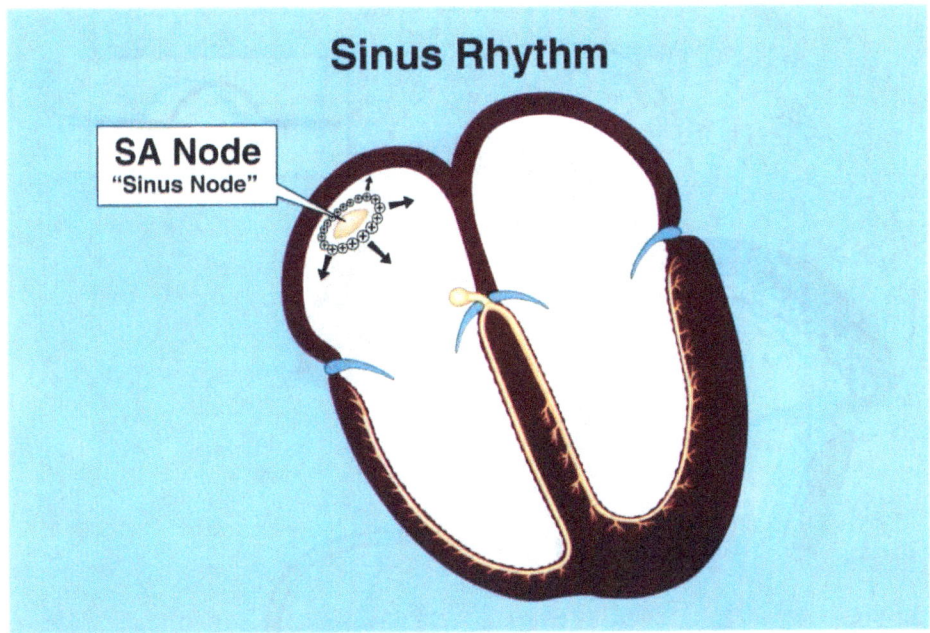

Sinus Rhythm

SA Node
"Sinus Node"

The heart's dominant pacemaker, the *SA Node*, initiates a wave of depolarization that spreads outward, stimulating the atria to contract as the circular wave advances.

Note: The SA Node ("Sinus Node") is the heart's dominant pacemaker, and its pacing activity is known as a "Sinus Rhythm." The generation of pacemaking stimuli is **automaticity**. Other focal areas of the heart that have automaticity are called "*automaticity foci.*"

The SA Node, located in the upper-posterior wall of the right
_____, initiates a depolarization wave at regular intervals   atrium
to accomplish its pacemaking responsibility.

Each depolarization wave of + charges (Na⁺ ions) proceeds outward
from the SA Node and stimulates both atria to _____.   contract

The ability of the SA Node to generate pacemaking stimuli
is known as _____.   automaticity

Note: The depolarization wave flows away from the SA Node in all directions. Imagine the atria as a pool of water. A pebble dropped in at the SA Node produces an enlarging, circular wave (depolarization) that spreads outward. Atrial depolarization (and contraction) is a spreading wave of positive charges within the atrial myocardial cells. Let's read this page again.

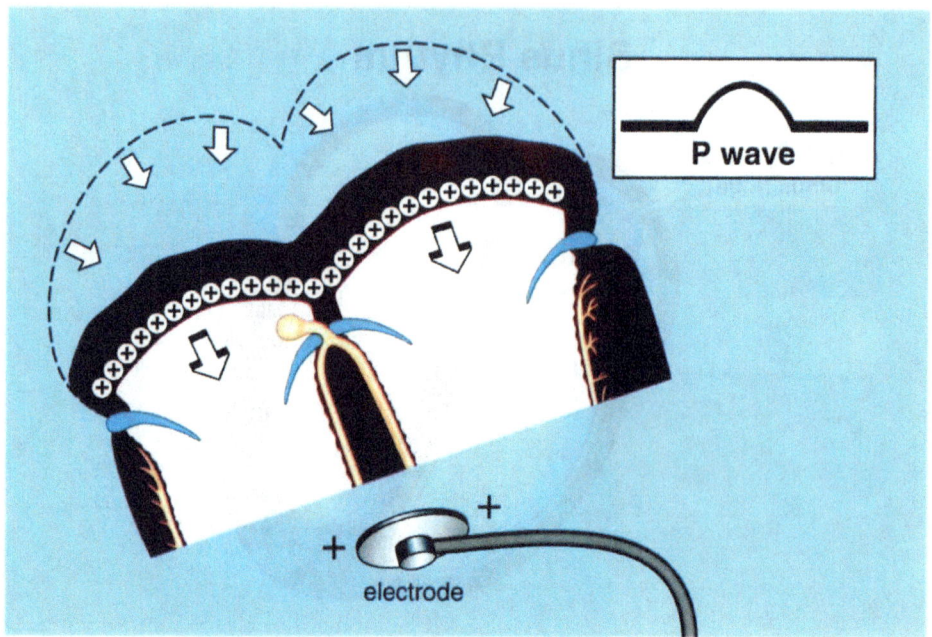

Each depolarization wave emitted by the SA Node spreads through both atria,
producing a **P wave** on the EKG.

Note: The illustration depicts the positive wave of atrial depolarization
advancing toward a positive skin electrode, producing an upward
(positive) P wave on EKG.

The wave of depolarization sweeping through the atria
can be detected by sensitive _____ electrodes.   skin

Atrial depolarization is recorded as a ___ wave on EKG.   P

So when we see a P wave on an electrocardiogram,
we know that, electrically speaking, it represents
atrial _____.   depolarization

Note: The atria have a specialized conduction system,
which we will examine later (page 101, if you're curious).

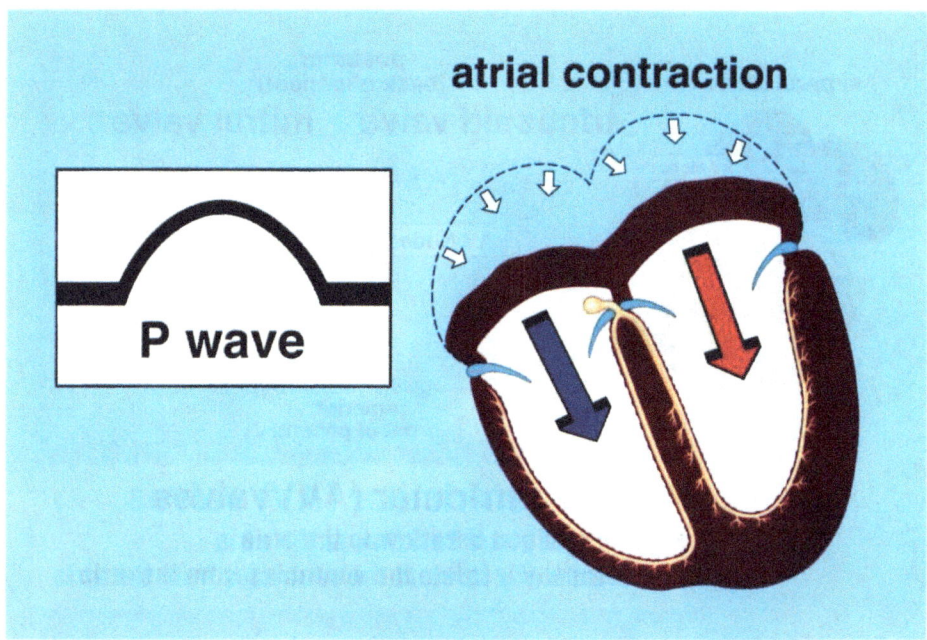

Thus the P wave represents the electrical activity (depolarization) of both atria, and it also represents the simultaneous contraction of the atria.

As the wave of depolarization moves through both atria, there is a simultaneous wave of atrial _____.   contraction

So the P wave represents the depolarization and contraction of both _____.   atria

Note: In reality, contraction of the atria lasts longer than the duration of the P wave. However, we'll still consider that a P wave = atrial contraction. This simultaneous contraction of the atria forces the blood they contain to pass through the Atrio-Ventricular (AV) valves between the atria and the ventricles.

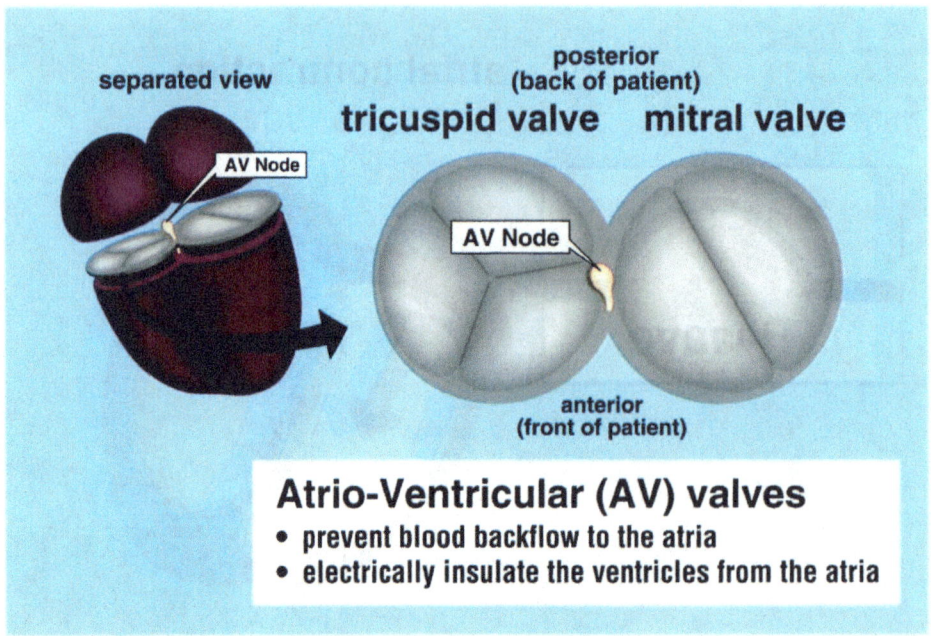

The **Atrio-Ventricular (AV) valves** prevent ventricle-to-atrium blood backflow, and they electrically insulate the ventricles from the atria… except for the **AV Node**, the only conducting path between the atria and the ventricles.

When the ventricles contract, the blood they contain cannot flow back into the atria due to the very efficient ___ valves.   AV

The **mitral** and **tricuspid (AV) valves** lie between the atria and the ventricles, thereby acting to electrically _____ the ventricles from the atria…   insulate

… leaving only the ___ Node as the sole pathway to conduct the depolarization stimulus through the fibrous AV valves to the ventricles.   AV

Note: The AV Node is just above, but continuous with, a specialized "ventricular conduction system" that distributes depolarization to the ventricles very efficiently. Next we will review the movement of blood through the heart's chambers.

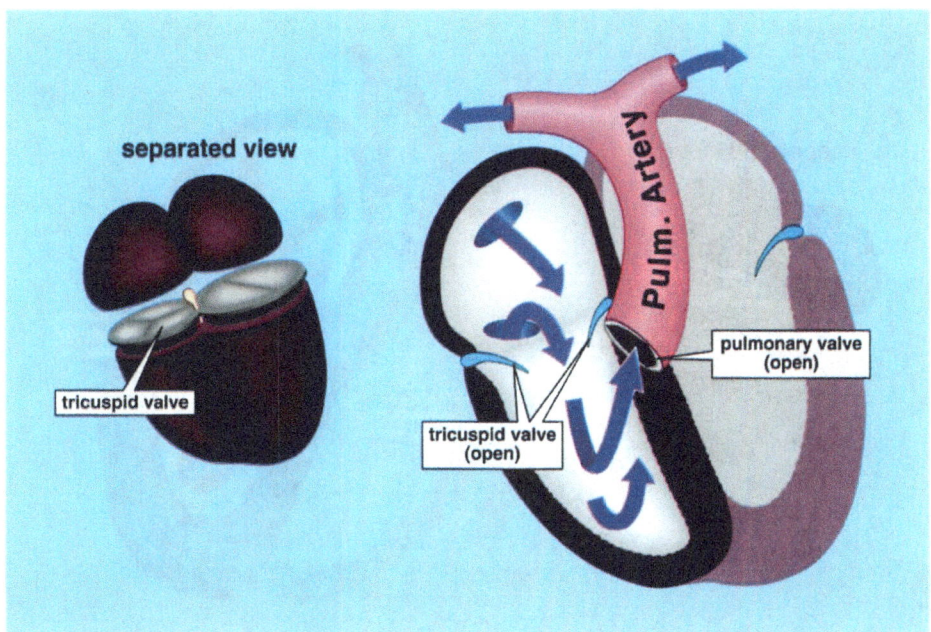

Oxygen-depleted venous blood enters the right atrium. Atrial contraction forces blood through the *tricuspid valve* into the right ventricle, which pumps it into the lungs.

Note: T<u>ri</u>cuspid is <u>ri</u>ght side.

The right side of the heart (right atrium and right ventricle) receives under-oxygenated venous blood from all over the body, and pumps it into the _____.   lungs

The right ventricle contracts, forcing the under-oxygenated venous blood through the **pulmonary valve** into the *pulmonary* _____, and thence to the lungs.   *artery*

Note: Remember, both atria contract simultaneously, and also both ventricles contract together. However, the right and left sides of the heart have different responsibilities.

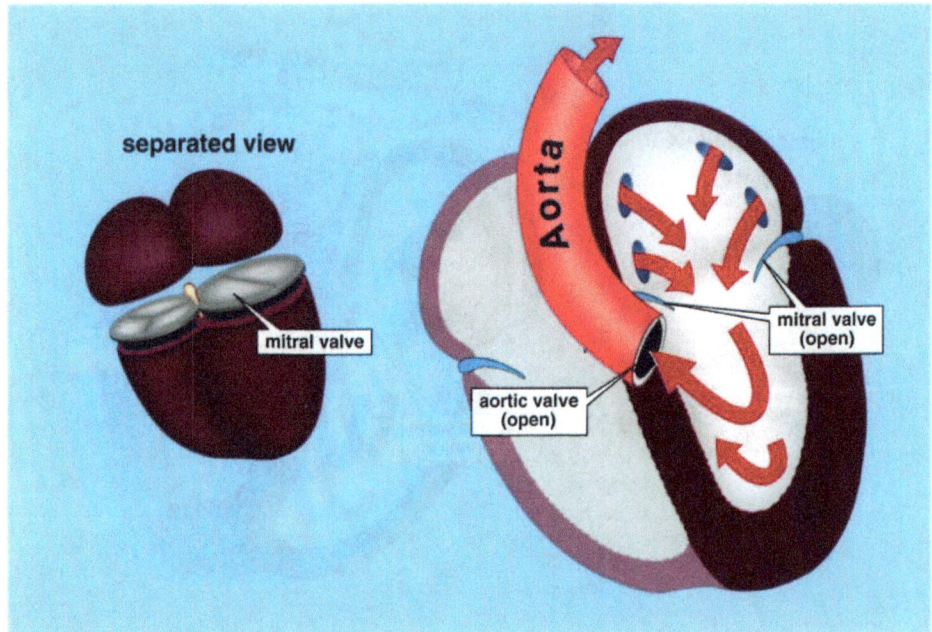

Oxygenated blood from the lungs enters the left atrium, which contracts to force blood through the *mitral valve* into the left ventricle. The powerful left ventricle, in turn, pumps blood through the **aorta** to all areas of the body.

Note: Mitral is left side.

The left atrium contracts, forcing oxygenated blood
through the _____ valve into the left ventricle.   mitral

Then the muscular left ventricle contracts, forcing oxygenated blood
through the **aortic valve** into the _____. (That's too easy!)   aorta

Both atria contract simultaneously, then both _____   ventricles
contract simultaneously.

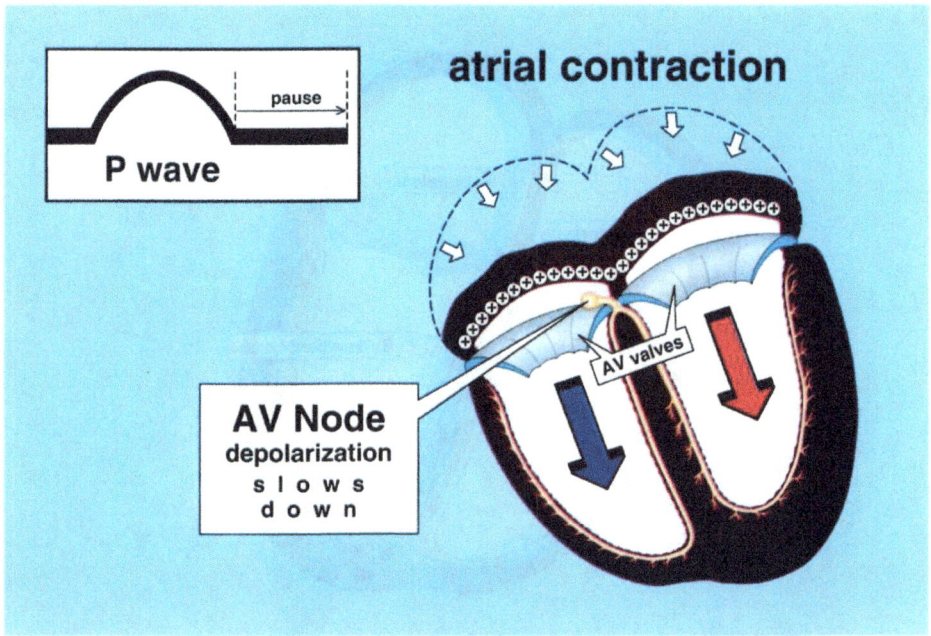

When the wave of atrial depolarization enters the AV Node, depolarization slows, producing a brief pause, thus allowing time for the blood in the atria to enter the ventricles. Slow conduction through the AV Node is carried by calcium (Ca^{++}) ions.

Note: Of course you remember that the AV Node is the only electrical conduction pathway between the atria and the ventricles.

Because depolarization slows within the AV Node, there is a brief delay or _____ before   pause
depolarization is conducted to the ventricles.

This brief pause allows the blood from the atria to pass through the AV valves and into the _____.   ventricles

Note: At this point, we are correlating electrical activity with mechanical physiology. The atria contract, forcing blood through the AV valves, but it takes a little time for the blood to flow through the valves into the ventricles (hence the necessary pause that produces a short piece of flat baseline after each P wave on the EKG). Please review the illustration again.

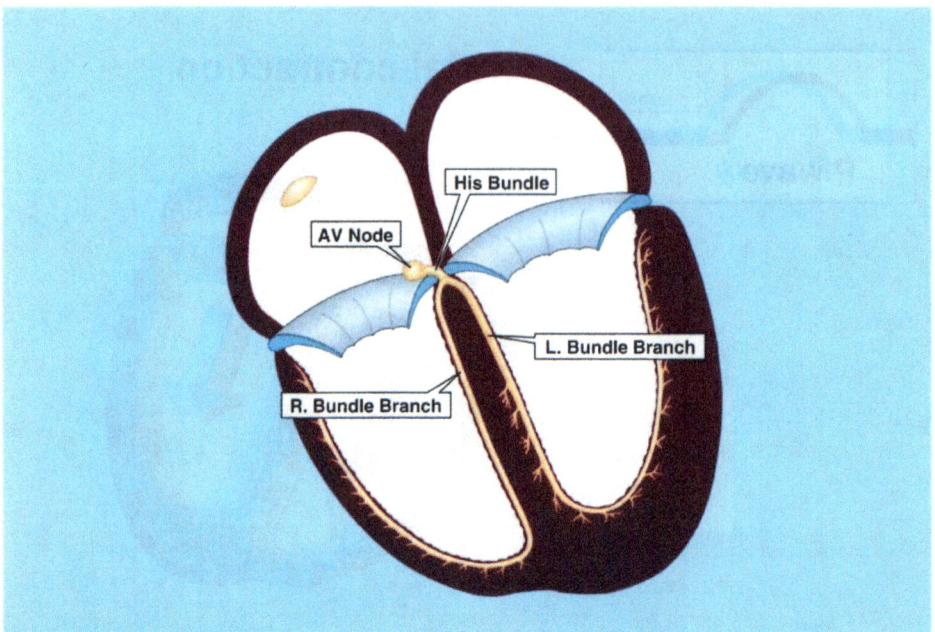

Depolarization conducts slowly through the AV Node, but upon reaching the
ventricular conduction system, depolarization rapidly shoots through the
His Bundle and the **Left** and **Right Bundle Branches** and their subdivisions.

Depolarization conducts slowly through the AV Node, since it is
carried by slow-moving Ca^{++} ions, but depolarization shoots rapidly
through the ventricular conduction system beginning in the _____ Bundle.   His

Depolarization conducts slowly through the AV Node,
then rapidly through the His Bundle to the Right and
Left _____ Branches.   Bundle

Depolarization shoots rapidly through the His Bundle and the
Bundle Branches and their subdivisions, so depolarization is
quickly distributed to the myocytes of the _____.   ventricles

Note: The ventricular conduction system originates at the His Bundle,
which penetrates the AV valves, then immediately bifurcates (in the
interventricular septum) into the Right and Left Bundle Branches. The
His "Bundle" and both "Bundle" Branches are "bundles" of rapidly
conducting **Purkinje fibers***. Like the myocardium, Purkinje fibers use
fast-moving Na^+ ions for the conduction of depolarization.

* Texts in the past (including this one) have *incorrectly* implied that only the
  terminal filaments were Purkinje fibers. Not so! Study "Note" and learn it correctly.

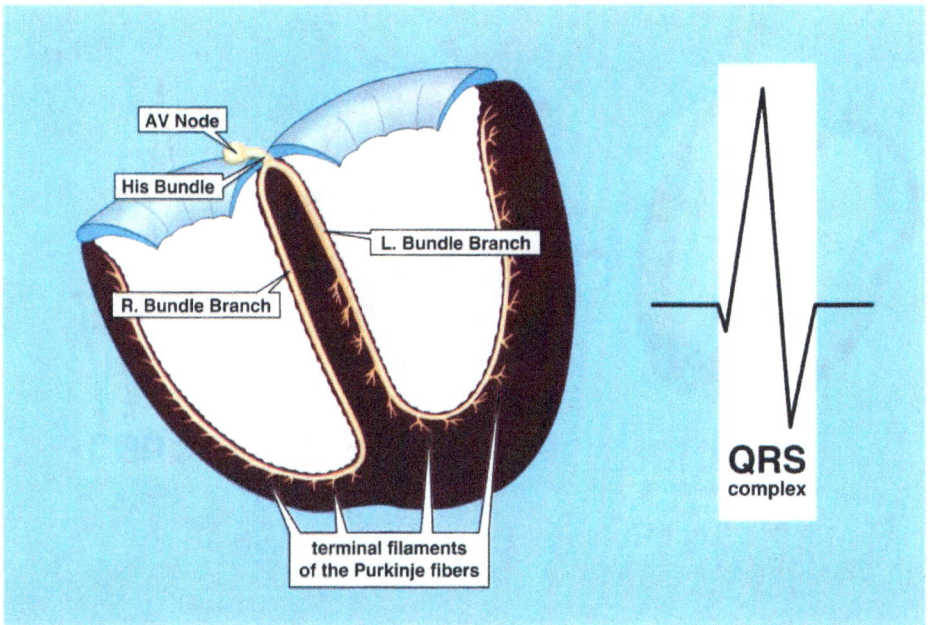

The terminal filaments of the Purkinje fibers rapidly distribute depolarization to the ventricular myocytes. Depolarization of the entire ventricular myocardium produces a **QRS complex** on EKG.

Note: The ventricular conduction system is composed of bundles of rapidly-conducting Purkinje fibers that carry depolarization away from the AV Node at high speed. The Purkinje fibers terminate in tiny filaments that directly depolarize the ventricular myocytes. The (rapid) passage of depolarization down the ventricular conducting system is too weak to record on EKG; however, depolarization of the ventricular myocardium records as a QRS complex.

Depolarization conducts slowly through the AV Node (using Ca^{++} ions), and then conducts rapidly (using Na^+ ions) through the His Bundle to the Right and Left Bundle Branches into the terminal filaments of the Purkinje fibers, which depolarize the _____ myocytes.   ventricular

Note: The terminal filaments of the Purkinje fibers spread out just beneath the **endocardium** that lines both ventricular cavities, therefore ventricular depolarization begins at the lining and proceeds toward the outside surface (**epicardium**) of the ventricles. The Purkinje fibers branch and subdivide just beneath the endocardial lining, but they barely penetrate into the myocardium. Since that's almost impossible to depict in a two-dimensional drawing, please recognize the limits of the illustration and remember it correctly.

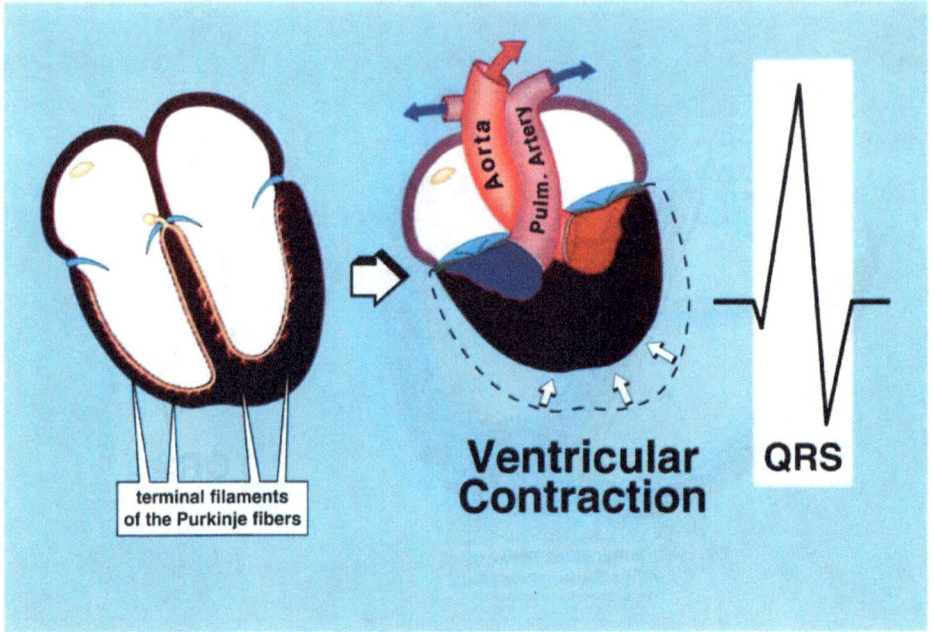

The entire ventricular conduction system consists of rapidly conducting Purkinje fibers. The terminal filaments of the Purkinje fibers depolarize the ventricular myocardium, initiating ventricular contraction while inscribing a QRS complex on EKG.

The terminal filaments of the Purkinje fibers rapidly conduct
_____ to the myocytes that lie just beneath the　　　depolarization
the endocardial lining of both ventricles.

Note: Remember, the entire ventricular conduction system, i.e., the His Bundle through the terminal filaments, is composed of Purkinje fibers that use fast-moving Na^+ ions for conduction.

Depolarization of the ventricular myocytes produces
a ____ complex on the electrocardiogram and initiates　　　　　　QRS
contraction of the ventricles.

Note: The QRS complex actually represents the beginning of ventricular contraction. The physical event of ventricular contraction actually lasts longer than the QRS complex, but we will still consider the QRS complex as generally representing the occurrence of ventricular contraction. So the QRS complex is an electrocardiographic recording of ventricular depolarization, which causes ventricular contraction. Still with me?

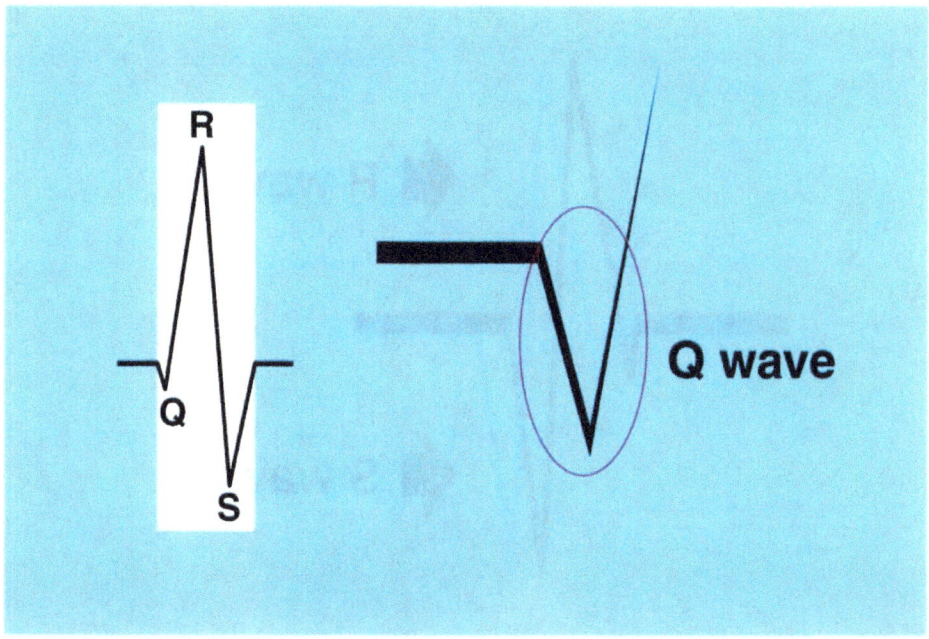

The **Q wave** is the first downward wave of the QRS complex, and it is followed by an upward **R wave**, however the Q wave is often absent on EKG.

The Q* wave, when present, always occurs at the _____ of the QRS complex and is the first downward deflection of the complex.

beginning

The downward Q wave is followed by an upward ___ wave.

R

Note: If there is any upward deflection in a QRS complex that appears before a "Q" wave, it is not a Q wave, for by convention, when present, the Q wave is always the first wave in the complex.

* It is now popular to use small (non-capital) letters to designate small waves in the QRS complex, for instance a "q" (small, lower case q) wave is a small wave.

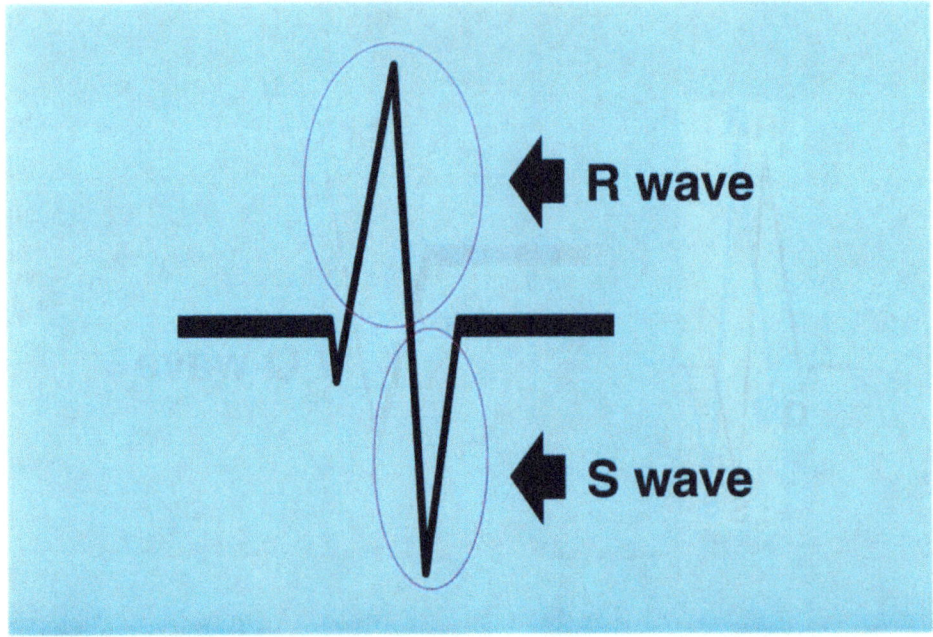

The upward R wave is followed by a downward **S wave**. The entire QRS complex represents ventricular depolarization.

The first upward wave of the QRS complex is
the _____.   R wave

Any downward wave PRECEDED by an upward
wave is an _____.   S wave

The complete QRS complex can be said to represent
_____ depolarization (and the initiation   ventricular
of ventricular contraction).

Note: An upward wave is always called an R wave. Distinguishing between the downward Q and downward S waves really depends on whether the downward wave occurs before or after the R wave. The Q occurs before the R wave, and the S wave follows the R. Just remember your alphabet.

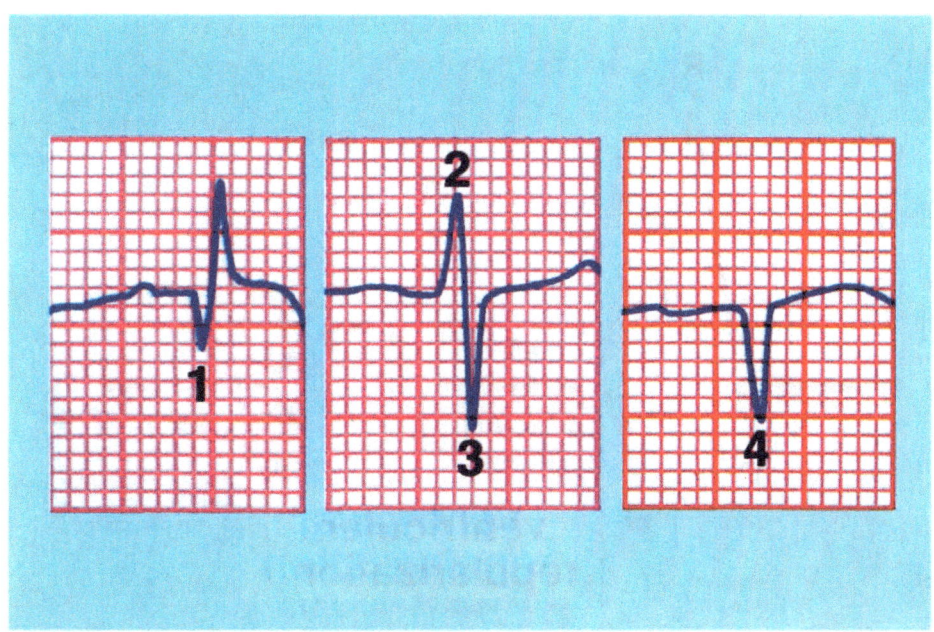

Name the numbered waves in each QRS complex.

1. _____   Q wave

2. _____   R wave

3. _____   S wave

4. _____   QS wave

Note: Number 4 is a little unfair. Because there is no upward wave, we cannot determine whether number 4 is a Q wave or an S wave. Therefore it is called a **QS wave**, and it is considered to be a Q wave when we look for Q's.

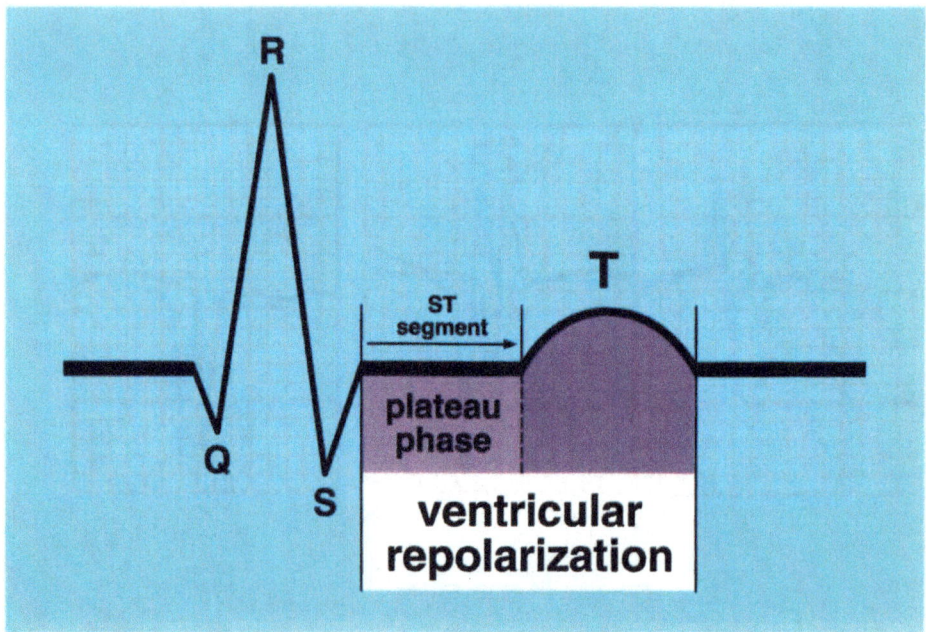

Following the QRS complex, there is a segment of horizontal baseline known as the **ST segment**, and then a broad **T wave** appears.

The horizontal segment of baseline that follows
the QRS complex is known as the _____ segment.   ST

After the QRS there is a segment of horizontal baseline,
followed by a broad hump called the _____ wave.   T

Note: The ST segment is horizontal, flat, and most importantly, it is
normally level with other areas of the baseline. If the ST segment is
elevated or depressed beyond the normal baseline level, this is usually
an sign of serious pathology that may indicate imminent problems.

Note: The ST segment represents the "plateau" (initial) phase of
ventricular repolarization. Ventricular repolarization is rather
minimal during the ST segment.

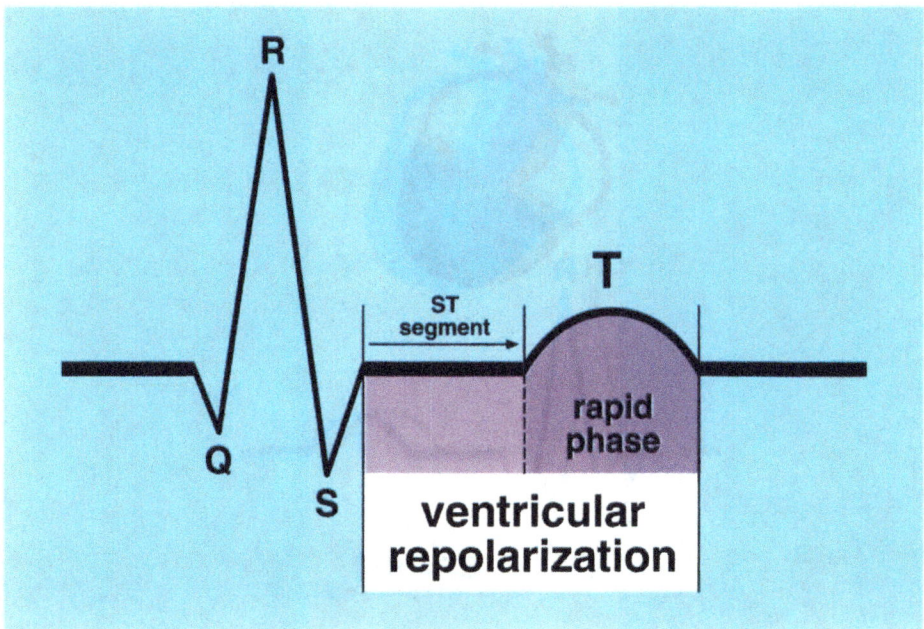

The T wave represents the final, "rapid" phase of ventricular repolarization, during which ventricular repolarization occurs quickly and effectively.

Repolarization occurs so that the ventricular myocytes
can recover their interior, resting _____ charge,   negative
so they can be depolarized again.

Even though the T wave is usually a low, broad hump,
it represents the _____ phase of ventricular repolarization.   rapid

Repolarization of the ventricular myocytes begins immediately
after the QRS and persists until the end of the ____ wave.   T

Note: Repolarization (both phases) is accomplished by
potassium (K^+) ions leaving the myocytes.

Note: Ventricular **systole*** (contraction) begins with the QRS
and persists until the end of the T wave. So ventricular contraction
(systole) spans depolarization and repolarization of the ventricles.
This is a convenient physiological marker.

* Pronounced "SISS-toe-lee"

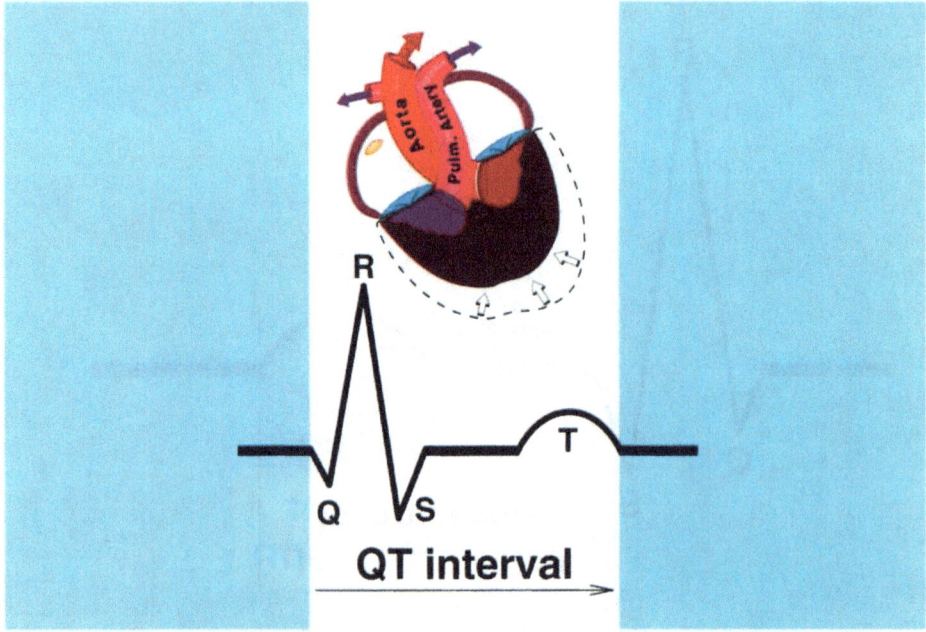

Since ventricular systole lasts from the beginning of the QRS until the end of the T wave, the *QT interval* has clinical significance.

The QT interval represents the duration of ventricular
_____ and is measured from the beginning of the   systole
QRS until the end of the T wave.

Note: The QT interval is a good indicator of repolarization, since repolarization comprises most of the QT interval. Patients with hereditary *Long QT interval* ("LQT") *syndromes* are vulnerable to dangerous (or even deadly) rapid ventricular rhythms. If you routinely examine the QT interval in all EKG's, eventually you will detect this anomaly, and probably save a patient's life during your career.

Note: With rapid heart rates both depolarization and repolarization occur faster for greater efficiency, so the QT interval varies with heart rate. Precise QT interval measurements are corrected for rate, so they are called QTc values. As a simple rule of thumb, the QT interval is considered normal when it is less than half of the R-to-R interval at normal rates.

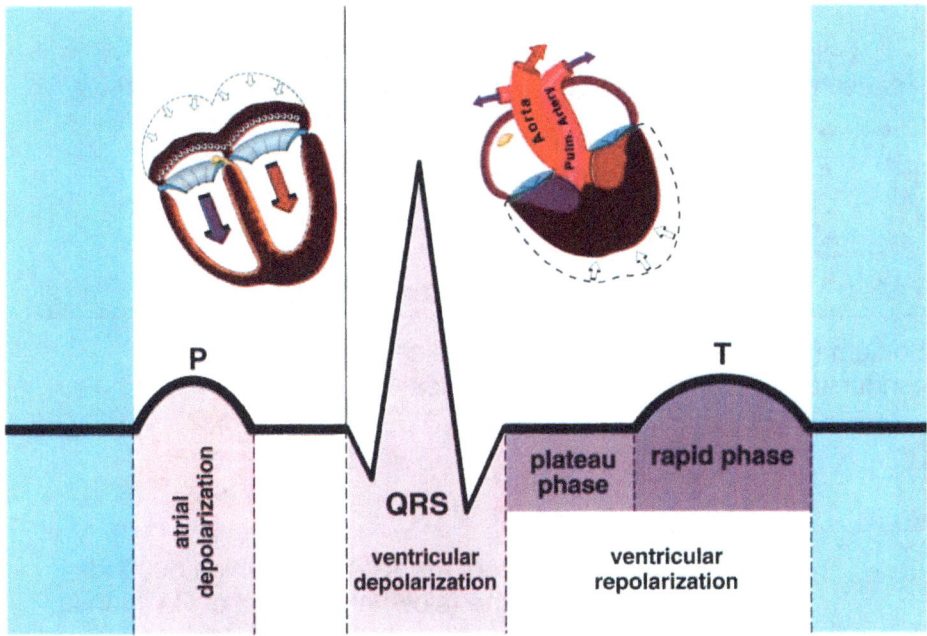

A *cardiac cycle* is represented by the P wave, the QRS complex, the T wave, and the baseline that follows until another P wave appears. This cycle is repeated continuously. Please study the illustration to make certain that you understand every event in sequence.

Note: Physiologically, a cardiac cycle represents atrial systole (atrial contraction), followed by ventricular systole (ventricular contraction), and the resting stage that follows until another cycle begins.

Atrial depolarization (and contraction) is represented
by the ___ wave.   P

Ventricular depolarization (and contraction) is represented
by the _____ complex.   QRS

Note: In reality, atrial contraction lasts longer than the P wave, and ventricular contraction lasts longer than the QRS complex, but you already knew that.

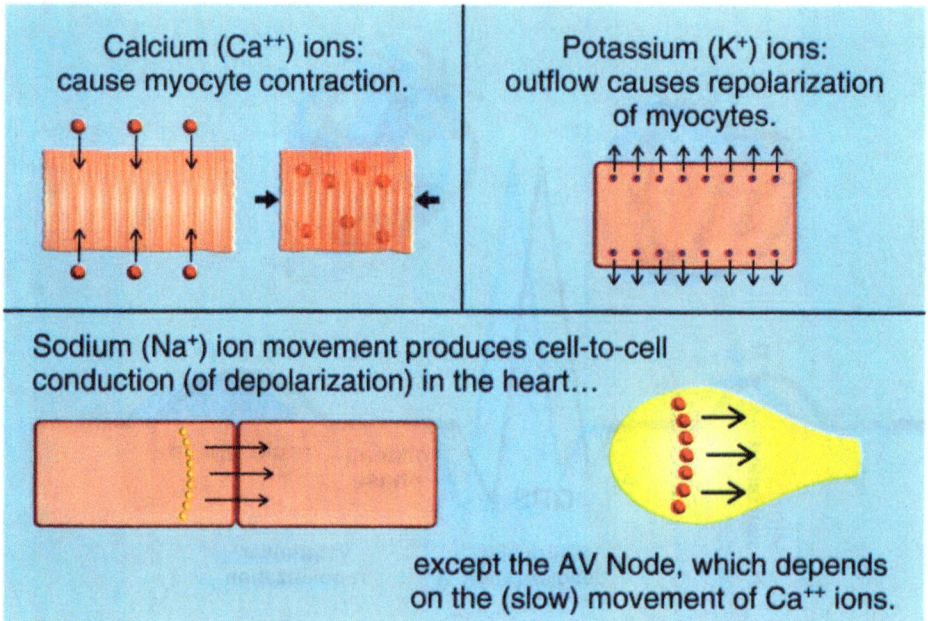

The movement of three types of ions determines all aspects of cardiac conduction, contraction, and repolarization.

The release of free Ca^{++} ions into the interiors of the myocytes produces myocardial _____.   contraction

Following depolarization, repolarization is due to the controlled outflow of ___ ions from the myocytes. K^+

Cell-to-cell conduction (of depolarization) through the myocardium is carried by Na^+ ions, however, AV Node conduction is due to the slow movement of ___ ions. Ca^{++}

Note: This information may seem incongruous in an EKG text, however, during this millennium this page will prove to be the most important of all. Movement of these three ions is the very basis of cardiac physiology; this knowledge will serve you well in the future.

Note: Very soon, all health care professionals will understand (so easy!) cardiac function on the ionic-molecular level by reading *Ion Adventure in the Heartland*, which demonstrates how and why the electrical messages of the heart are displayed on EKG. See pages 331 and 332.

Chapter 2: Recording the EKG

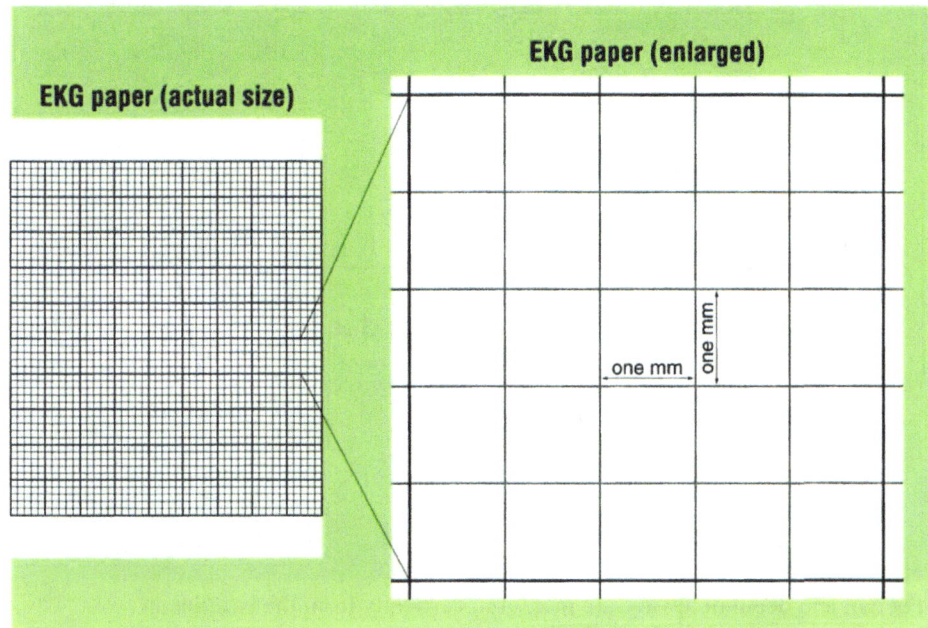

EKG paper (enlarged)

EKG paper (actual size)

one mm

one mm

The EKG is recorded on ruled (graph) paper. The smallest divisions are one millimeter (mm) squares.

The EKG is recorded on a long strip of _____   ruled (graph)
paper, although some EKG machines record many
different leads simultaneously on a large sheet.

The smallest divisions are one _____   millimeter
long and one _____ high.   millimeter

Between the **heavy** black lines there are ___ small squares.   5
Each large square is formed by **heavy** black lines on each side,
and each side measures five mm.

Note: As with all graphs, the time axis is horizontal and moves
left to right, like we read. So timed events on EKG are measured
left to right and similarly, cardiac monitors display a time axis that
reads from left to right.

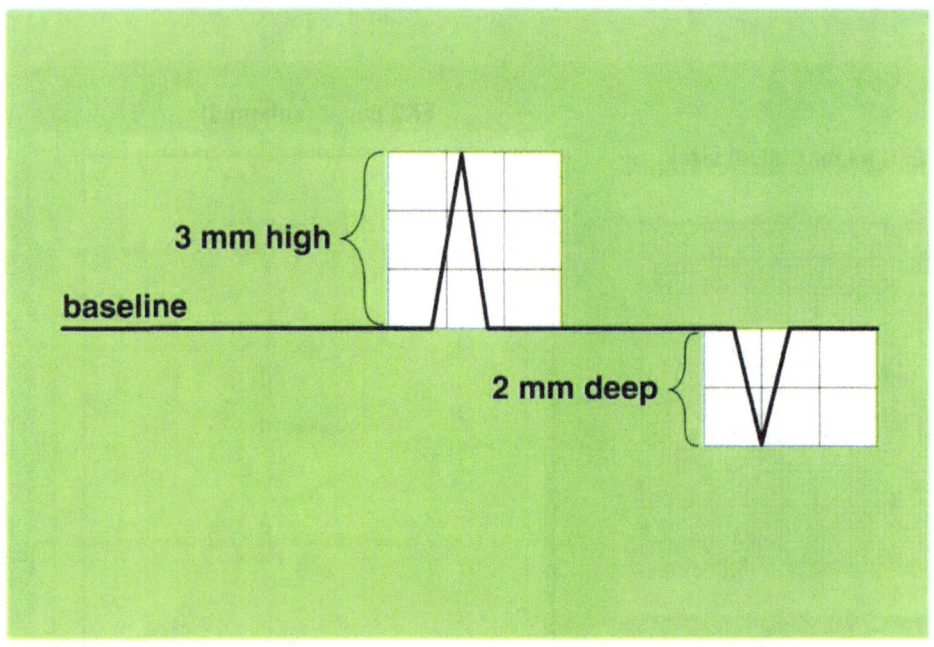

The height and depth of a wave are measured vertically from the baseline in millimeters, and this vertical amplitude represents a measure of voltage.*

The height or depth of waves is measured from the
baseline in millimeters and is a measure of _____.   voltage

Note: The *deflection* of a wave is the <u>direction</u> in which it records on
EKG; for instance, the "upward deflection" or "downward deflection"
of a wave. However, the *amplitude* of a wave is the <u>magnitude</u>
(in millimeters) of upward deflection or downward deflection. The
height or depth of a wave (i.e., its amplitude) is a measure of voltage.

The first wave in the illustration has an upward
deflection of 3 mm in _____.   amplitude

Note: The elevation or depression of segments of baseline is also
measured vertically in millimeters, just as we measure waves.

* Ten millimeters vertically represents one millivolt (mV), however, in practice, one usually
  speaks of "millimeters" of height or depth (waves) and the same for elevation or depression
  of baseline segments.

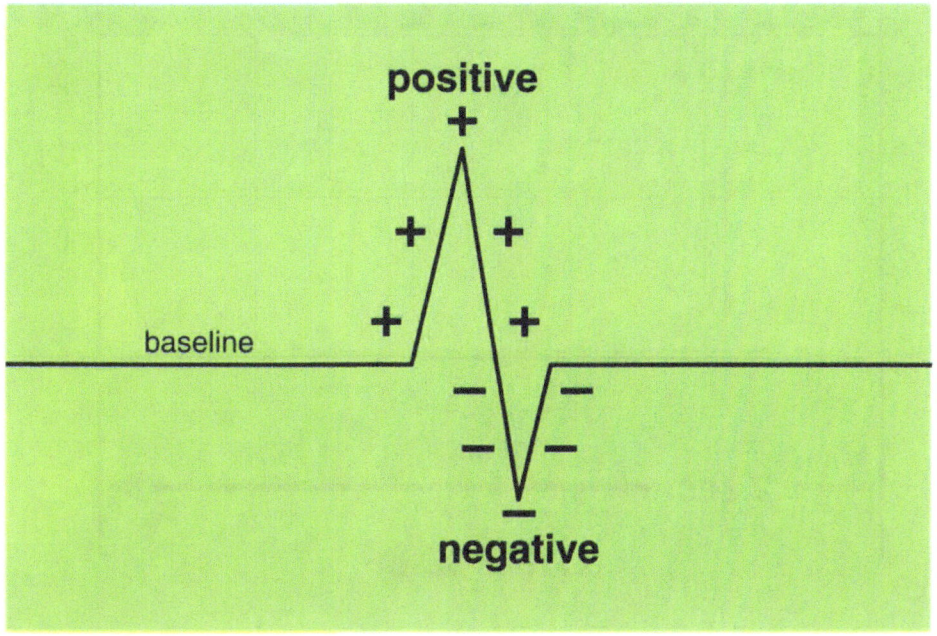

Upward deflections are called "positive" deflections. Downward deflections are called "negative" deflections.

Positive deflections are _____ on the EKG.   upward

Negative deflections are _____ on the EKG.   downward

Note: When a wave of stimulation (depolarization) advances toward a positive skin electrode, this produces a positive (upward) deflection on EKG. You will recall that depolarization is an advancing wave of positive charges (Na^+ ions) within the cardiac myocytes. So with depolarization, the advancing wave of positive intracellular charges produces a positive deflection on EKG as this wave moves toward a positive electrode. Be positive!

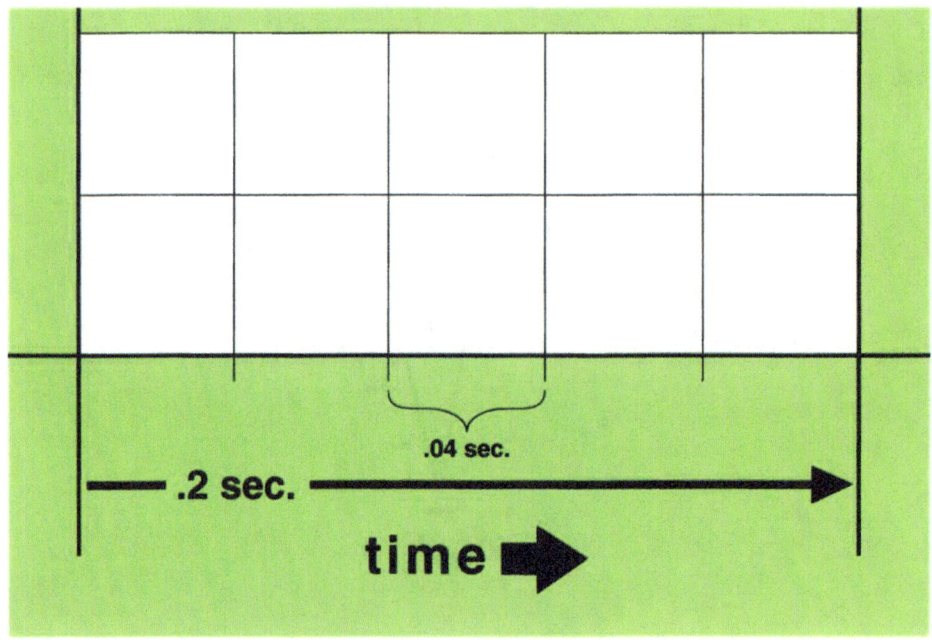

The horizontal axis represents time.

Between the **heavy** black lines there are __ small squares.   5

The amount of time represented by the distance between
two **heavy** black lines is _____.   .2 of a second

Each small division (measured horizontally between
two fine lines) represents _____.   .04 of a second
(that's four hundredths!)

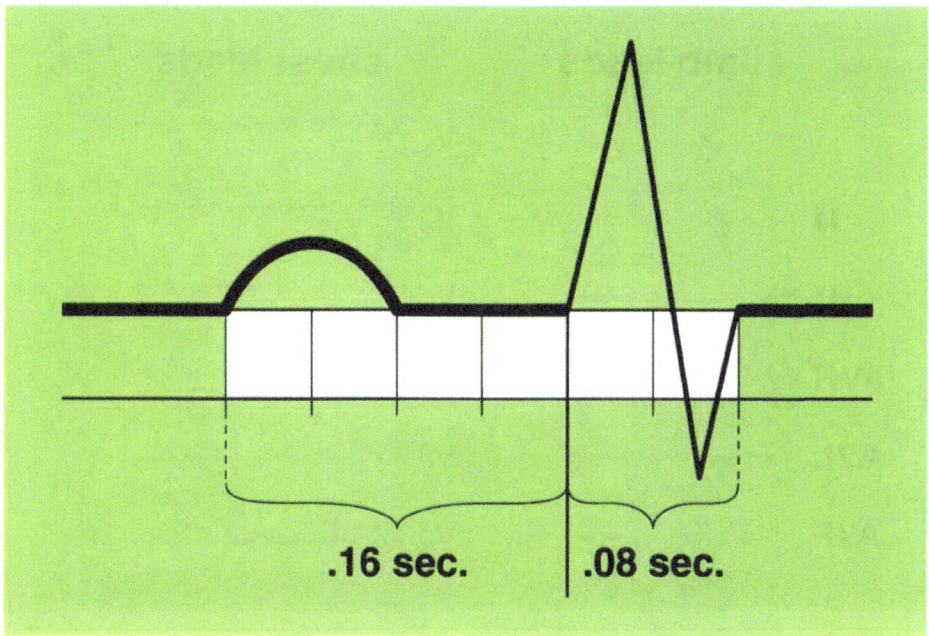

.16 sec.   **.08 sec.**

By measuring along the horizontal axis, we can determine the duration of any part of a cardiac cycle. Remember, each small (one mm) square is .04 second in duration.

The duration of any wave may be determined by
measuring along the horizontal _____.   axis

Four of the small squares represents _____ of a second.   .16
                                                                    (sixteen hundredths)

The amount of EKG graph paper that passes out of the
EKG machine in .12 second is _____ small squares.   three (3)
(You don't have to be a mathematician to read EKG's.)

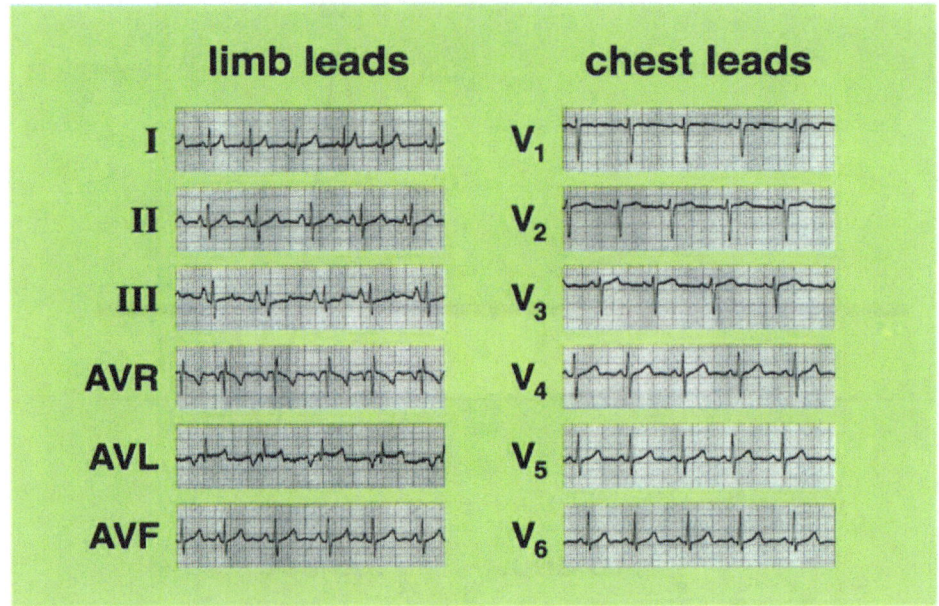

The standard EKG is composed of 12 separate **leads**.*

A standard EKG is composed of six limb _____,   leads
recorded by using arm and leg electrodes and…

… there are also six _____ leads obtained by placing   chest
an electrode at each of six different positions on the chest.

Note: Leads not considered "standard" may be monitored from various
locations on the body as required for special diagnostic purposes.

* Rhymes with seeds.

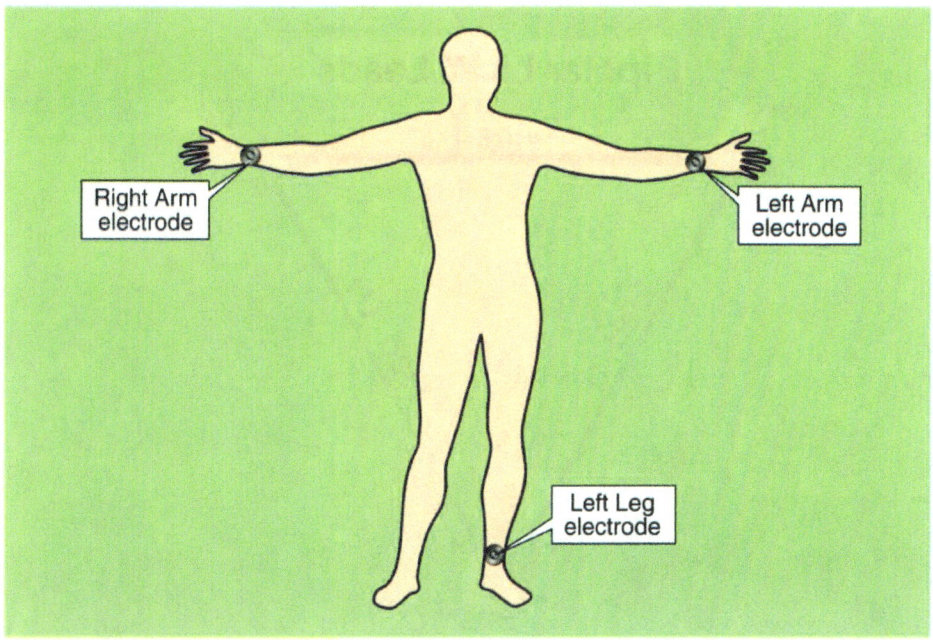

To obtain the **limb leads**, electrodes are placed on the right arm, the left arm, and the left leg. A pair of electrodes is used to record a lead.

By placing electrodes on the right and left arms and the left leg, we can obtain and record the _____ leads.   limb

Note: Einthoven used these three locations for limb electrodes. They remain the conventional standard for recording the EKG.

The placement of these _____ is the same   electrodes
as originally used by Willem Einthoven.

Note: Two electrodes are used to record a lead. A different pair is used for each lead.

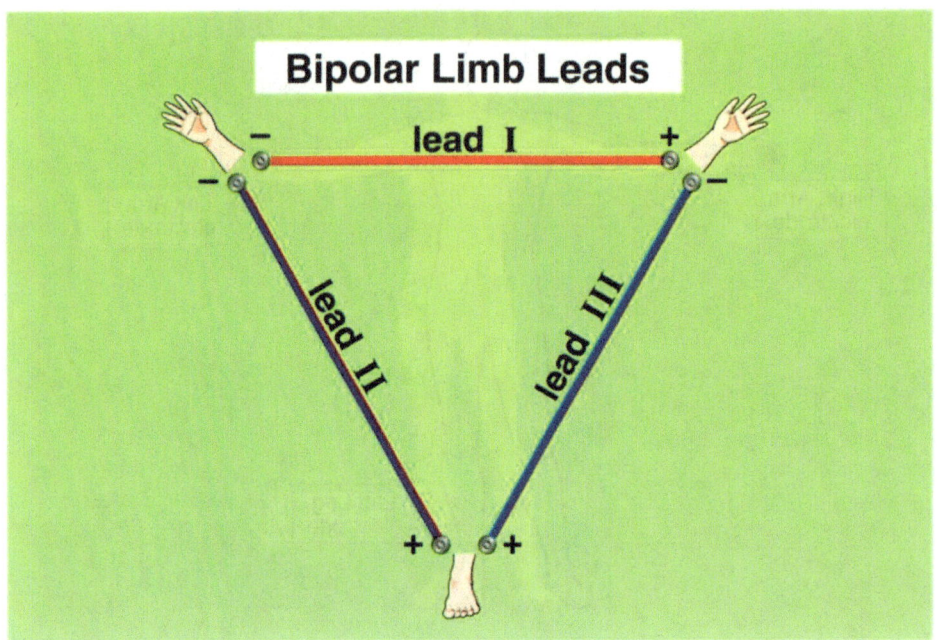

Each **bipolar limb lead** is recorded using two electrodes. So by selecting a different
pair of electrodes for each lead, we create three separate bipolar
limb leads (**lead I, lead II, and lead III**) for recording.

Each limb lead consists of a pair of electrodes,
one is positive and one is _____, so these   negative
leads are called "bipolar" limb leads.

Lead I is horizontal, and its left arm electrode is _____,   positive
while its right arm electrode is negative.

When we consider lead III, the left arm electrode
is now _____, and the left leg electrode is   negative
positive.

Note: The engineering wonders of the EKG machine permit us to
make any skin electrode positive or negative depending on which
pair of electrodes (that is, which lead) the machine is recording.

Note: The bipolar limb lead configuration is sometimes called
"Einthoven's triangle."

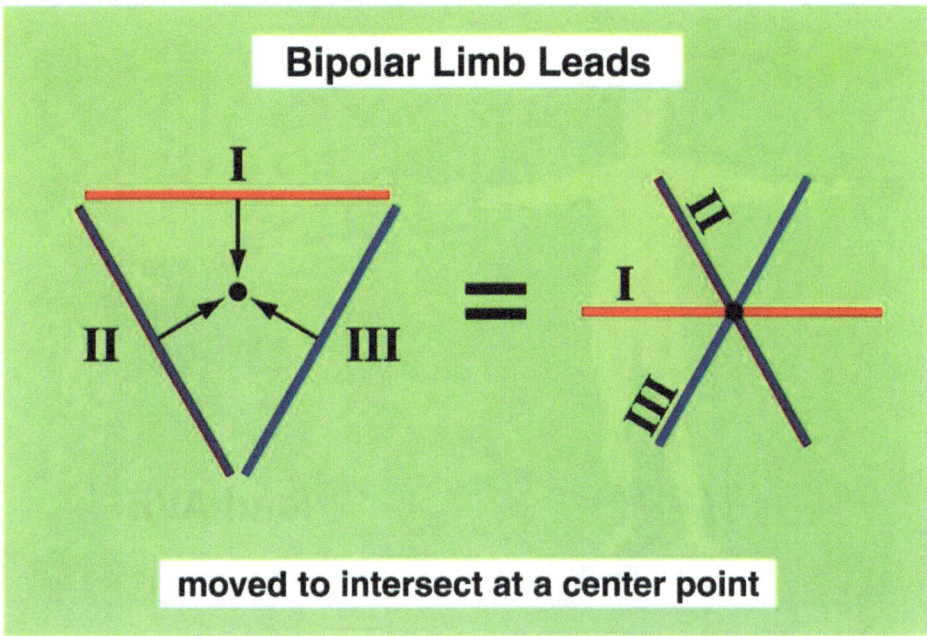

By pushing the three (bipolar) limb leads to the center of the triangle, we produce three intersecting lines of reference.

The triangle has a center, and each _____ may be moved to that center point.

lead

By pushing leads I, II, and III to the center of the triangle, three intersecting lines of _____ are formed.

reference

Although the three bipolar limb leads may be moved to the _____ of the triangle, they remain at the same angles relative to each other. (They're still the same leads, yielding the same information.)

center

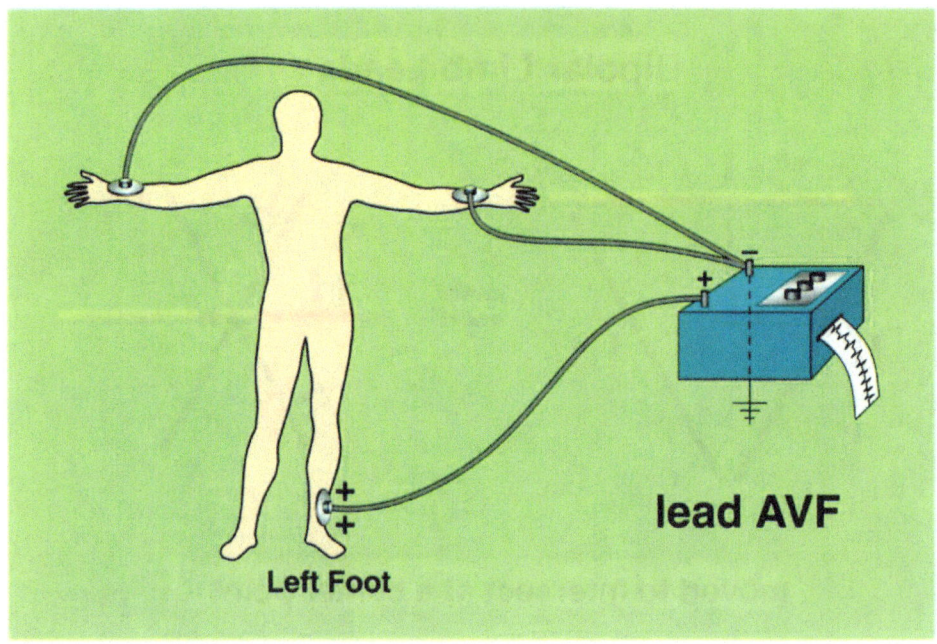

lead AVF

Left Foot

Another standard lead is the **AVF** lead. The AVF lead uses the left foot electrode as
positive and both arm electrodes as a common ground (negative).

The AVF lead uses the left foot electrode as _____.   positive

In AVF both the right and left arm electrodes are
channeled into a common ground that has a
_____ charge.   negative

Note: Dr. Emanuel Goldberger, who designed and introduced the
"Augmented" limb leads, discovered that in order to record a lead
in this manner, he had to amplify (Augment) the Voltage in the EKG
machine to match the wave magnitude of leads I, II, and III. He named
this lead: A (Augmented), V (Voltage), F (left Foot), and he went on to
produce two more leads using this same technique.

Aside: Your deductive mind tells you that lead AVF is a combination
of leads II and III... just what Dr. Goldberger was trying to accomplish!
Therefore lead AVF is a cross between (and oriented between) those
two bipolar limb leads. Now, let's create two more augmented leads.

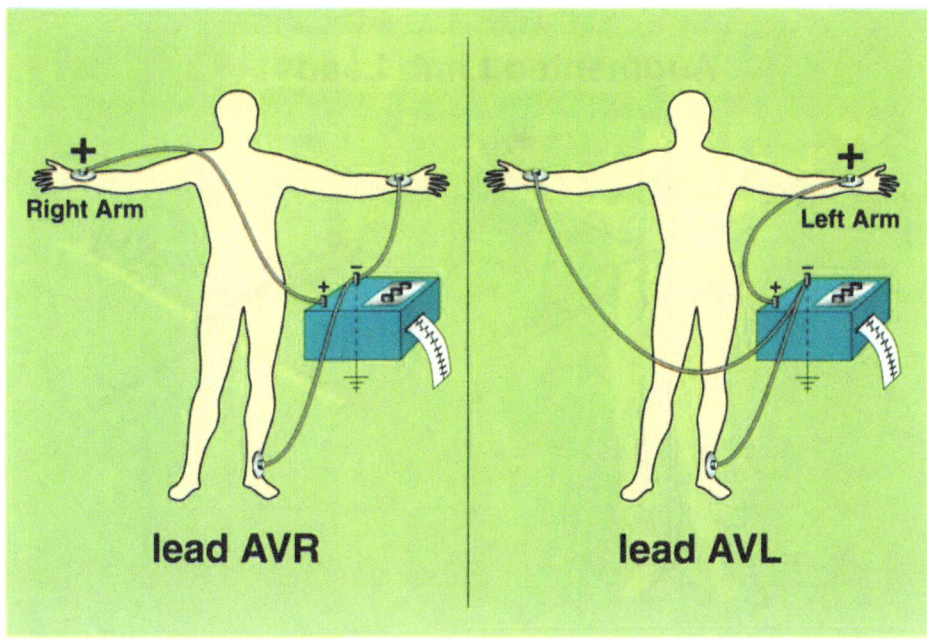

The remaining two augmented limb leads, **AVR** and **AVL**, are obtained in a similar manner.

For the AVR lead the <u>R</u>ight arm electrode is positive, and the remaining two electrodes are _____.   negative

To obtain the AVL lead, the <u>L</u>eft arm electrode is made _____; the other two electrodes are negative.   positive

Note: AV<u>R</u> — Right arm positive

AV<u>L</u> — Left arm positive

AV<u>F</u> — Foot (left foot) positive

(These augmented limb leads are sometimes called the "unipolar" limb leads, stressing the importance of the positive electrode.)

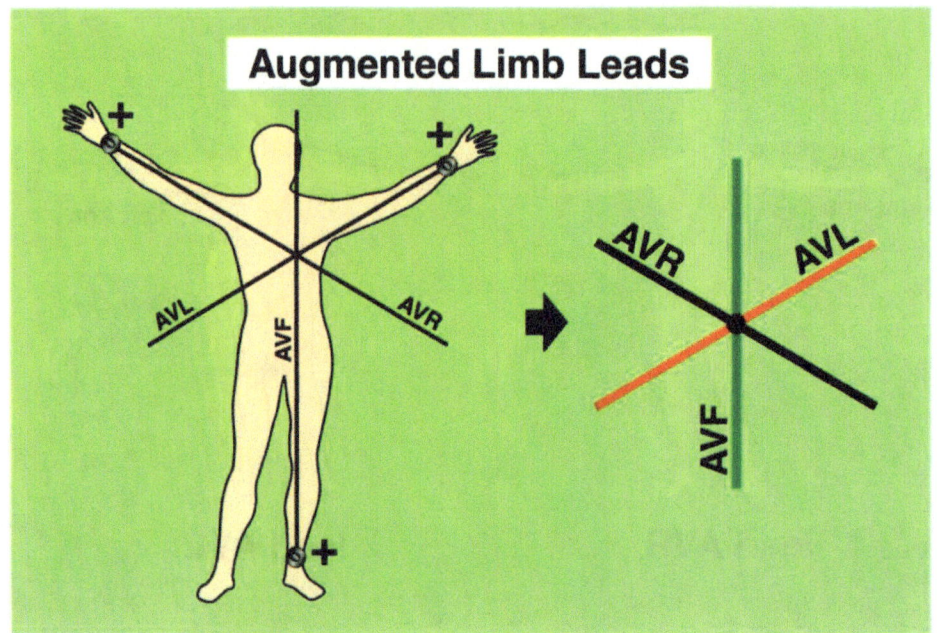

The **augmented limb leads**, AVR, AVL, and AVF, intersect at different angles than those produced by the bipolar limb leads, and they produce three other intersecting lines of reference.

AVR, AVL, and AVF are the augmented (or "unipolar")
_____ leads.   limb

These augmented limb leads _____ at   intersect
60 degree angles, but the angles differ from those
formed by bipolar limb leads, I, II, and III.

Leads AVR, AVL, and AVF intersect at angles _____   different
from leads I, II, and III. In fact, leads AVR, AVL, and AVF
split the angles formed by leads I, II, and III.

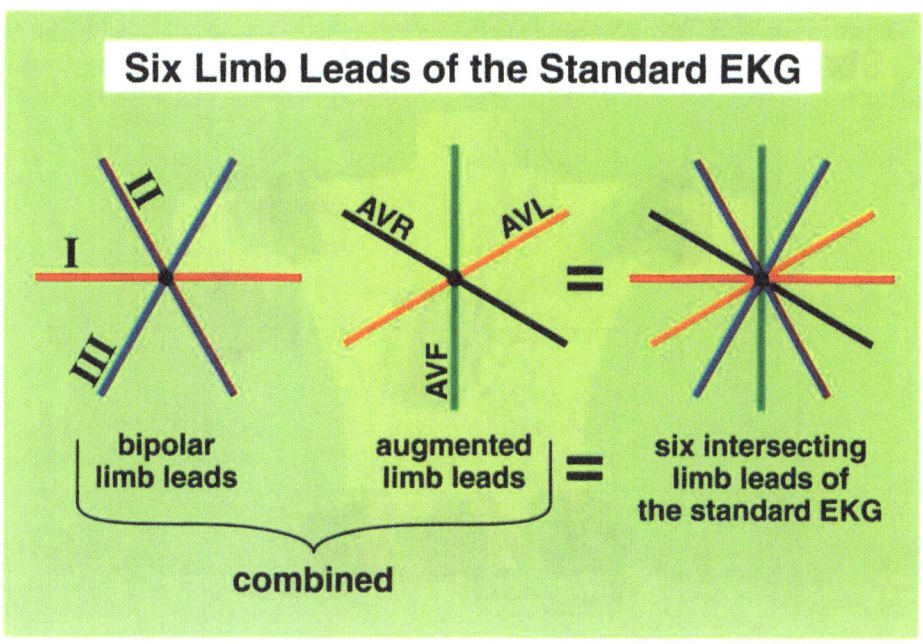

All six limb leads (I, II, III, and AVR, AVL, and AVF) meet to form six intersecting leads that lie in a flat "**frontal**" plane on the patient's chest.

The six limb leads consist of the three bipolar leads, I, II, III, and three augmented leads, _____, _____, and _____.

AVR, AVL, and AVF

If the bipolar limb leads I, II, and III are superimposed on augmented limb leads AVR, AVL, and AVF, we have six intersecting leads in a flat plane on the patient's _____.

chest

The flat plane of the limb leads is called the _____ plane.

frontal

Note: Don't get bedazzled by the kaleidoscope of limb leads. Bear with me for a few pages, and soon you will understand their utility, and a simplified way to visualize this concept.

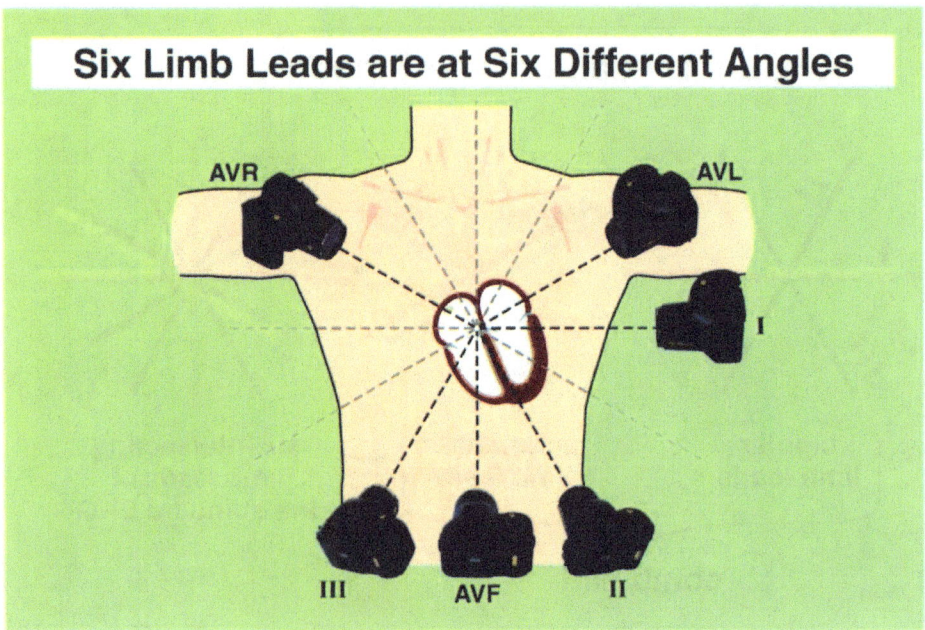

Six Limb Leads are at Six Different Angles

Each camera* position represents the positive electrode of a standard limb lead. Each limb lead (I, II, III, AVR, AVL, and AVF) records from a different angle (viewpoint), to provide a different view of the same cardiac activity.

Note: The heart's electrical activity remains constant, but the positive electrode position changes from lead to lead. Therefore the tracing looks slightly different in each lead, as the angle from which we record the electrical activity changes with each lead. Remember, a wave of depolarization is a progressive wave of POSITIVE charges passing through the myocardial cells. So, when a depolarization wave moves toward a POSITIVE electrode, a POSITIVE (upward) deflection is produced on the EKG (or monitor) for that particular lead. (A little repetitious, but it is *so* important!)

The EKG records the same cardiac _____ in   activity
each lead.

The waves look different in various leads because
the heart's electrical activity is recorded from a
different _____ for each lead.   angle
                                                                   (viewpoint)

* If this were a video camera, it could record the information for a cardiac monitor.

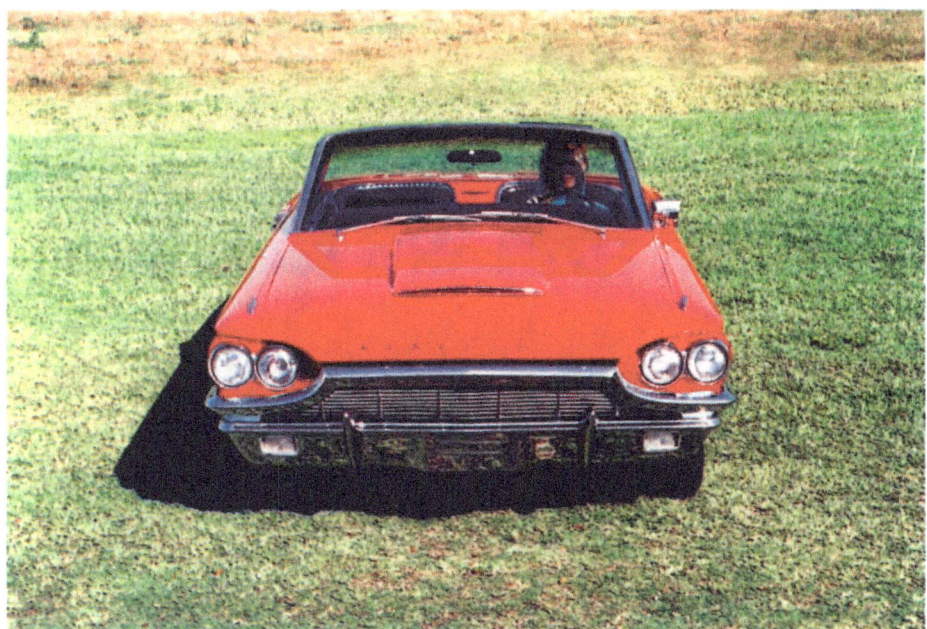

It is conceptually necessary for you to visualize the six intersecting limb leads. Why? Can you identify this car?

Note: This page sure seems empty, doesn't it?

Note: Automobile experts are encouraged not to recognize the car for the sake of understanding the concept.

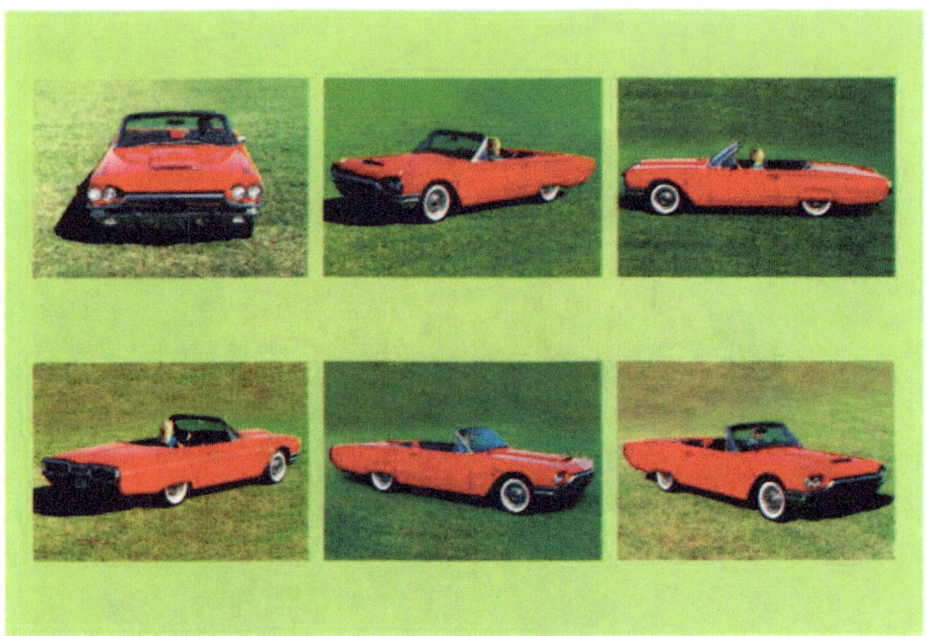

By observing the same object from six different angles, you will obtain a great deal of information, and in this case, perhaps even identify the car.

Note: You can't see the car's rear bumper in the photo at top left. But with progressively different views, you can determine more about the bumper (or even the driver). Similarly, it may be difficult to see a specific wave in a given lead, but with six different lead positions, it is certain to show up better in other leads.

Note: Observation from six different perspectives is better than one. Thus recording cardiac electrical activity from six different angles provides a more accurate and thorough examination. At this point you can take a sip of coffee and relax. By the way, the car is a 1965 Ford Thunderbird, but it is far more important that the concept (not the car) always remains in your mind.

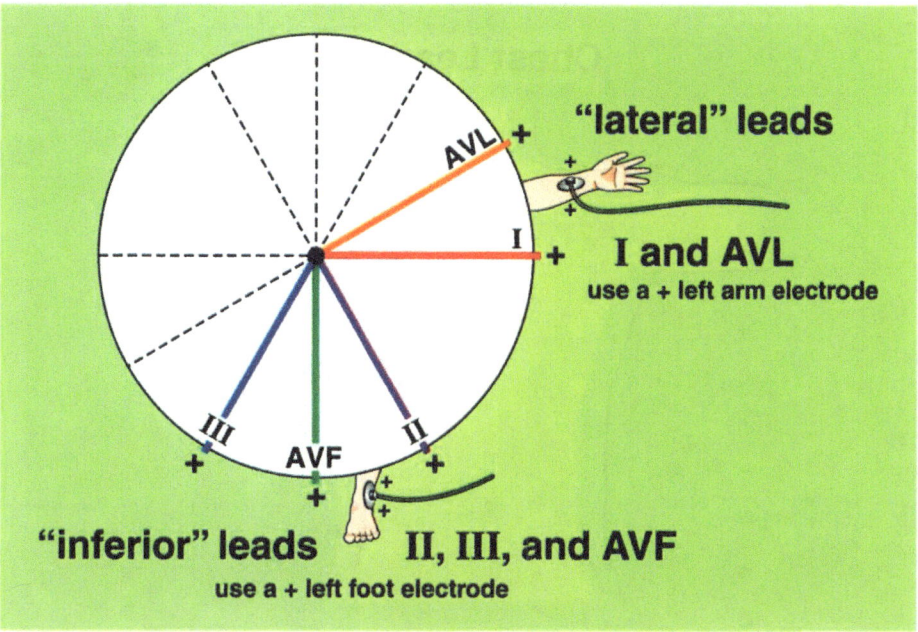

The importance of the positive electrode's position is emphasized by the conventional grouping of limb leads. A positive left arm electrode is used to record "**lateral leads**" I and AVL, and a positive left foot electrode is used to record "**inferior leads**" II, III and AVF. The location of the positive electrode is the key.

Leads I and AVL are called the *lateral leads* (*left* lateral understood) because each has a _____ electrode positioned laterally on the left arm.

positive

Leads II, III, and AVF are called the *inferior leads* because each of these leads has a positive electrode positioned inferiorly on the left _____.

foot

Note: So now you can determine if depolarization is moving toward (or even away from) the patient's left side, and the same for depolarization directed inferiorly toward (or even away from) the left foot. The "inferior leads" and the "lateral leads" include 5 of the 6 limb leads. These are not arbitrary designations. These terms are common cardiology parlance and have important clinical/diagnostic significance. Know and understand them.

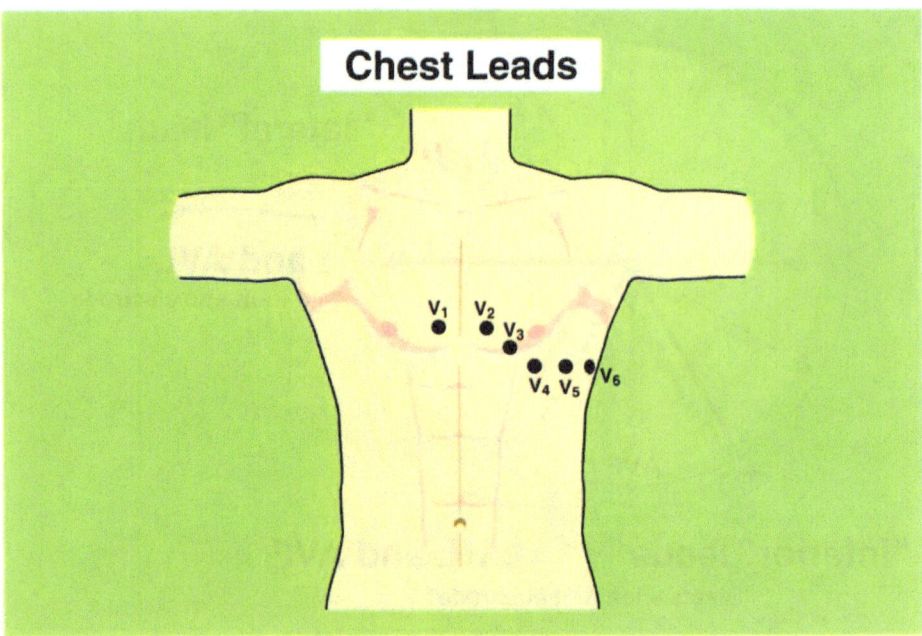

Chest Leads

To obtain the six standard **chest leads**, a positive electrode (suction cup) is placed at six different positions (one for each lead) on the chest.

The six chest leads are recorded from six progressively different positions around the _____. (See illustration.)   chest

For each of the chest leads, the suction cup electrode that is placed on the chest is considered _____.   positive

The chest leads are numbered from V_1 to V_6 and are positioned in successive steps from the patient's right to the left side of the chest. Notice how the chest leads cover the _____ in its normal anatomical position   heart within the chest.

Note: Traditionally a suction cup electrode records the chest leads, however adhesive electrodes are now commonly used. Because the electrode for the chest leads is always *positive*, a depolarization wave moving toward a given chest electrode produces a *positive* (upward) deflection in that chest lead of the EKG tracing.

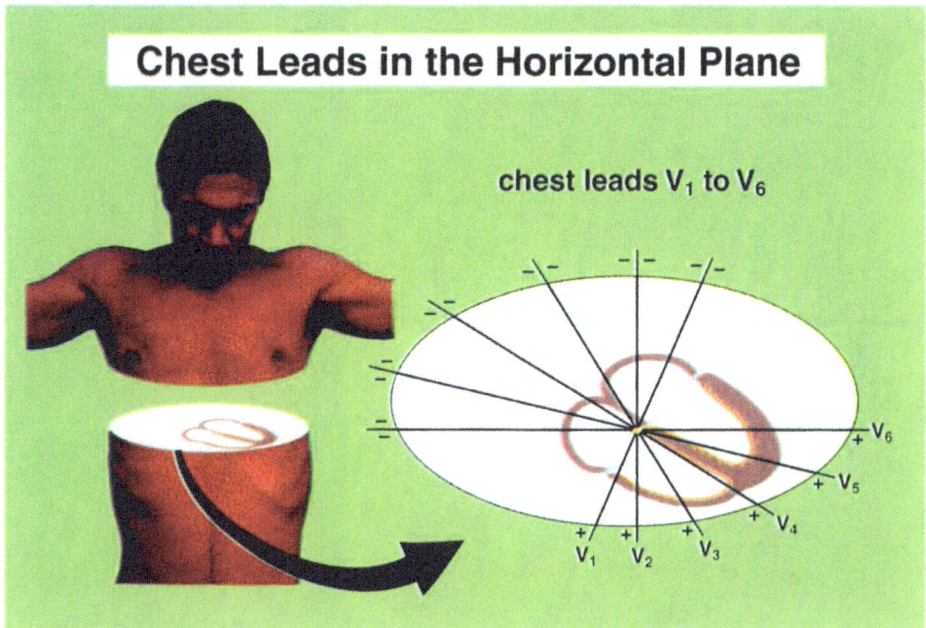

Chest Leads in the Horizontal Plane

chest leads V₁ to V₆

In general, each of the chest leads* is oriented through the AV node and projects through the patient's back, which is negative.

Note: The plane of the chest leads (called the "**horizontal**" plane) cuts the body into top and bottom halves.

The electrode for each of the chest leads is always considered _____ (positive or negative).   positive

If leads V_1 through V_6 are imagined to be the spokes of a wheel, the center of the wheel is the _____.   AV Node

Lead V_2 describes a straight line directly from the front to the back of the patient. In lead V_2 the patient's back is considered _____ (positive or negative).   negative

---

* The chest leads, also called the "precordial" (in front of the heart) leads, were introduced by Dr. Frank Wilson.

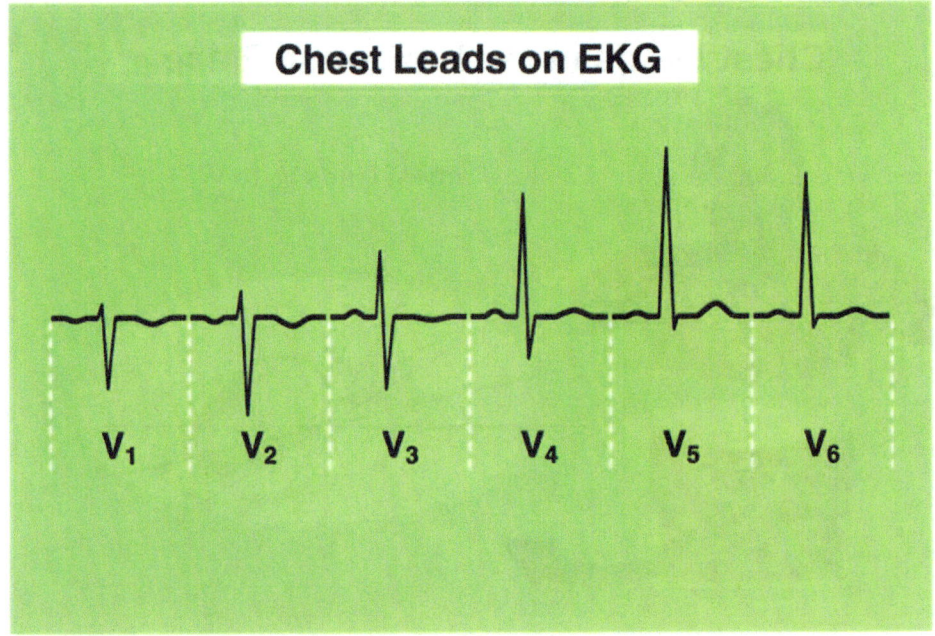

By examining an EKG, you will notice that the waves in the six chest leads show progressive changes from V_1 to V_6.

Note: When observing the chest leads from V_1 to V_6 you will see gradual changes in all the waves (as the position of the positive electrode changes for each successive lead).

In the illustration the V_1 chest lead, the QRS complex is mainly _____ (positive or negative) normally.   negative

In chest lead V_6 the QRS complex is usually mainly _____ (positive or negative). Understand why.   positive

Observing the V_6 chest lead, we know that the mainly positive QRS complex is produced by ventricular depolarization moving _____ the POSITIVE chest electrode of V_6 toward (if you're a little unsure about this concept, take another look at page 12).

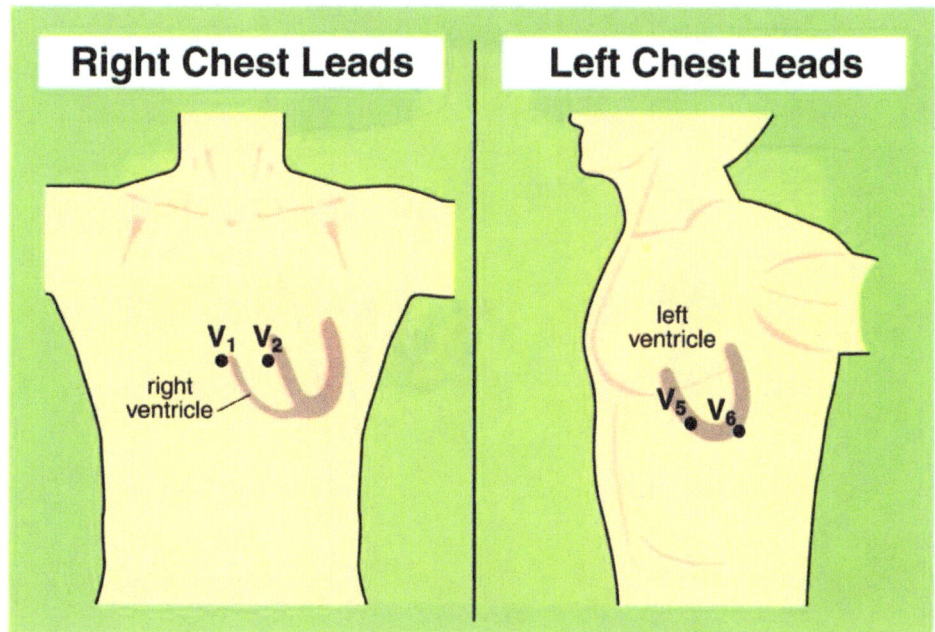

Leads V_1 and V_2 are oriented over the right side of the heart, while V_5 and V_6 are oriented over the left side of the heart.

Leads V_1 and V_2 are called the "_____" chest leads.   right

The two chest leads oriented over the left side of the heart are ____ and ____, (and are called the "left" chest leads). V_5 and V_6

A depolarization wave moving toward the (positive) chest electrode in lead V_6 causes an _____ deflection on the EKG tracing of this lead. (*Now you understand!*)   upward (positive)

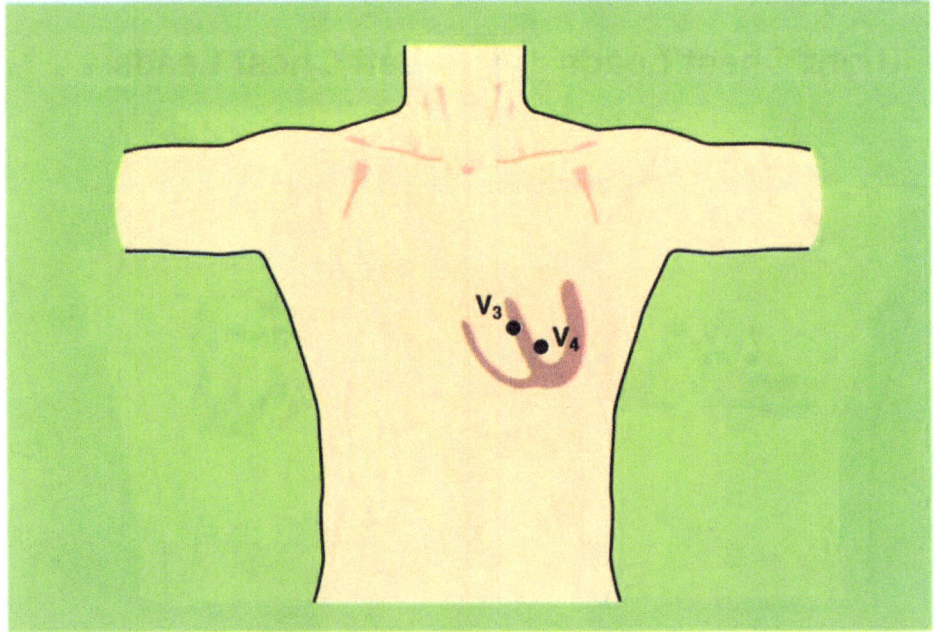

Leads V_3 and V_4 are generally oriented over the *interventricular septum*. V_3 is nearer the right ventricle, and V_4 is nearer the left ventricle.

Leads V_3 and V_4 are oriented over the area of
the interventricular _____.   septum

Note: The interventricular septum is a common wall shared by the right and left ventricles, so this septum separates the cavity of the right ventricle from the cavity of the left ventricle. The Right and the Left Bundle Branches course through the interventricular septum.

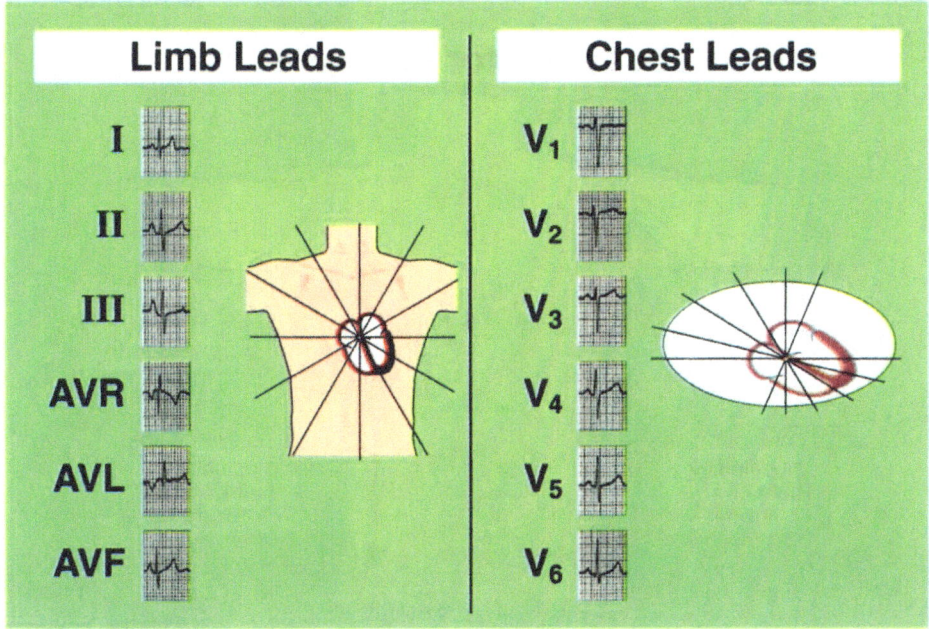

On the standard EKG tracing there are six chest leads and six limb leads. This is the 12 lead electrocardiogram.

The six limb leads all lie in the _____ plane, which can be visualized on the patient's chest.

frontal

The six chest leads lie in the horizontal plane and are arranged in progressive order from V_1 to ____.

V_6

The six chest leads are recorded using a positive electrode, which is placed at six specific anatomical positions on the chest, encircling the heart in the _____ plane.

horizontal

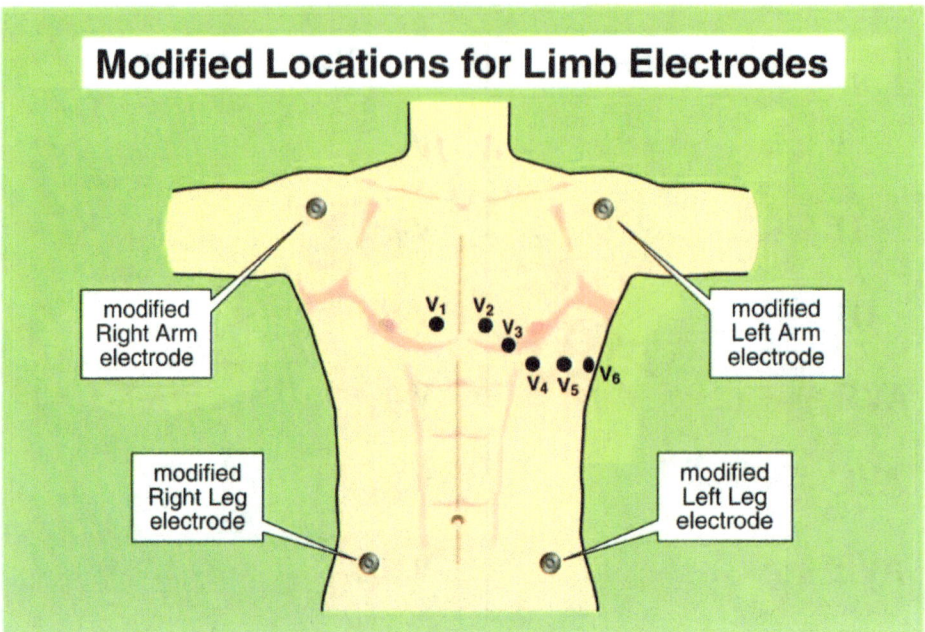

The six limb leads also can be recorded by using carefully positioned electrodes on the trunk of the patient. The special electrode placement (above) used for exercise ("stress") testing, can be used to record each of the twelve EKG leads.

Note: An EKG recorded from a carefully positioned trunk* electrode can record the same information (same accuracy and same amplitude) as an ankle or wrist electrode for a given limb lead. In this way, a standard twelve lead EKG can be recorded using trunk electrodes.

Cardiac monitoring in hospital rooms, as well as in the emergency department, surgery, recovery room, coronary care, and intensive care, is carried out using modified electrode positions on the patient's _____ to monitor classical limb (and other) leads.   trunk

Paramedics and many Emergency Medical Technicians (EMT's) use trunk* _____ for diagnostic purposes and also for   electrodes telemetry transmission.

        Now we're ready to tackle the autonomic nervous system... O.K.?

* These are "trunk" but not truly "chest" electrodes, for they often use the shoulders
  and abdomen as electrode locations. A variety of modifications are commonly used
  to monitor patients in various settings and circumstances (see page 346).

Chapter 3: Autonomic Nervous System

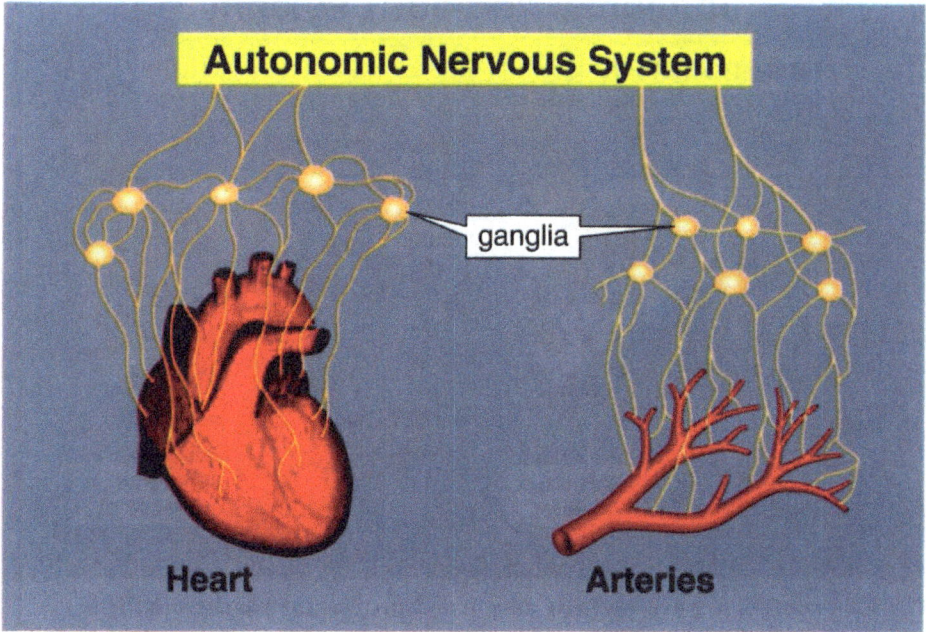

The **Autonomic Nervous System** (ANS) regulates vital functions of all organs by both reflex and central nervous system control, but *not* by conscious control.

Although the ANS controls all organs and organ systems, our main concern is autonomic control of the _____,   heart and also of the systemic arteries as they relate to blood pressure.

Note: The ANS has two divisions that sometimes seem difficult to comprehend, because one division may stimulate an organ, yet inhibit another organ. However, these two divisions have well defined roles in the heart and the systemic arteries; *one division stimulates, and one division inhibits*. It's that simple! One division stimulates cell function, while the other division opposes that stimulation. Each division operates like an electrical system that controls its own terminal switches called "receptors" that modulate the function of heart cells, via the ion-moving structures of those cells.

Note: A stimulus originating in the ANS is transmitted to a **ganglion*** of secondary nerve cells for processing. The nerves of the ganglion relay the stimulus to their nerve ends, each of which terminates as a disc called a **bouton** (bouton is French for button) that covers the receptors of a cardiac cell (or an arterial muscle cell). See next page.

* "Ganglion" is singular, "ganglia" is plural.

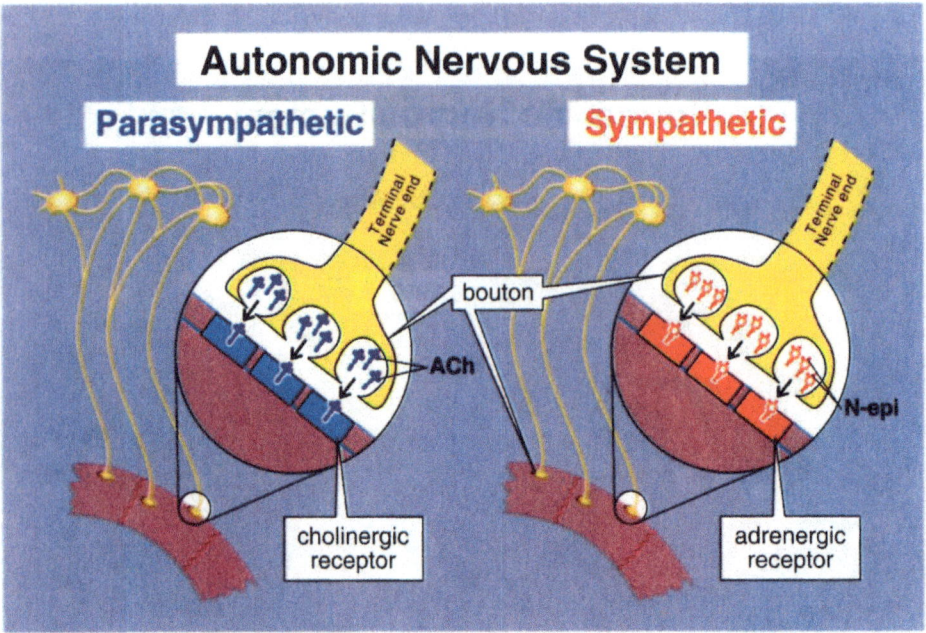

The ANS consists of a **sympathetic** system and an opposing **parasympathetic** system. Each of these two systems secretes its own *neurotransmitter* from its terminal boutons in order to activate specific cell receptors in the cell membrane.

The terminal ends (boutons) of *sympathetic* nerves secrete **Nor-epinephrine*** (N-epi), an adrenaline-like neurotransmitter that activates specific _____ receptors called *adrenergic* receptors.   cell

Note: In the heart, the sympathetic and parasympathetic nervous systems have opposite functions. Interestingly, the parasympathetic exercises some direct control of the sympathetic.

The terminal *parasympathetic* nerve ends (boutons) secrete the neurotransmitter **Acetylcholine** (ACh), which exclusively activates cell _____ called *cholinergic* receptors.   receptors

* Nor-epinephrine, hyphenated for recognition purposes, will be "Norepinephrine" from now on. Although the abbreviation "N-epi" is used here, some texts use "NE."

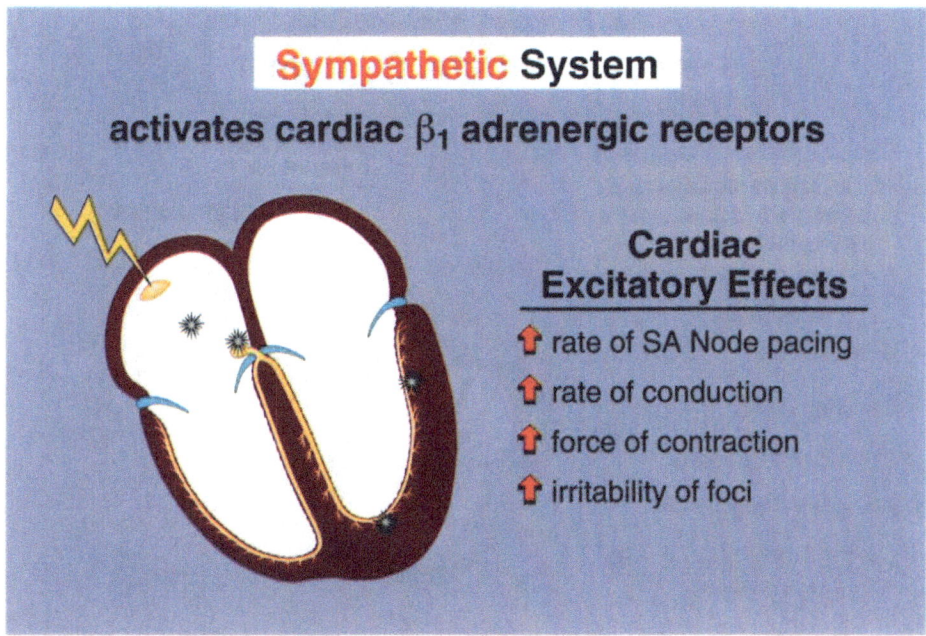

The heart is stimulated by the sympathetic system through its terminal boutons. The boutons deliver N-epi to the β_1 (**adrenergic**) receptors; this activates the β_1 receptors,* producing an *excitatory* response at the cellular level.

Norepinephrine (N-epi), the neurotransmitter of the sympathetic system, activates the heart's β_1 (adrenergic) receptors, stimulating the SA Node to _____ faster. N-epi also:

pace

...improves AV Node conduction and accelerates conduction through the atrial and ventricular _____,

myocardium

...increases the force of myocardial _____,

contraction

...and increases the irritability of atrial and Junctional (page 123) automaticity _____ and minimally affects ventricular foci.

foci

Note: N-epi's brother, **epinephrine** ("adrenaline") is secreted into the blood by the adrenal glands. Epinephrine is an even *more potent* stimulator of the heart's β_1 receptors.

* "β_1 adrenergic receptors" is often shortened to "β_1 receptors," but *adrenergic* is understood.

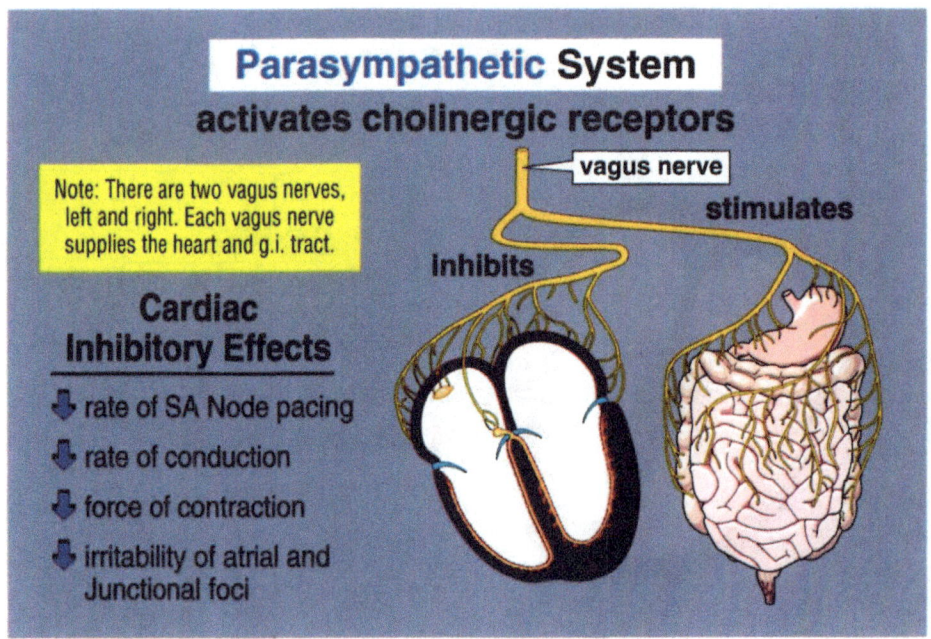

Parasympathetic nerves release the neurotransmitter acetylcholine (ACh), which activates cardiac cholinergic receptors (most are within the atria) to produce a cardiac *inhibitory* effect. Conversely, the gastrointestinal tract is stimulated by its parasympathetic innervation.

Parasympathetic activation of cholinergic receptors by ACh:

…inhibits the SA Node, decreasing the heart _____,   rate

…decreases the speed of myocardial conduction,
and depresses the AV _____,   Node

…diminishes the force of myocardial _____,   contraction

…and depresses irritability of automaticity _____,   foci
mainly those in the atria and AV Junction.

Note: The **vagus** nerves are the body's main parasympathetic pathway, so "vagal" stimulation means parasympathetic stimulation, with the understanding that vagal "stimulation" of the heart is <u>inhibitory</u>.

Note: Despite the parasympathetic system's inhibiting effect on the heart, parasympathetic activation of cholinergic receptors stimulates the gastro-intestinal tract. Recalling the agony of severe vomiting or an episode of painful, crampy diarrhea will help you remember the effect of excessive parasympathetic stimulation of the stomach and the bowel.

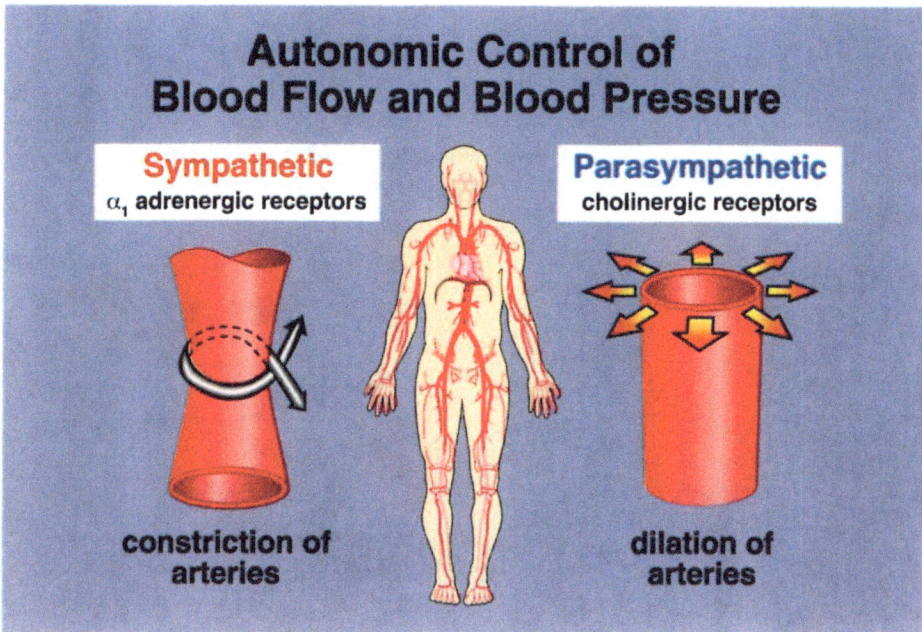

Besides controlling the SA Node's pacing rate, the Autonomic Nervous System controls blood flow and blood pressure by regulating constriction and dilation of arteries throughout the body.

Sympathetic stimulation of arterial α_1 (adrenergic) receptors constricts arteries throughout the body, increasing blood pressure and blood _____. The α_1 receptors are more responsive   flow to the neurotransmitter N-epi than to circulating epinephrine.

Note: By pulling both ends of the Greek *alpha*, the center loop of the "α" constricts the artery (see arrows on the α in the illustration). Now you will always remember alpha adrenergic sympathetic effects on systemic arteries.

Parasympathetic activation of arterial (cholinergic) receptors dilates the same arteries as above, reducing blood _____   pressure and blood flow. Besides the direct cholinergic inhibition of the arteries, there is also an indirect inhibitory parasympathetic effect on the sympathetic ganglia that send nerve fibers to the vessels.

Note: Blood flow is also very dependent on the heart rate: sympathetic stimulation increases the SA Node pacing rate, while the parasympathetic decreases it. Autonomic control of the heart rate and systemic blood pressure involves delicate regulation of the parasympathetic–sympathetic balance to maintain circulatory **homeostasis** (the ideal status quo).

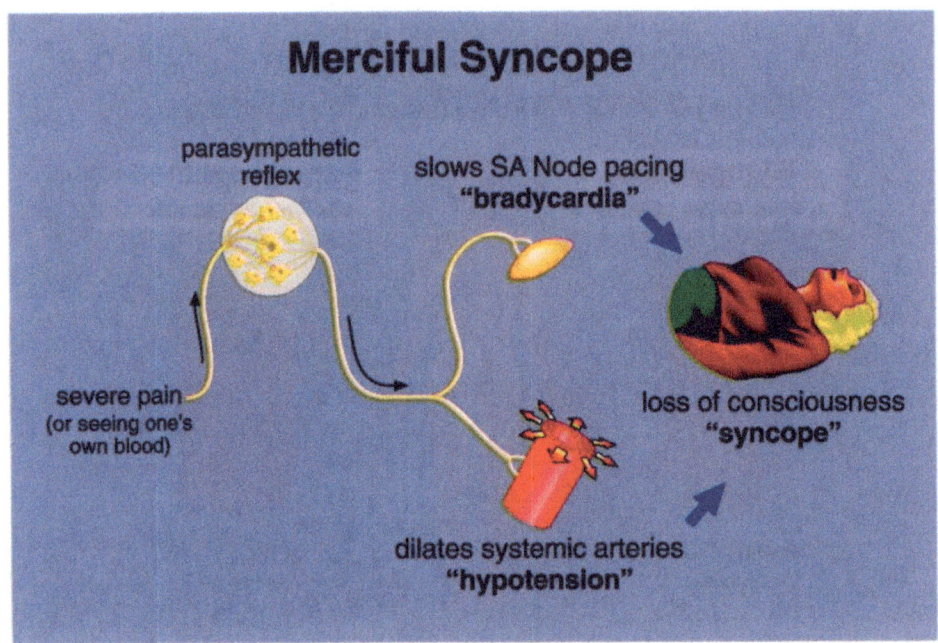

Severe pain and/or seeing one's own blood may induce a reflex parasympathetic response that causes **syncope*** (loss of consciousness).

Severe pain and/or seeing one's own blood often initiates
reflex parasympathetic activity that slows SA Node
pacing, known as _____-cardia.   brady

The same reflex parasympathetic response dilates systemic
arteries causing hypotension, as the blood _____ falls.   pressure

Note: A devastating injury, which causes excruciating pain/awareness
of bleeding, can induce a parasympathetic response that dramatically
lowers the blood pressure and slows the heart. This merciful reflex
effectively reduces the brain's blood supply to the point of syncope.

Aside: Perhaps you have encountered (oversensitive) patients who
lose consciousness upon seeing their own blood drawn for lab tests,
or if they experience minimal pain. Be compassionate; their body is
only responding to a normal parasympathetic reflex.

* This and other types of vagally mediated syncope are sometimes
    called "**vaso-vagal syncope**." Syncope is pronounced "SINK-oh-pee."

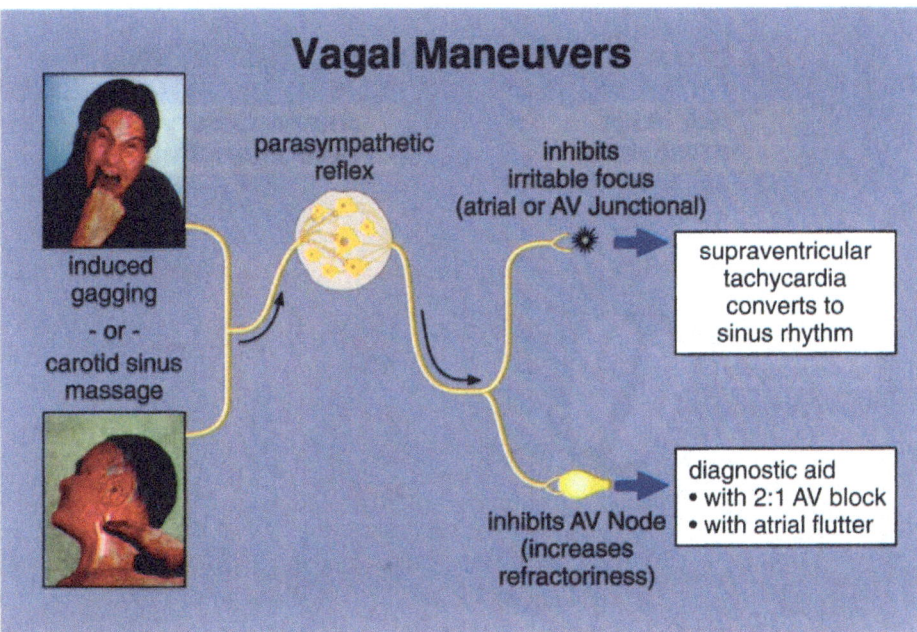

Cardiovascular sensors provide ("afferent") input for parasympathetic reflexes that counterbalance sympathetic effects. **Vagal maneuvers** may be employed to produce a reflex parasympathetic response for both diagnostic and therapeutic purposes.

Gastrointestinal stimulation (e.g., gag reflex) may be employed to produce a parasympathetic _____.   response

Carotid sinus massage may be used in carefully selected patients* to produce a _____ response.   parasympathetic

Note: An induced parasympathetic response may be used therapeutically to depress an irritable focus in the atria or AV Junction. An induced parasympathetic response may be diagnostically employed to transiently slow AV Node conduction, or to make the AV Node more refractory to depolarization (see pages 160 and 183).

* Injudicious use of carotid sinus massage in some patients can dislodge a piece of atheromatous plaque, sending plaque emboli to the brain (careful!). Use discretion when employing diagnostic procedures that can cause iatrogenic stroke, which can disable a patient and incite a feeding frenzy of lawyers.

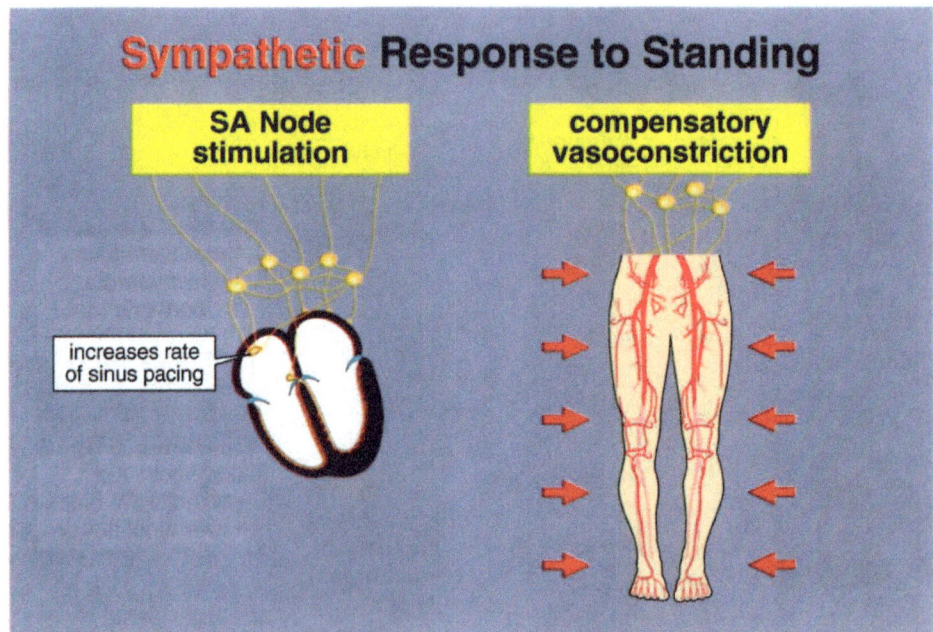

It seems as though standing would allow blood to gravitate into the lower extremities. However, standing produces a compensatory *sympathetic* response that constricts peripheral arteries to prevent distal blood pooling, and stimulates sinus pacing.

Note: The body has "pressure" receptors* that detect low blood pressure, particularly with standing. These pressure receptors initiate a sympathetic reflex that constricts peripheral arteries and increases the heart rate slightly, thereby conserving blood flow to the brain.

Impaired function of this normal sympathetic response to standing can diminish blood flow to the brain, causing _____.   syncope

Orthostatic hypotension is an abrupt fall in blood pressure caused by failure of these compensatory sympathetic mechanisms upon _____.   standing

* Careful! These "receptors" are cardiovascular sensors, called *baroreceptors*, that the body uses to detect changes in blood pressure. Please don't confuse them with the cell membrane receptors that are activated by N-epi or ACh.

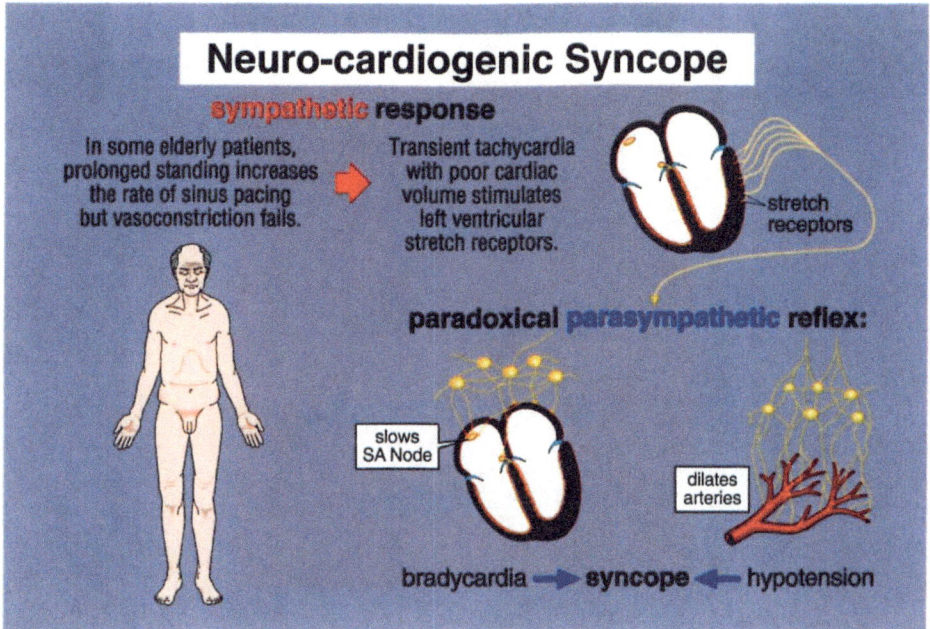

Standing produces a sympathetic vasoconstriction response to maintain adequate circulation. This compensatory mechanism may fail with prolonged standing in *certain* elderly patients, triggering a *paradoxical* parasympathetic response causing syncope.

Note: Pooling of blood in the lower extremities from prolonged standing is normally compensated by a reflex sympathetic increase in both blood pressure and heart rate. However, in some elderly patients, sinus pacing accelerates, but peripheral vasoconstriction is inadequate. So, the partially filled ventricles contract rigorously, stimulating parasympathetic *mechanoreceptors* in the left ventricle. This initiates an undesirable parasympathetic reflex that slows SA Node pacing and reduces blood pressure; so blood flow to the brain is reduced, causing syncope. This is **neuro-cardiogenic syncope**.

Neuro-cardiogenic syncope, a (paradoxical) parasympathetic response to prolonged standing, causes vasodilation and slowing of the pulse, resulting in a loss of _____.   consciousness

Under controlled circumstances, a Head Up Tilt ("HUT") test confirms the diagnosis of neuro-cardiogenic _____.   syncope

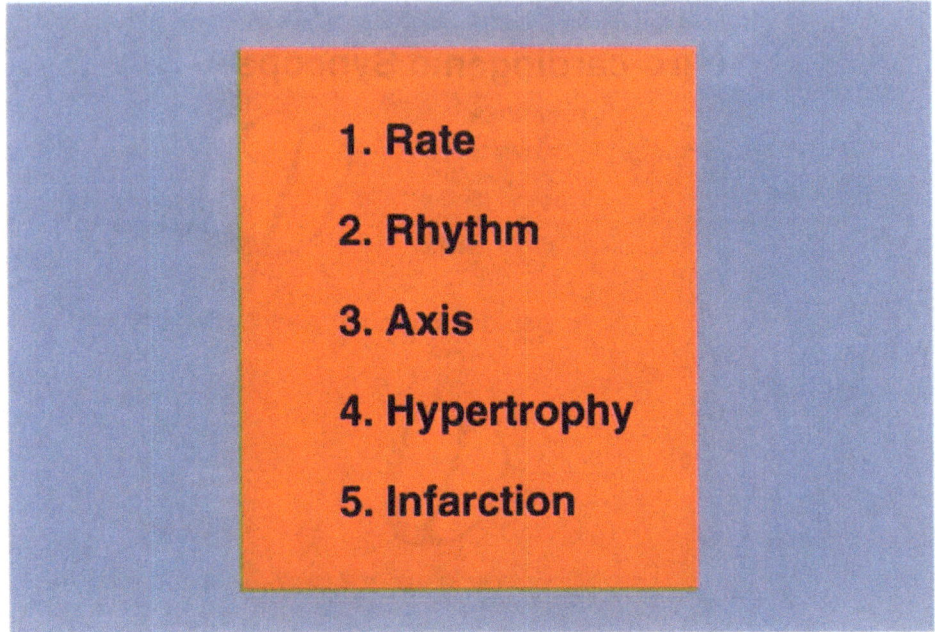

1. Rate

2. Rhythm

3. Axis

4. Hypertrophy

5. Infarction

Knowing basic cardiac principles and understanding the autonomic nervous system ensures mastery these five general areas of routine EKG interpretation.

Proper interpretation of an _____ requires consideration of   EKG
Rate, Rhythm, Axis, Hypertrophy, and Infarction. They are
all equally important.

Note: Take a moment and examine page 334 to observe the
simple methodology that will become your routine.

Before you begin each chapter, preview its summary (pages 335 to 346).
Then, as you progress through the chapter, little "aha's" of recognition
will flash in your brain, and you will appreciate how each concept is
carefully woven into this simplified methodology. Your **understanding**
evolves rapidly; this is the foundation of your permanent **knowledge**.

Ready? Let's go!

Chapter 4: Rate

65

Before you begin, look at this chapter's summary on pages 334 and 335.

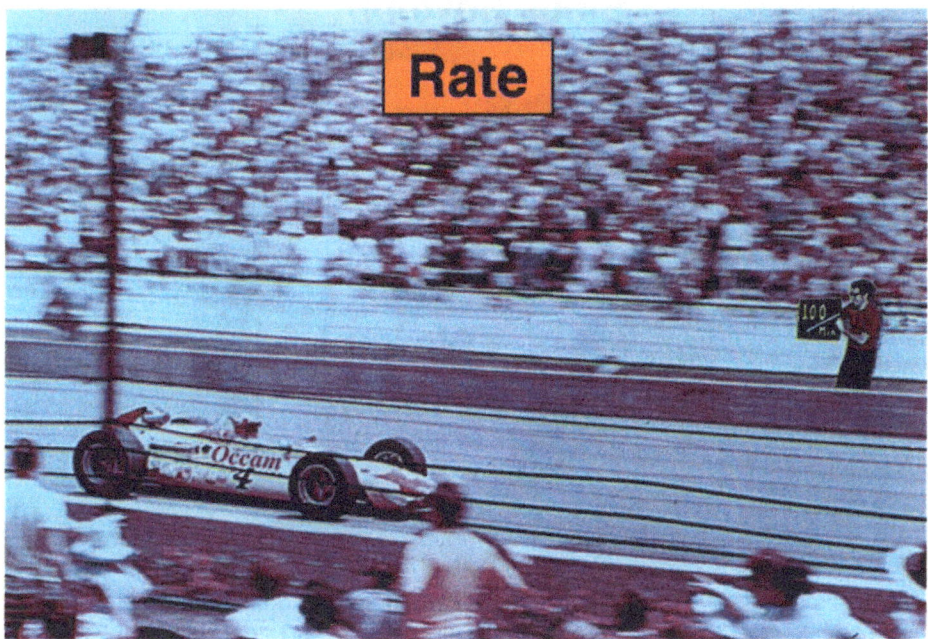

When reading an EKG, you should first consider the rate.

Note: The sign in this picture is not informing the driver* about the rate of his race car. The man holding the sign is a physician who has been monitoring the driver's transmitted EKG. The sign is telling the driver about his current heart rate (he's a little excited).

When examining an EKG, you should determine the _____ first.

rate

The rate is read as cycles per _____.

minute

Now, let's examine where and how the normal heart rate originates…

* With a sincere dedication to Billy Occam, deceased long ago, who made simplicity a virtue of science.

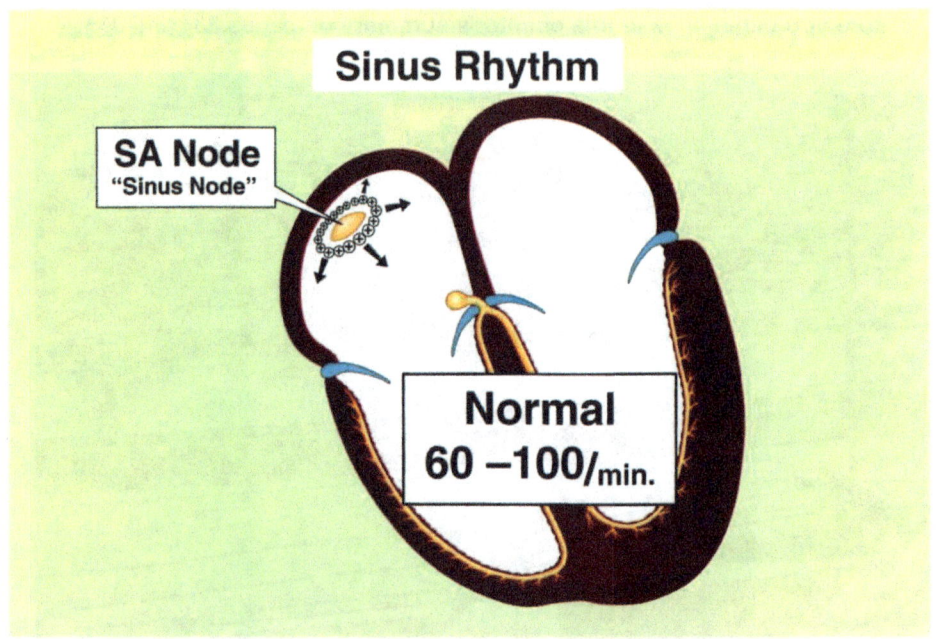

The SA Node (Sinus Node), the heart's pacemaker and the dominant center of
automaticity, generates a **Sinus Rhythm**. The SA Node paces the heart in the normal
rate range of 60 to 100 per minute.

The heart's normal pacemaker, the _____, generates   SA Node
a continuous series of regular, pacemaking stimuli
(this is its "**automaticity**").

The SA Node is located within the upper-posterior wall of
the right _____. The SA Node emits a regular series of   atrium
pacemaking (depolarization) stimuli.

Note: The Sinus Node (SA Node) is the heart's dominant center
of automaticity, and the normal, regular rhythm that it generates
is called the Sinus Rhythm.

At rest, the Sinus Rhythm maintains a rate of 60
to _____ beats per minute, which is the normal range   100
of the pacing rate.

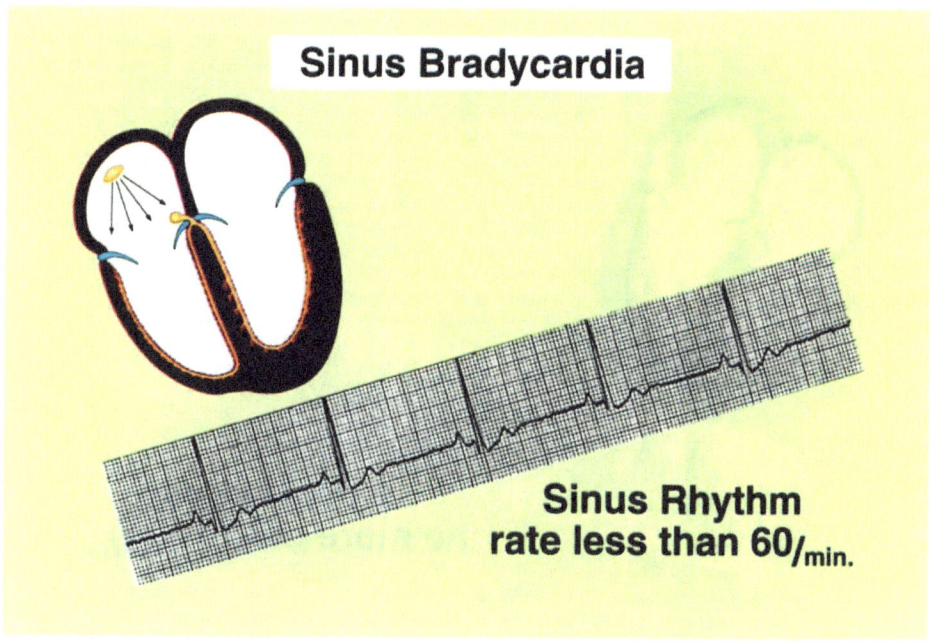

If the Sinus Node (SA Node) paces the heart at a rate slower than 60 per minute, this is **Sinus Bradycardia**.

Note: "Brady" = slow; "cardia" = heart.

A rhythm originating in the heart's normal pacemaker, the
SA Node, with a rate slower than 60 per minute is called
Sinus _____.   Bradycardia

Note: Sinus Bradycardia most often results from parasympathetic
excess, as we see in conditioned athletes at rest. Sometimes an
extremely slow heart rate may reduce blood flow to the brain
causing loss of consciousness (**syncope**). See pages 60 and 63.

Sinus Bradycardia is present if the SA Node produces
a heart rate of less than one beat per _____.   second
                                                                      (careful!)

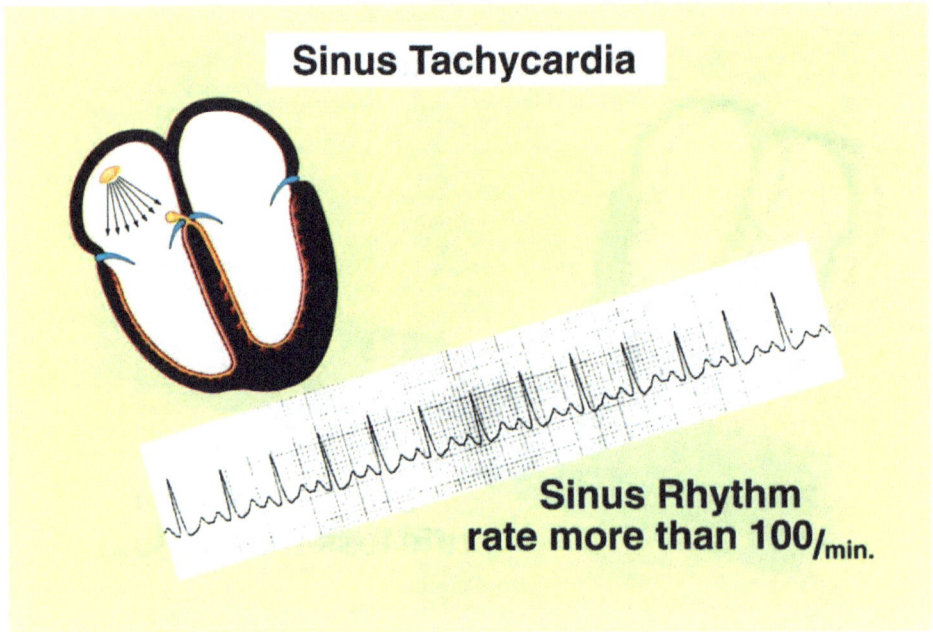

If the Sinus Node (SA Node) paces the heart at a rate greater than 100 per minute, this is **Sinus Tachycardia**.

Note: "Tachy" = fast; "cardia" = heart.

A rhythm originating in the SA Node (Sinus Node)
is called Sinus Tachycardia if the rate is greater
than _____ per minute.   100

Exercise produces sympathetic stimulation of the SA Node;
this is the most common cause of Sinus _____.   Tachycardia

Note: There are focal areas of automaticity in the heart known as
automaticity foci. * They are potential pacemakers that are capable
of pacing in emergency situations. Under normal circumstances,
these foci are electrically silent (that's why they are referred to as
"potential" pacemakers).

* *"Automaticity foci"* refers to more than one *"automaticity focus"*; in fact, when the word
  "foci" is used alone, *"automaticity foci"* is understood. Foci is pronounced "FOE-sigh."

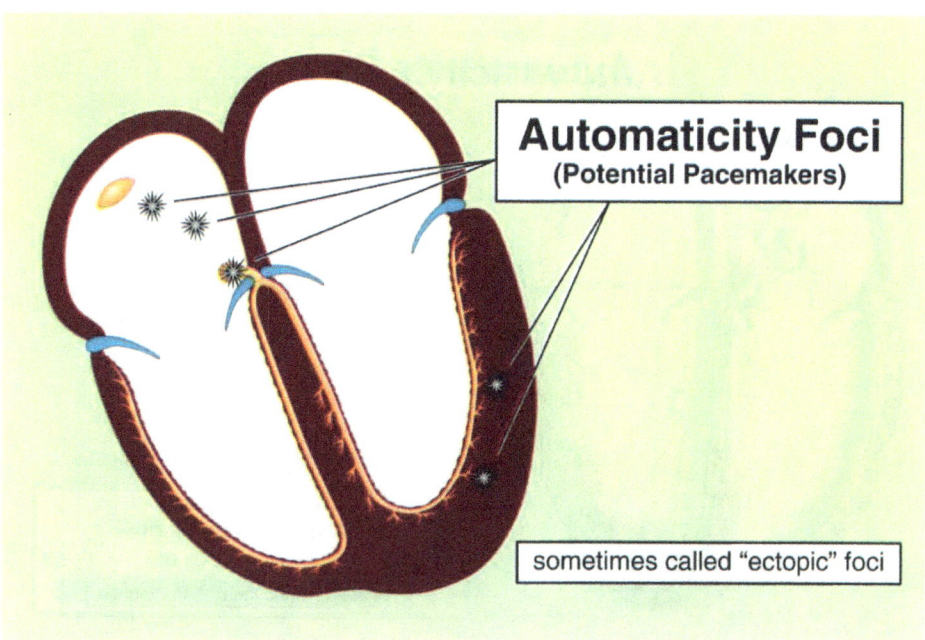

If normal SA Node pacemaking fails, other potential pacemakers known as *automaticity foci* (also called "ectopic" foci) have the ability to pace (at their **inherent rate**). They are in the atria, the ventricles, and the AV Junction.

If the SA Node ceases to function, one of the potential pacemakers, known as an *automaticity focus*, will assume pacemaking activity at its inherent _____ (only one focus assumes pacing responsibility).   rate

The atria have automaticity _____ of potential pacemakers   foci
that are within the atrial conduction system (see page 101),
and they are called *atrial automaticity foci*.

Note: The proximal end of the AV Node has no automaticity foci, however the middle and distal regions of the AV Node, an area known as the *AV Junction* <u>does have</u> automaticity foci that are called *Junctional automaticity foci*.

Purkinje fibers have automaticity foci, so there are foci of
these potential _____ in the His Bundle and in   pacemakers
the Bundle Branches and their subdivisions; these foci
are called *ventricular automaticity foci*.

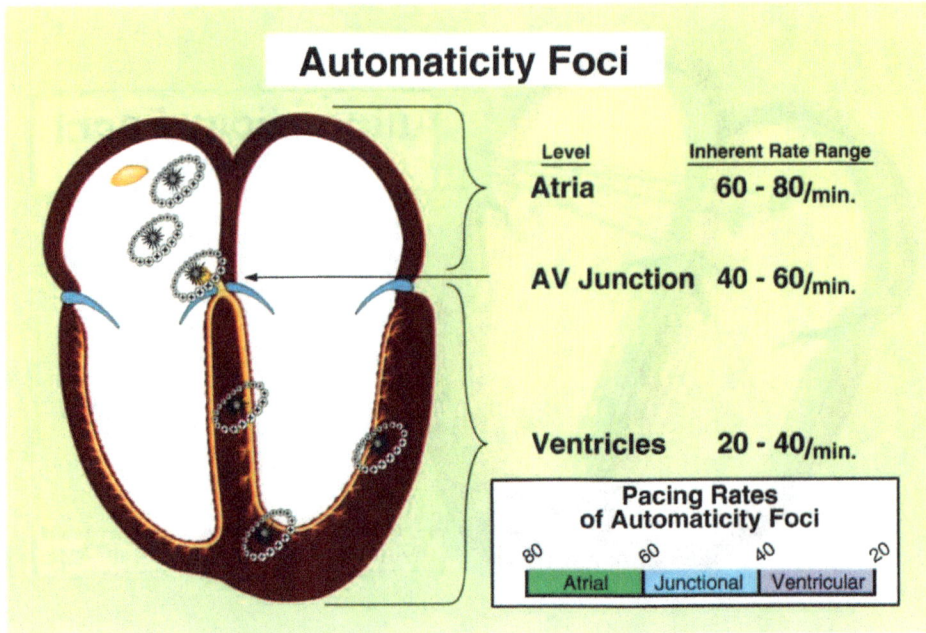

The automaticity foci of each "level" (the atria, the AV Junction, and the ventricles are each a "level") have a general range of pacemaking rate. Although all foci of a given level pace within a general rate range, each individual automaticity focus has its own precise *inherent rate* at which it paces.

Each automaticity focus of the atria has a specific inherent rate at which it paces, but its inherent rate falls within the general range of ___ to 80 per minute.

60

The automaticity foci of the AV Junction all pace in the range of ___ to 60 per minute, but any single Junctional focus paces at its individual inherent rate.

40

Ventricular automaticity foci all pace in the ___ to 40 per minute range, but any specific ventricular focus has a distinct inherent rate of pacing.

20

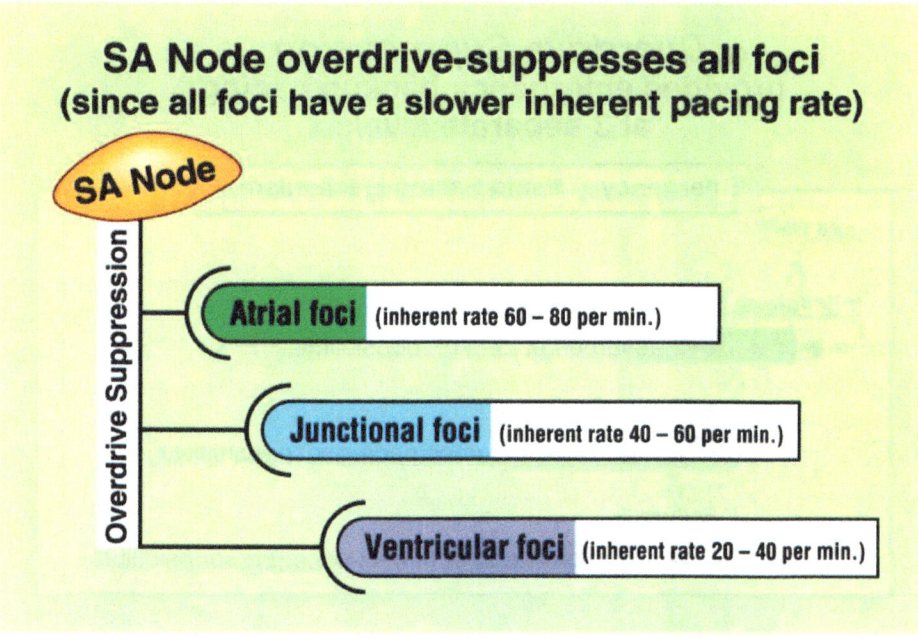

Rapid automaticity (pacemaking activity) suppresses slower automaticity (pacemaking activity) – this is **overdrive suppression**, a very important fundamental characteristic of all automaticity centers.

Note: Overdrive suppression is characteristic of all centers of automaticity (including the SA Node and all automaticity foci). Simply stated: any automaticity center will overdrive-suppress* all others that have a slower inherent pacemaking rate.

The SA Node overdrive-suppresses the (slower) inherent pacemaking activity of all the automaticity _____ below it; this provides the SA Node with the luxury   foci of not having to compete with slower pacemaking activity of lower automaticity foci.

In fact, once an automaticity focus actively begins pacing, it will overdrive-_____ all lower (slower) foci,   suppress including slower foci at the same level…

…eliminating any competition. Well Designed!

* When used as a verb, "overdrive-suppress" is hyphenated… so says the publisher.

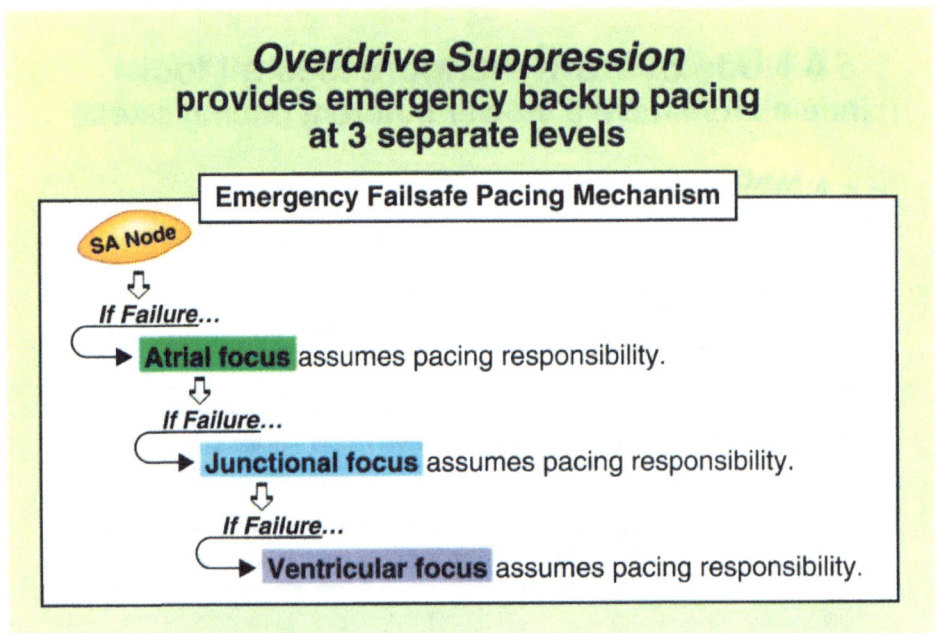

Overdrive suppression is the heart's failsafe pacing mechanism, providing three separate levels of backup pacing, by utilizing automaticity foci in the atria, the ventricles, and the AV Junction.

Note: An automaticity focus actively pacing at its inherent rate, overdrive-suppresses all slower foci including slower foci at its own level.

Should normal SA Node pacing fail (pacemaker failure), a backup pacemaker (i.e., an automaticity focus from a lower level) – no longer overdrive-suppressed – will emerge to pace at its inherent rate; and it conveniently overdrive-suppresses potential pacemaking activity at all levels that are _____ it.   below

Therefore, an automaticity focus only emerges to function as a pacemaker when it is no longer _____-suppressed.   overdrive
For instance, in SA Node failure…

…a focus from a lower level – no longer overdrive-suppressed by regular pacing stimuli from above – can emerge to pace.
Very well Designed!

Let's do that once again, slowly.

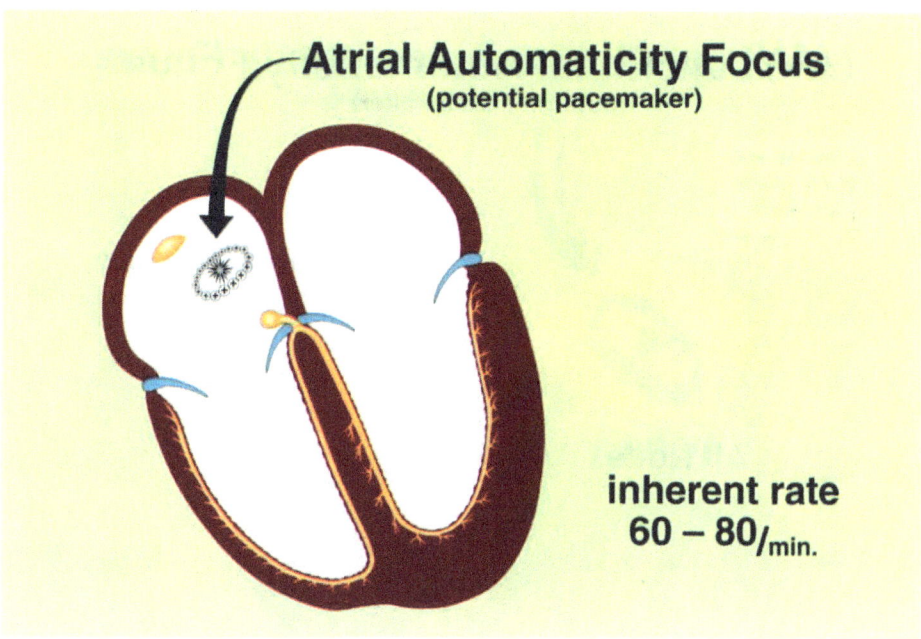

Atrial Automaticity Focus
(potential pacemaker)

**inherent rate
60 – 80/min.**

The atria have automaticity foci of potential pacemakers, any one of which can assume active pacemaking responsibility in its inherent rate range of about 60 to 80 per minute, if normal pacemaking fails.

If SA Node pacing fails, an atrial automaticity focus can assume the active pacemaking responsibility in its inherent rate range of about 60 to ___ per minute (close to the SA Node's normal rate).

80

If the SA Node fails, an atrial automaticity _____ (within the atrial conduction system) may then assume active pacing responsibility to become the *dominant pacemaker*. (The last sentence on this page explains "dominant" pacemaker.)

focus

So without SA Node pacing, an atrial automaticity focus can emerge as an active backup pacemaker, and it becomes the *dominant pacemaker* by overdrive-suppressing all lower levels of foci, since they have slower_____ rates.

inherent

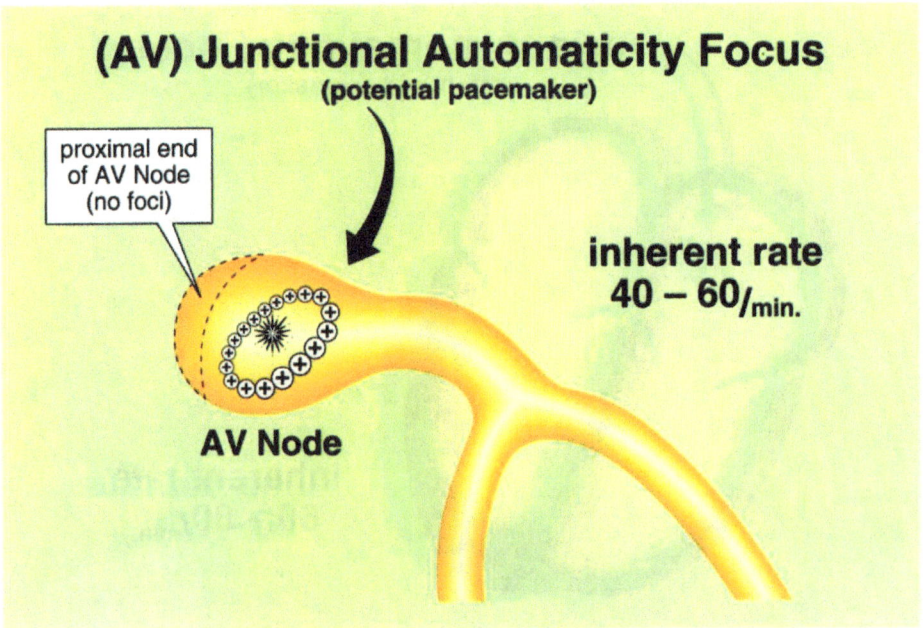

(AV) Junctional Automaticity Focus
(potential pacemaker)

proximal end
of AV Node
(no foci)

**inherent rate
40 – 60/min.**

AV Node

The AV Junction has automaticity foci (potential pacemakers), one of which will emerge to actively pace in its inherent rate range of 40 to 60 per minute if there is an <u>absence</u> of regular pacing stimuli progressing down from the atria.

Note: The AV Junction is that portion of the AV Node that has foci of automaticity. The proximal end of the AV node has no foci. The AV Junction has foci of automaticity called "*Junctional foci.*"

An automaticity focus in the AV Junction begins active backup pacing only in the absence of pacing stimuli coming down from the atria. Then, no longer overdrive-suppressed, it emerges to actively pace in its inherent _____ range of 40 to 60 per minute, and it overdrive-suppresses all   rate
lower (slower) automaticity foci, becoming the dominant pacemaker.

A Junctional focus actively pacing at its inherent rate
(___ to 60 per minute range), produces an *idio-junctional** rhythm.   40

Note: A Junctional focus (that is, an automaticity focus in the AV Junction) emerges as the active pacemaker if it is no longer overdrive-suppressed by regular pacing stimuli from above. This can occur if the SA Node and all atrial foci fail. But wait — something else can prevent a Junctional focus from being depolarized by regular pacing stimuli from above. Next page!

* The prefix "idio" is of Greek origin, and it means "one's own."
  Idiojunctional is usually <u>not</u> hyphenated.

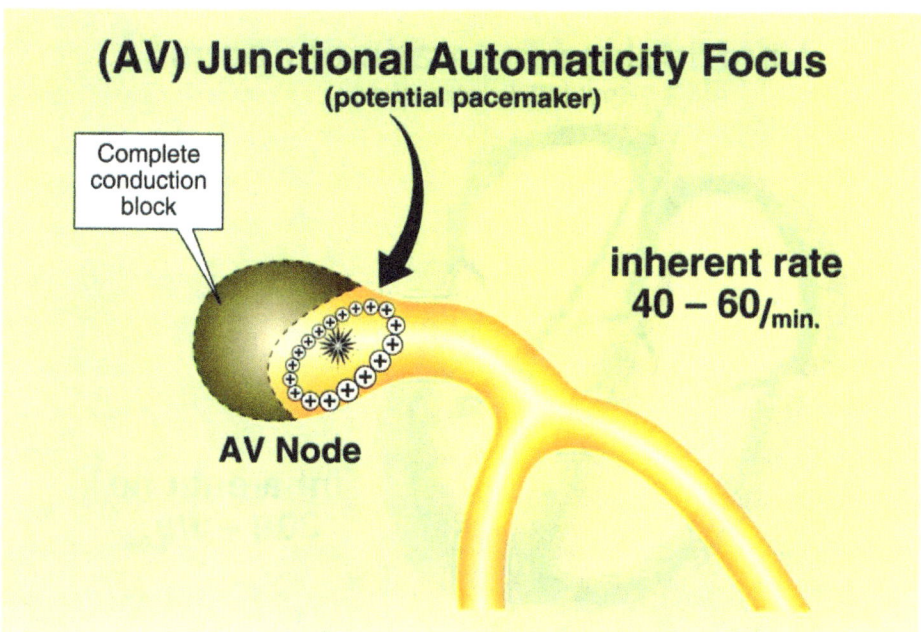

If there is a complete conduction block in the AV Node above the AV Junction, then no regular paced depolarization stimuli from above reach the automaticity foci in the AV Junction.

Note: You will recall that the AV Node is the only conduction link between the atria and the ventricular conduction system below.

With a complete conduction block in the AV Node above the AV Junction, an automaticity _____ in the AV Junction   focus
just below, receives no pacing stimuli from above…

… so, no longer overdrive-suppressed, the Junctional focus escapes to become the active pacemaker for the ventricles. And that Junctional focus paces the ventricles at its inherent rate of ___ - ___ per minute while overdrive-suppressing lower,   40 - 60
(slower) ventricular foci.

Note: It is possible for the AV Junction (together with all its automaticity foci) to suffer a complete block. In that instance, only an automaticity focus in the Purkinje fibers of the ventricles can come to the rescue to pace the ventricles. Let's see how…

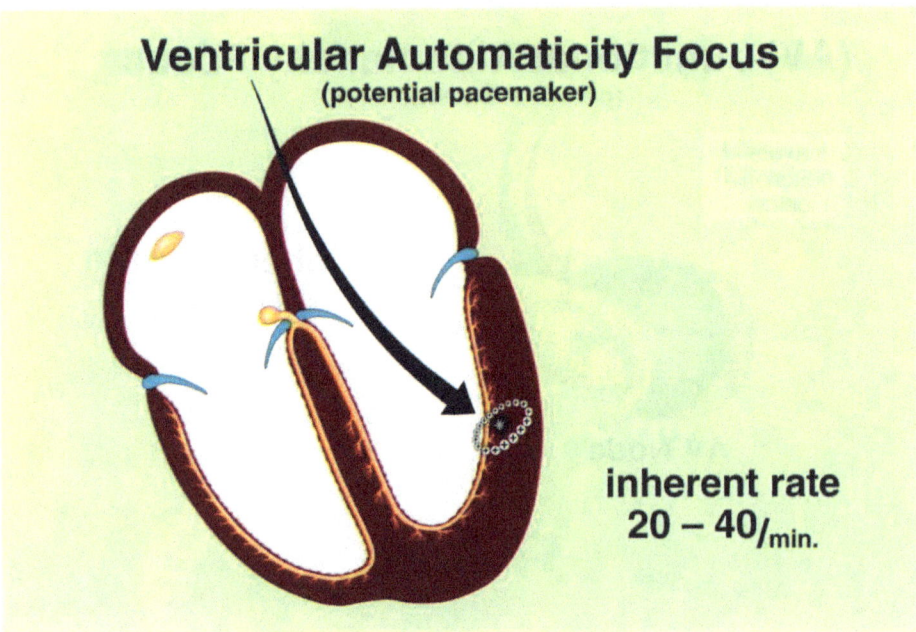

Ventricular Automaticity Focus
(potential pacemaker)

inherent rate
20 – 40/min.

The ventricles have automaticity foci (potential pacemakers), any one of which will assume pacing in its inherent rate range of 20 to 40 per minute, if the usual overdrive suppression (due to regular pacing stimuli from above) is absent.

Note: *Ventricular automaticity foci* are composed of specialized Purkinje fibers. These pacemaking foci are in the His Bundle, the Bundle Branches, and all their subdivisions, since they are all composed of Purkinje fibers.

Without overdrive suppression from above, a ventricular automaticity focus emerges to actively pace in its inherent rate range of ___ to 40 per minute; this is an *idio-ventricular** rhythm.

20

Note: A ventricular focus emerges as the active ventricular pacemaker *only* if it is no longer overdrive-suppressed by regular, paced stimuli from above. This occurs:
- if all pacemaking centers above it have failed.
          -or-
- if there is a complete block of conduction below the AV Node (including the AV Junction) that prevents any pacing stimulus above it (i.e., from the SA Node, an atrial focus, or a Junctional focus) from reaching the ventricles.

*Hyphenated here for ease of recognition, *idioventricular* should <u>not</u> be hyphenated.

OVERDRIVE SUPPRESSION
provides emergency backup pacing at 3 separate levels

Emergency Failsafe Pacing Mechanism

SA Node

If Failure...
→ **Atrial focus** assumes pacing responsibility.

If Failure...
→ **Junctional focus** assumes pacing responsibility.

If Failure...
→ **Ventricular focus** assumes pacing responsibility.

Range of Inherent Pacing Rates of Automaticity Foci

80   60   40   20

| Atrial | Junctional | Ventricular |

If normal SA Node pacing fails, an automaticity focus in the atria, or in the AV Junction, or even in the ventricles (in that order) is available to assume the pacemaking responsibility at its own inherent rate. This provides three levels of backup pacing.

If the SA Node should cease pacing, an atrial automaticity focus can pace in its inherent rate range of 60 to 80 per minute; failing that, backup pacing by a Junctional focus will assume the active _____ responsibility in its (slightly slower) inherent rate range of 40 - 60 per minute.

pacing

The ventricles can be paced by a ventricular automaticity focus in its _____ rate range of 20 to 40 per minute, if the focus is not regularly depolarized by paced stimuli. The lack of properly paced stimuli to the ventricular focus can be due to failure of all automaticity centers above, or due to an intervening complete conduction block that prevents pacing stimuli (from above) from conducting to the ventricles. What a miracle of Nature!

inherent

Note: In a physiological or pathological emergency, an irritable automaticity focus may suddenly discharge at a rapid rate. This emergency rate (150 to 250 per minute) is approximately the same for foci of all levels.

Now let's try something real easy...

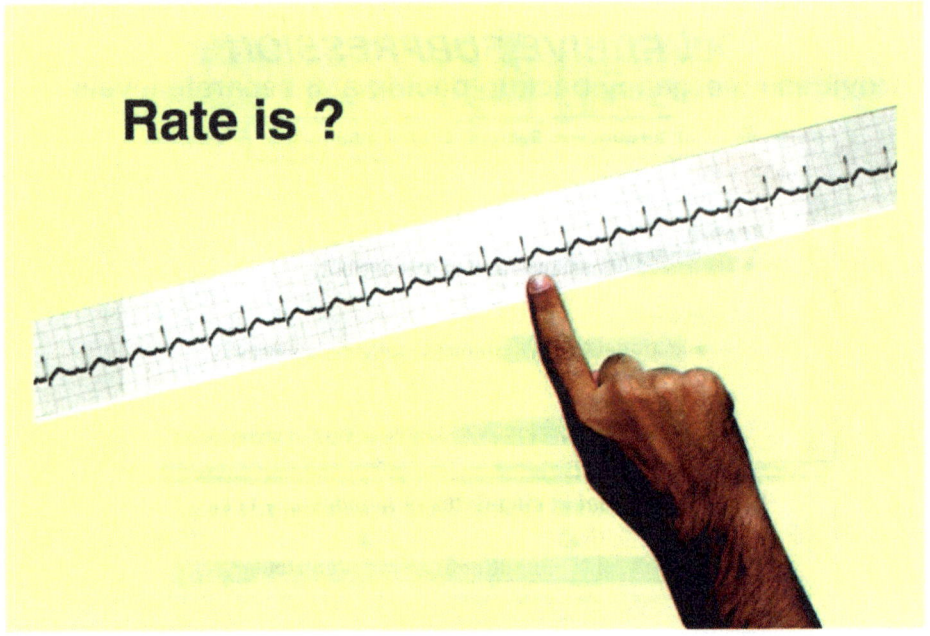

Rate is ?

Our main objective is to rapidly determine the heart rate.

After finishing this chapter you will be able to
determine the _____ rapidly.   rate

No special devices, calculators, rulers, or awkward
mathematical computations are needed in order to
_____ the rate.   determine

Note: In emergency situations, you probably will not be able
to find, much less use a calculator; and you may not have the
presence of mind (or the time) to do mathematical calculations.

Observation alone can give us the _____.   rate

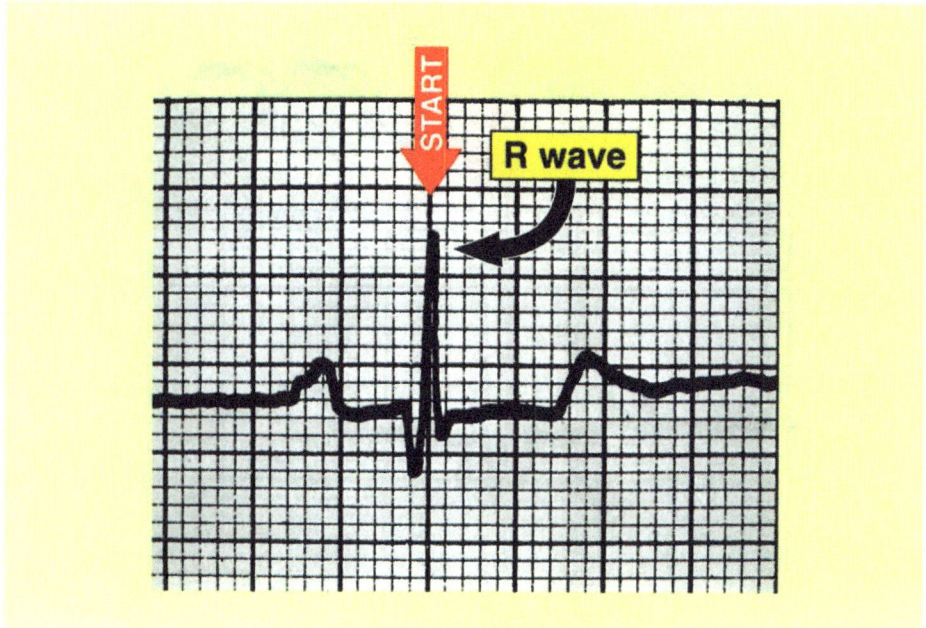

First: Find an R wave that peaks on a **heavy black line** (our "start" line).

To calculate rate, you should first look at the ___ waves.   R

Now find one that peaks on a heavy black line,
and we will call it the "_____" line.   start

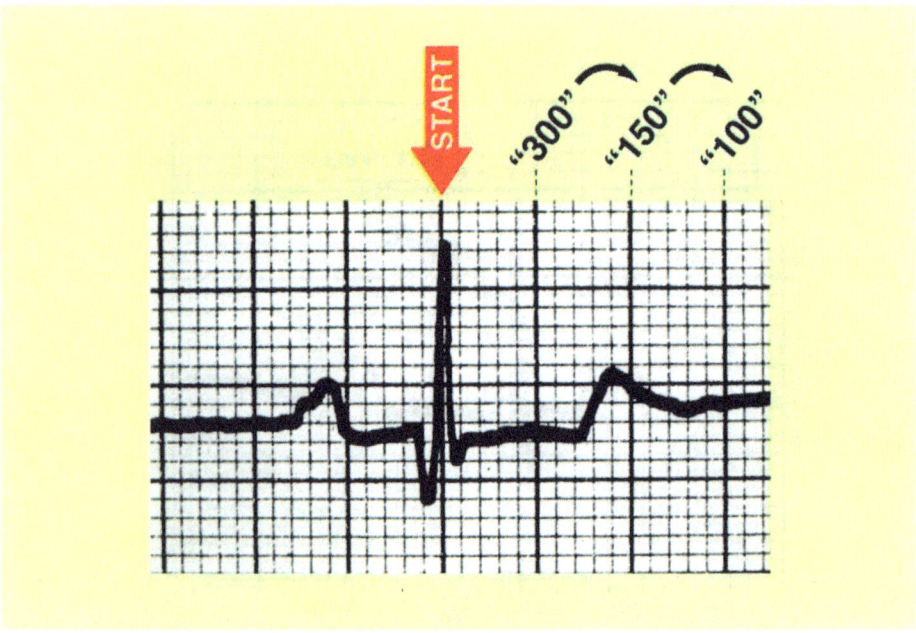

Next: Count off "300, 150, 100" for the three thick lines that follows the start line, naming each line as shown. <u>Memorize these numbers</u>.

An R wave peaks on a heavy black start line...

...the <u>next</u> heavy black line is named "_____"... followed by   300

"_____" and "_____" for the next two heavy black lines.   150, 100

Note: The line that the R wave peaks upon is the start line; we only name the heavy lines that follow the start line.

The three lines following the start line (where the R wave falls) are named "_____, _____, _____" in succession. (Say them out loud!)   300, 150, 100

Again!

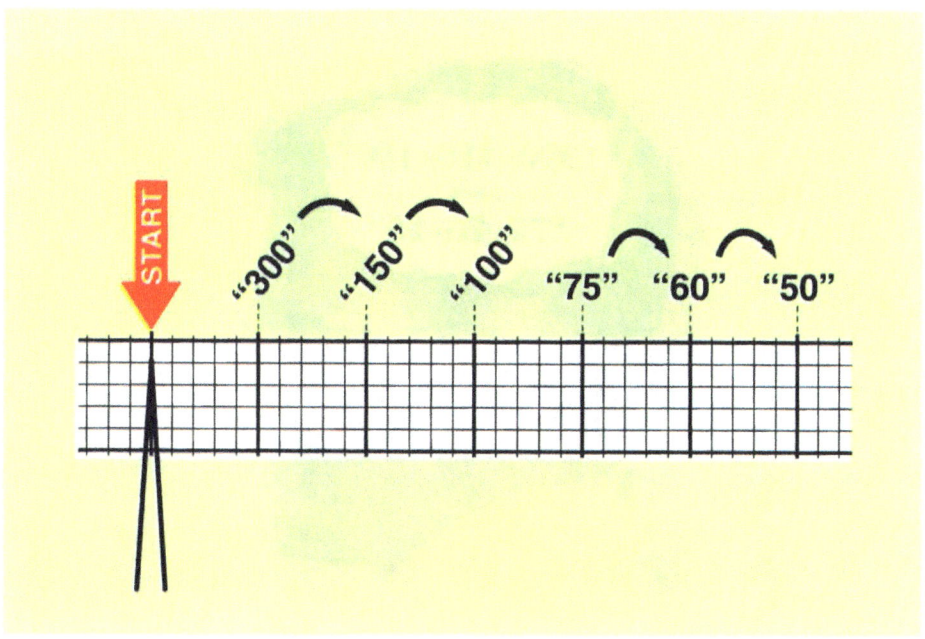

Then: Count off the next three lines after "300, 150, 100" as "75, 60, 50."

The next three lines after "300, 150, 100" are
named "_____, 60, 50."

75

Remember the next three lines together as:
"_____, _____, _____."

75, 60, 50

Once more out loud, please.

Very good!

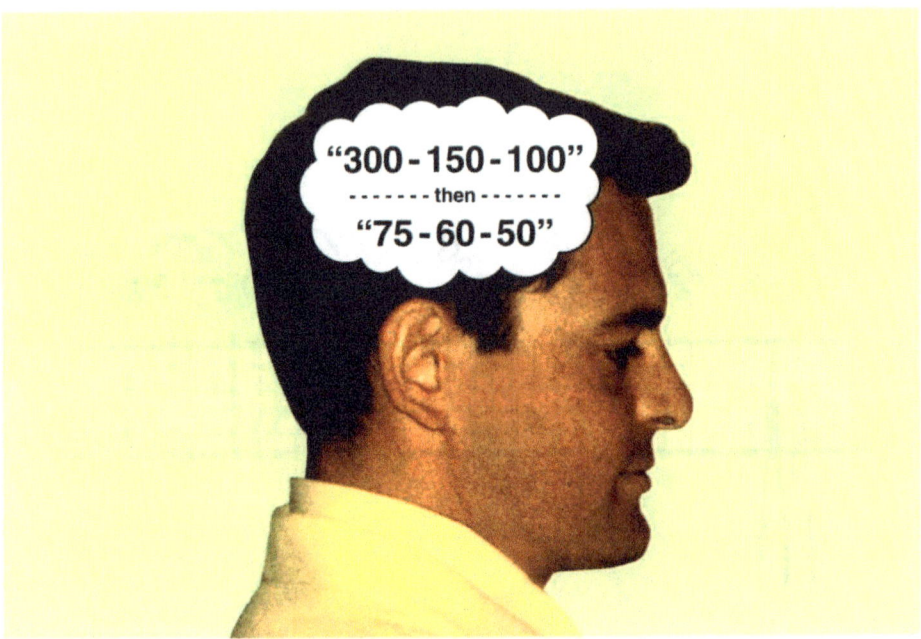

Now: Memorize these triplets until they are second nature. Make certain that you can *say* the triplets without using the picture.

These triplets, "300, 150, 100" and "75, 60, 50"
must be _____.   memorized

Be able to name the lines that follow the start line on which
an R wave _____; it is easy to remember them as   peaks
triplets, and so easy to use immediately. (Can hardly wait!)   (falls)

Do not count those lines that follow the start line -
name them with the _____ as you go.   triplets

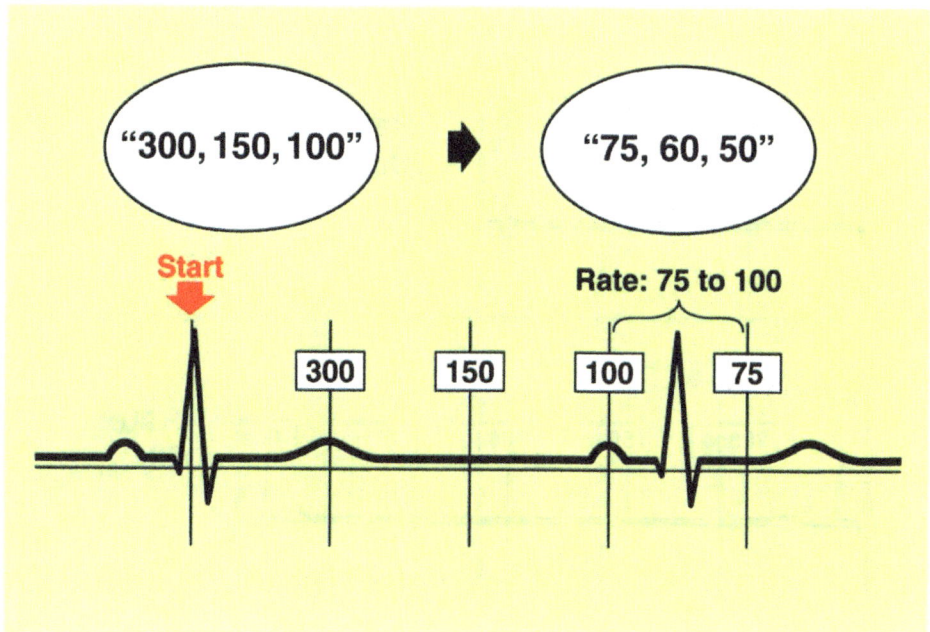

Where the next R wave falls, determines the rate. It's that simple.

Find an R wave peaked upon a heavy black (start) line,
then look for the _____ R wave.   next

Where the next R wave falls gives the _____.   rate
There is no need for mathematical computations.

If the next R wave falls on "75"…
the rate is 75 per _____.   minute

Note: You may have noticed that the illustration shows the
normal rate range of 75 to 100.

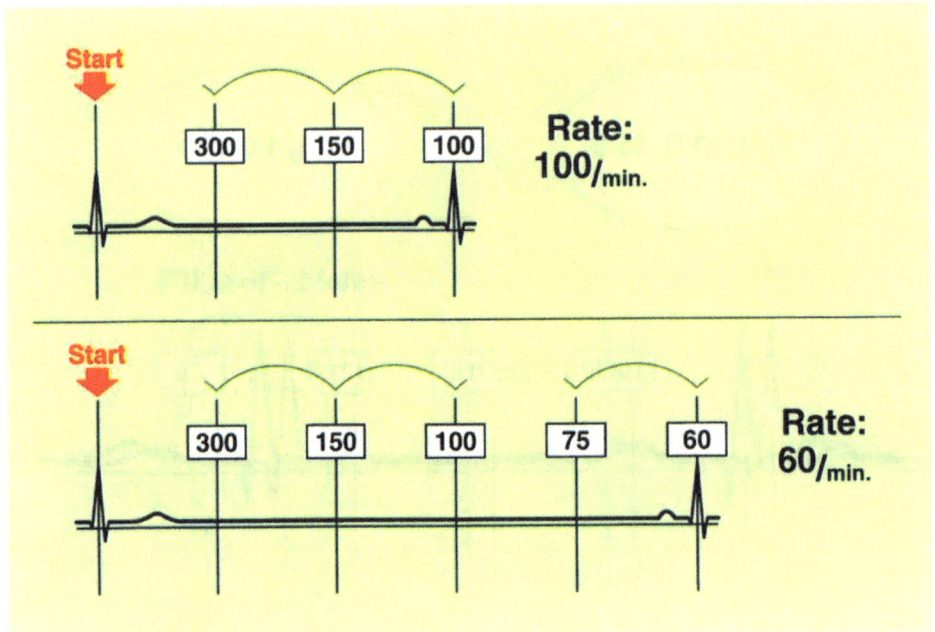

By knowing the triplets "300, 150, 100" then "75, 60, 50" you can merely look at an
EKG and tell the approximate rate immediately.

The triplets are: first "_____, _____, _____."   300, 150, 100

                   then "_____, _____, _____."   75, 60, 50

By simply naming the lines following the start line,
you can identify the rate immediately using the _____.   triplets

Practice Tracing

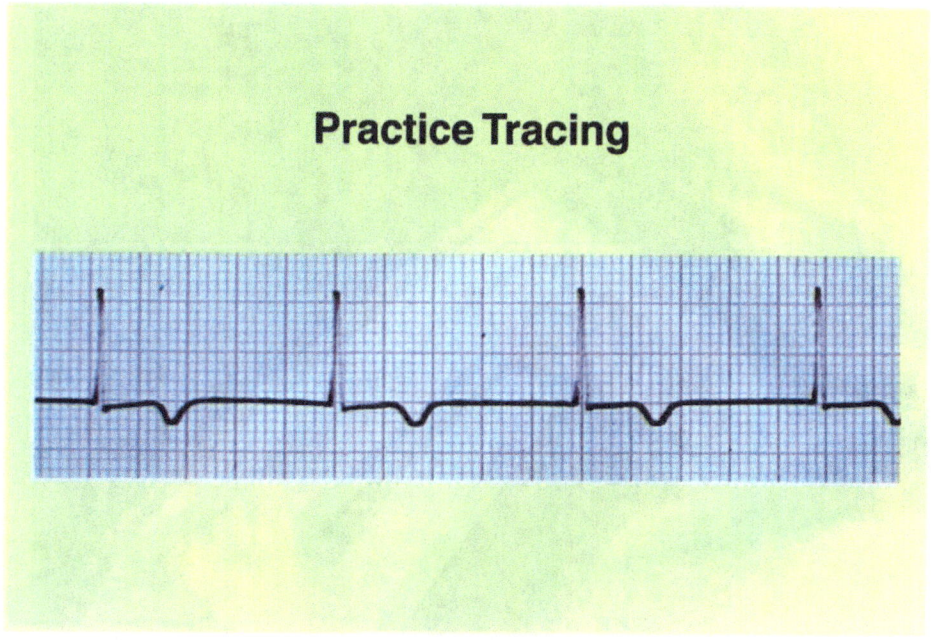

This is an EKG tracing from a resting patient, whose heart rate is slower than the usual rate one would see with a Sinus Rhythm. Let's examine the rate.

The rate in the above tracing is about _____ per minute.   60

If you were told that this rhythm probably originated in an automaticity focus, by the rate alone, you would suspect the origin (pacemaker) to be in the ___ _____.   AV Junction

Note: This is indeed a rhythm originating in the AV Junction, and that's why you don't see P waves. This elderly woman has a very diseased heart. Her SA Node failed, then all the atrial automaticity foci failed. Fortunately, a Junctional focus came to the rescue. This natural pacing backup system is wonderfully effective.

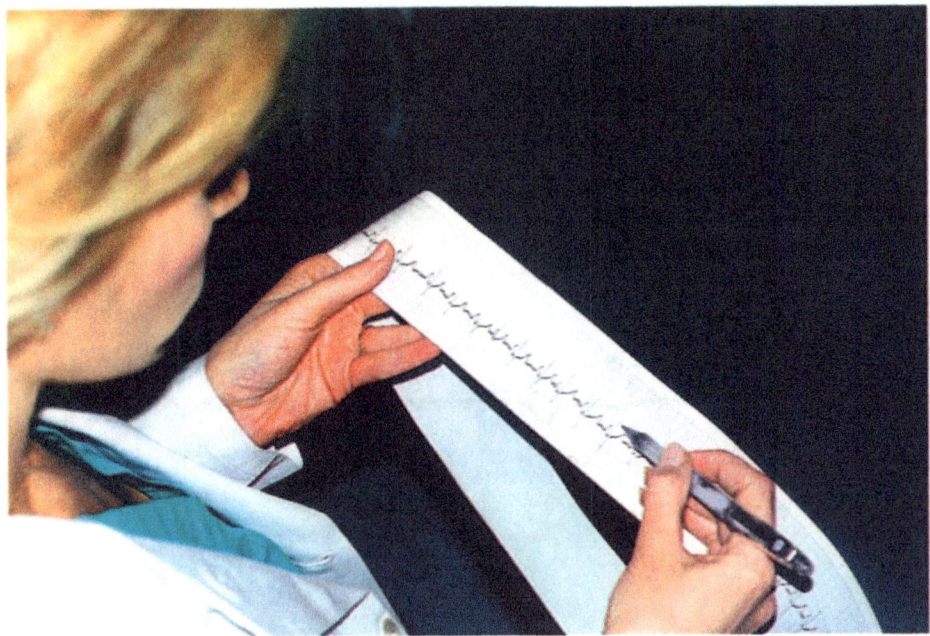

You do not need to depend on mathematical computations in order to calculate the rate. Observation alone will do it!

You can rapidly determine the rate on an EKG tracing
by _____ alone.   observation

There is no need to depend on annoying math, rate rulers,
or calculators (where did I put that darn thing?)
in order to determine the _____.   rate

Note: You will always have your brain with you (at least until that time
when brain transplants would provide you with someone else's brain).
Just remember to name the lines that follow the *start* line using the
triplets, and say: "300, 150, 100" then "75, 60, 50."
Enough, enough... let's try it!

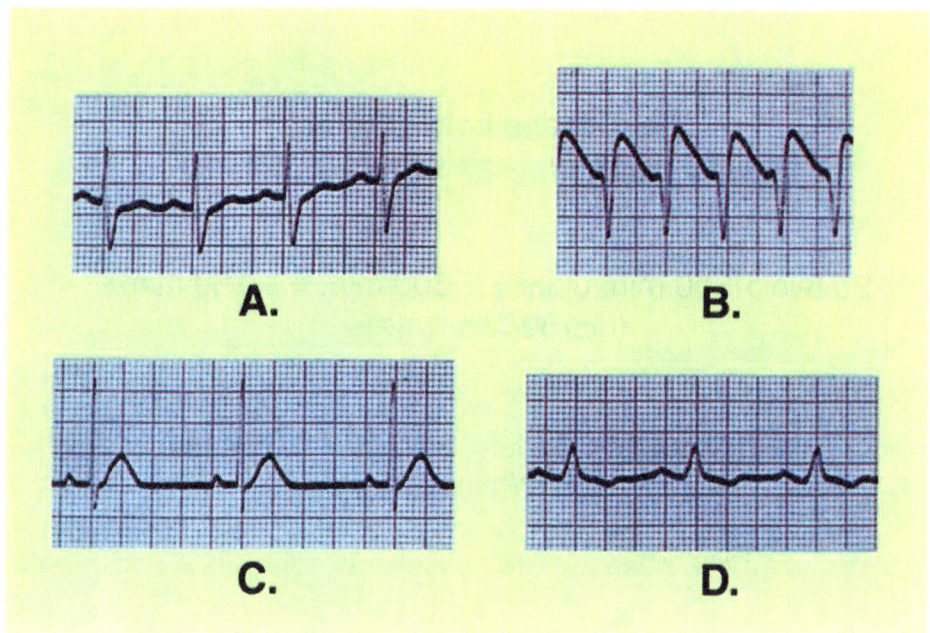

Now, let's determine the approximate rates of these EKG tracings.

A. _____   100

B. _____   150 or so

C. _____   60

D. _____   75

Note: As you may have discovered for yourself, any prominent wave
(like the S wave in example B.) can be used to determine the rate.

The distance between the
heavy black lines represents 1/300 min.

So two 1/300 min. units = 2/300 min. = 1/150 min.
(or 150/min. rate)

and three 1/300 units = 3/300 = 1/100 min.
(or 100/min. rate)

There is a logical explanation for the seemingly unusual rate determinations using the triplets.

Note: The unit of time (duration) between two heavy black lines is .2 sec., which is 1/300th of a minute.

The number of time units between five consecutive
heavy black lines is ___.   4

So this represents 4/300 minute or a rate
of ____ per minute.   75

Therefore if a heart contracts 75 times per minute, there
will be a span equal to the distance between five heavy
black lines between the _____ complexes.   QRS

Note: Reasonable instructors should not require students to master this page. As author, I have not personally memorized the text material on this boring page. Let's keep it simple and practical.

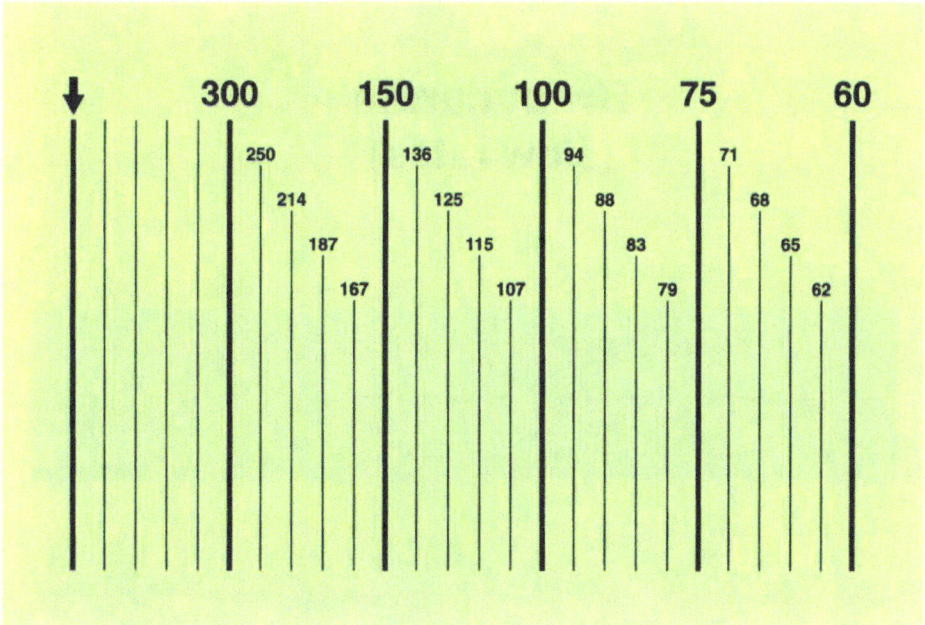

The fine line divisions can provide more precise rate determination. Memorizing them is impractical, so when determining fast rates, most of us use a reference like the one provided in the **P**ersonal **Q**uick **R**eference **S**heets (page 335).

Note: It is admittedly a great task to memorize the fine line subdivisions, so you can use page 335 as a personal reference when you need it. Determining the rate range using the triplets is more than adequate in most cases.

Note: For rates less than sixty per minute, see the next few pages for a simple way to determine rate when you see a bradycardia.

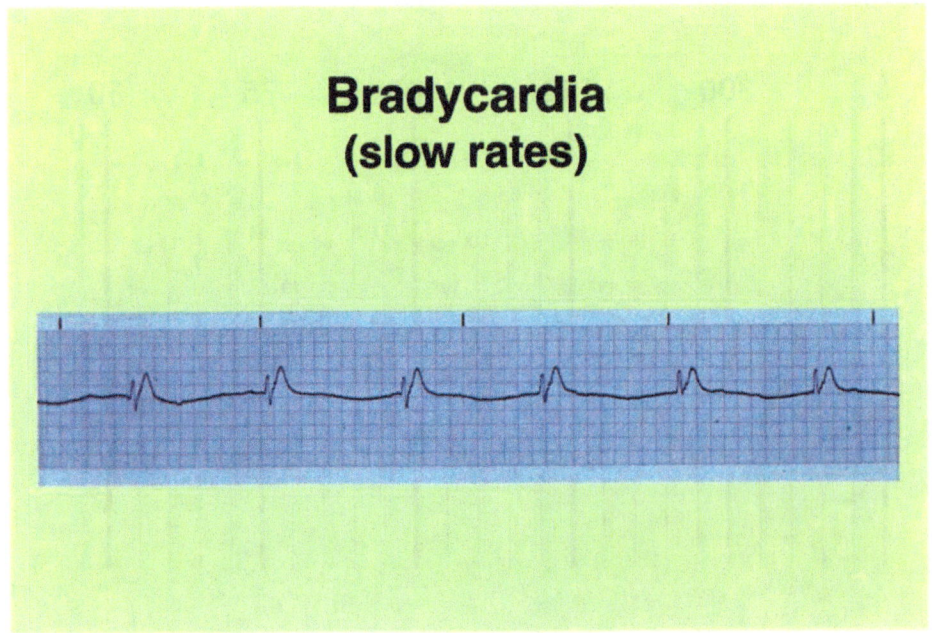

Bradycardia
(slow rates)

For very slow rhythms, there is an easy method for quickly determining the rate.

The proper term for slow heart rate is _____.   bradycardia

Note: The triplets give us a very large range of rates. By using
the triplets "300, 150, 100" then "75, 60, 50" you can determine
rates ranging from 300 to 50. Bradycardia means a rate slower
than 60 per minute.

For bradycardia you can use another easy method
to determine the _____. I'll show you on the next page...   rate

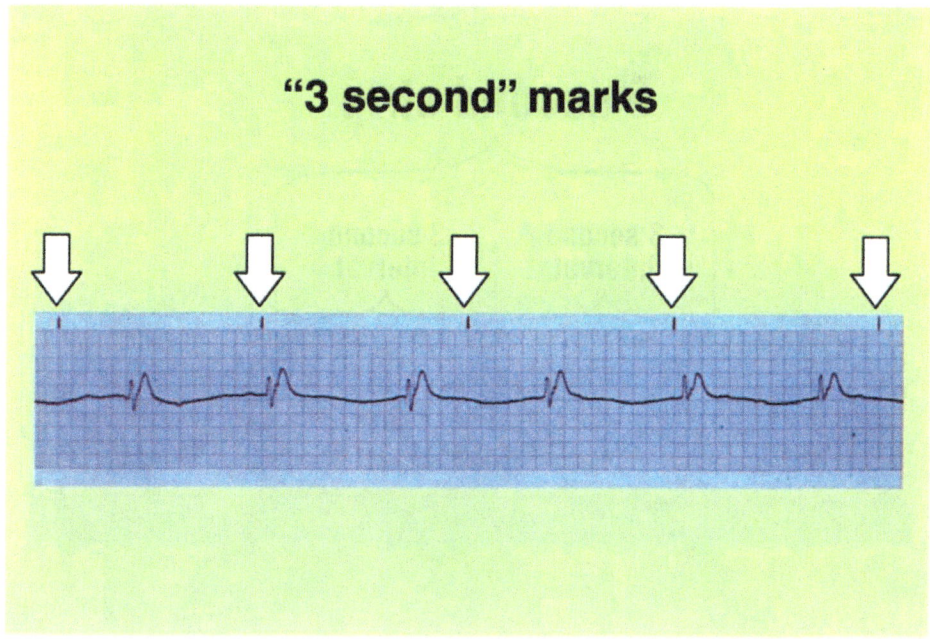

On the top margin of every EKG strip, there are small marks that identify the "three second" intervals.

There are small marks above the graph portion of the _____ tracing. Find a strip of EKG tracing and examine it.

EKG

Two of these marks enclose a three second _____.

interval

Note: Some EKG paper has "3 second intervals" that are marked with a dot, circle, triangle, or a vertical line.

When an EKG machine is running, the span of paper between two of these "3 second interval" marks passes under the stylus needle in _____.

3 seconds

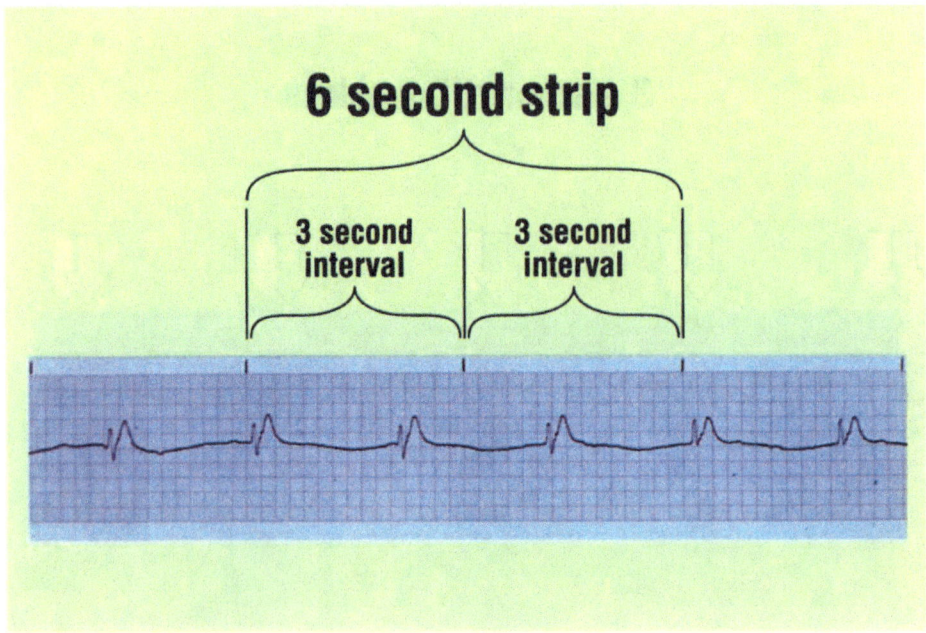

Taking two of the three second intervals, we have a 6 second strip.

Note: A three second interval is obviously the distance
between two consecutive 3 second interval marks.

Taking two of the three second intervals gives us
a 6 second _____.   strip

This 6 second strip represents the amount of paper used
by the machine in six seconds (one-_____ of a minute).   tenth

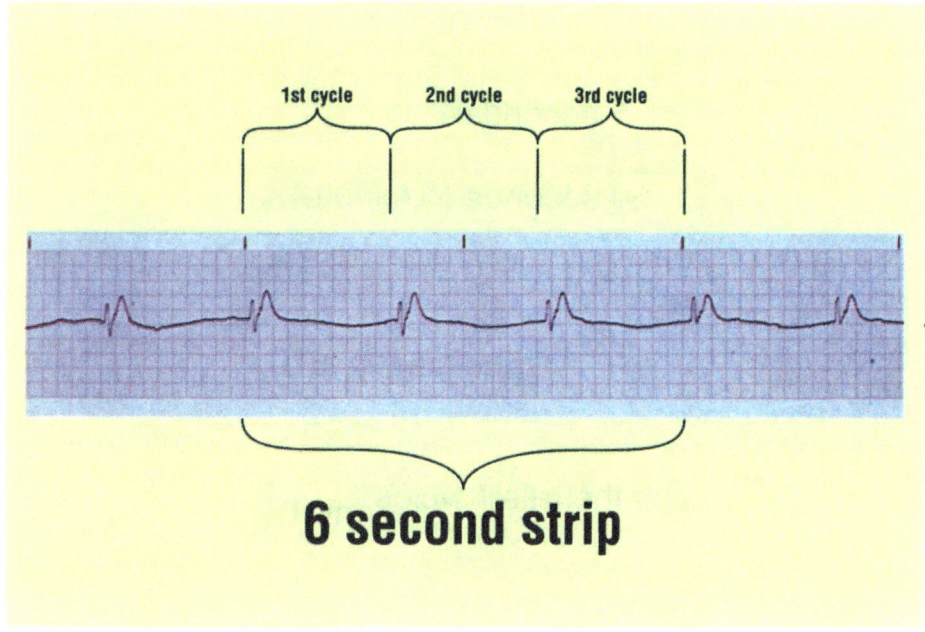

1st cycle   2nd cycle   3rd cycle

6 second strip

Count the number of complete (R wave to R wave) cycles in this 6 second strip. With marked bradycardia, there will be few cycles per 6 second strip.

The length of a cardiac _____ can be measured from a specific wave until the wave is repeated again.

cycle

So R wave to ___ wave gives us the duration (length) of one cardiac cycle.

R

Count the number of cycles in the 6 second _____.
Next page…

strip

6 seconds
x 10
——————
60 seconds (1 minute)

So:
cycles/6 sec. strip x 10...

gives the rate $\left(\text{cycles}/\text{min}\right)$

Find the rate by multiplying the number of cycles in the six second strip by ten (10).

Ten of the 6 second strips equals one _____ (time)   minute
of EKG tracing.

The number of cycles per minute is the _____.   rate

So cycles per 6 second strip multiplied by ___   10
equals the rate. Simple!

So, if there are 4 cycles per six sec. strip...

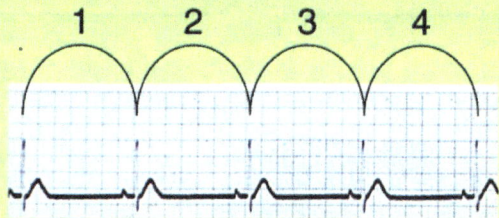

the rate is 40

You can just place a zero on the right of the number of cycles per six second strip, and you have the rate.

For very slow heart rates (bradycardia), you should
first find a six second _____,   strip

... count the number of _____ in this strip,   cycles

... and multiply by ___ to get the rate.   10

Note: Multiplying by ten may be done by placing a zero on the
right side of the number of cycles per six second strip. For instance,
5 cycles (per six second strip) gives a rate of 50.

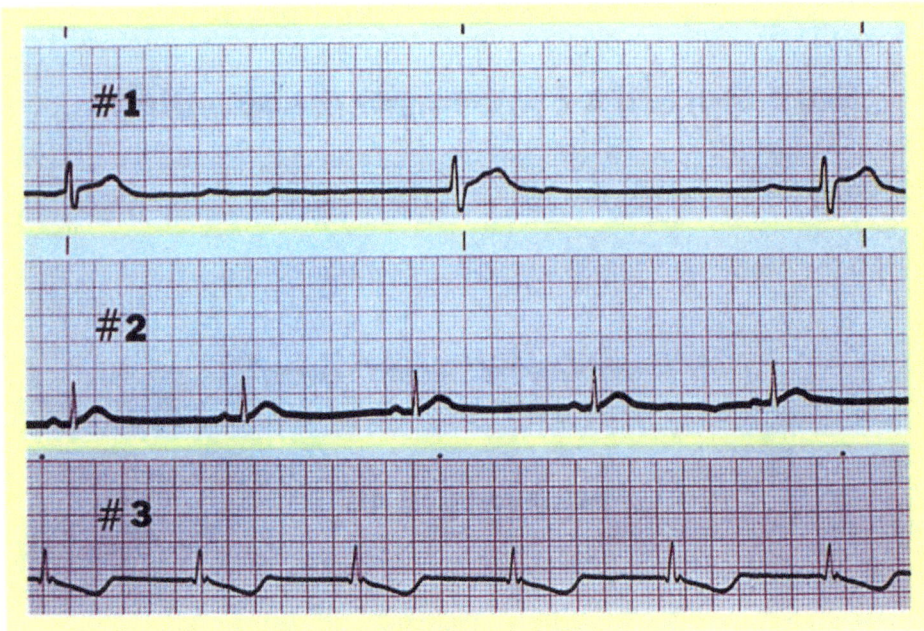

Let's determine the approximate rates of these EKG's.

Rates: No. 1. _____ per minute   20

         No. 2. _____ per minute   about 45

         No. 3. _____ per minute   50

Note: The general, average rates of *irregular* rhythms are usually determined using this method.

Why don't you obtain some EKG tracings and amaze yourself (and your friends) at how easily you can determine the rate.

Note: Take a minute to review the illustrations in this chapter, then turn to the **Personal Quick Reference Sheets** at the end of this book for a simplified summary of determining rate (page 335).

Before you begin, look at this chapter's summary on pages 334 and 336-338.

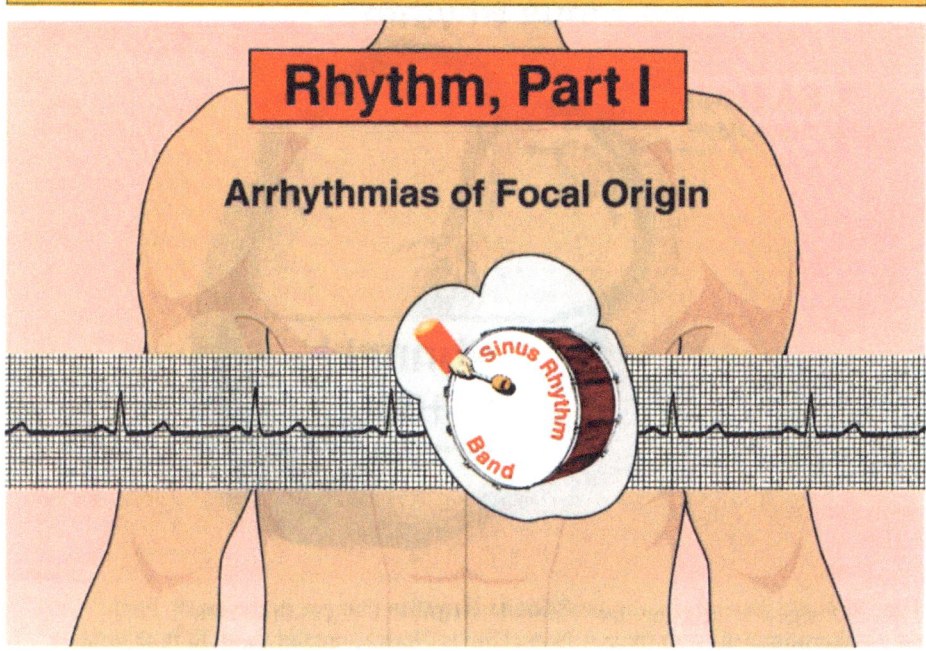

The EKG provides the most accurate means of identifying a cardiac **arrhythmia** (abnormal rhythm), which can be diagnosed easily, once we understand the electrophysiology of the heart.

"Arrhythmia" literally means without _____, however it is used to denote any abnormal rhythm. The term "dysrhythmia" (bad rhythm) has the same meaning, and also is commonly used in medical literature.

rhythm

The EKG records the heart's electrical phenomena that may not be seen, felt, or heard on physical examination, so the EKG is a very accurate means of recording _____ disturbances.

rhythm

Note: To understand the arrhythmias, you must first become familiar with the normal electrophysiology of the heart, including the normal conduction pathways. Let's begin…

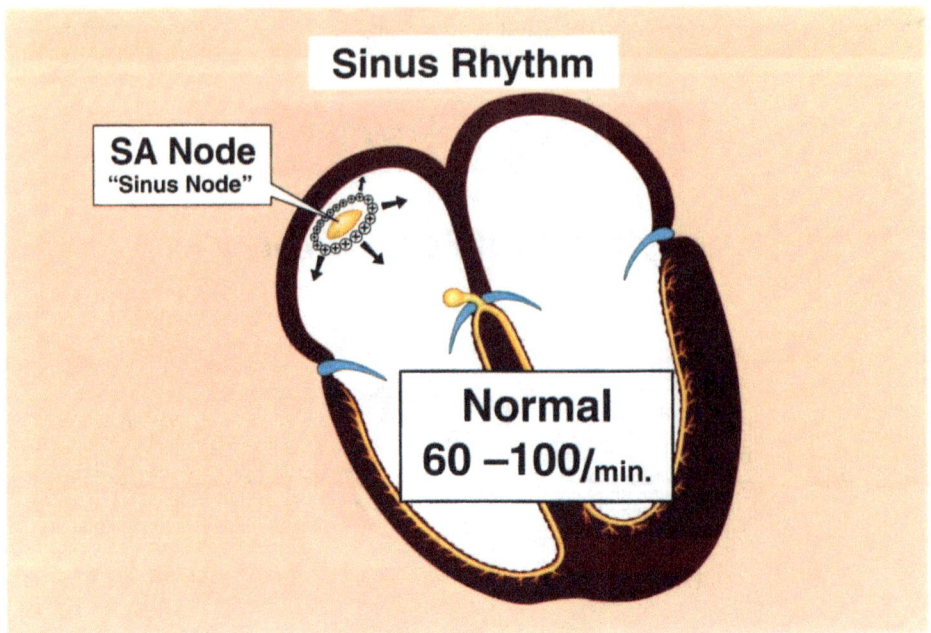

The SA Node generates a regular* **Sinus Rhythm** that paces the heart. Each
pacemaker impulse from the SA Node (Sinus Node) spreads through both atria as
an advancing wave of depolarization.

It is the <u>automaticity</u> of the Sinus Node (SA Node)
that generates the regular* cadence of depolarization
stimuli for pace-_____ activity.   making

Normally, the SA Node discharges regular pacing
impulses (60 to 100 per minute) that depolarize the _____.   atria

Note: We know that the SA ("<u>S</u>ino-<u>A</u>trial") Node is the same as the
Sinus Node, so we understand that the terms "Sinus" and "Sino" imply
SA Node origin.

* The term "regular" indicates a rhythm of constant rate. See next page...

Normal (Regular) Rhythm

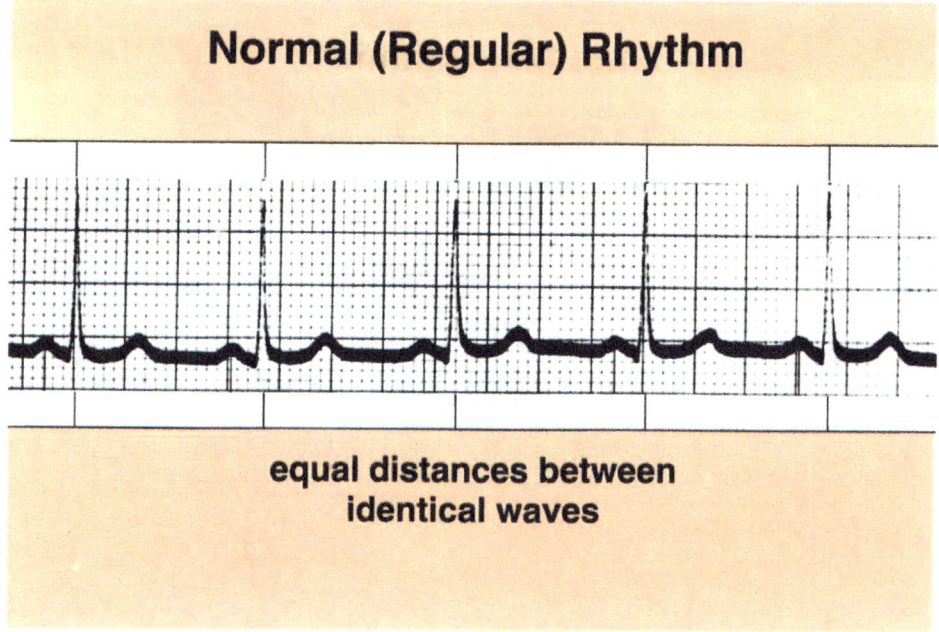

equal distances between identical waves

On EKG there is a consistent distance (duration) between similar waves during a normal, **regular** cardiac rhythm, because the SA Node's automaticity precisely maintains a constant cycle duration between the pacing impulses that it generates.

Note: All **automaticity foci** pace with a regular rhythm. This is a characteristic of all automaticity centers.

The SA Node generates pacing impulses at a constant, unvarying rate, producing cycles of equal length, so the rhythm of the heart is said to be _____. This characteristic pattern of regularity is typical of SA Node pacing.*

regular

And, because the sequence of depolarization is the same in each repeating cycle, there is a predictable regularity of all similar (named) waves. Therefore, irregularities in _____ are easy for you to spot on EKG.

rhythm

Note: We can visually scan an EKG and appreciate the repetitive continuity of a regular rhythm. But breaks in that continuity, such as a pause, the presence of too-early (premature) beats, or sudden, dramatic rate change, immediately catch our attention, warning us of a rhythm disturbance.

* In reality, a Normal **S**inus **R**hythm varies imperceptibly with respiration.

Sinus "Arrhythmia"

SA Node's pacing rate
normally varies with respiration

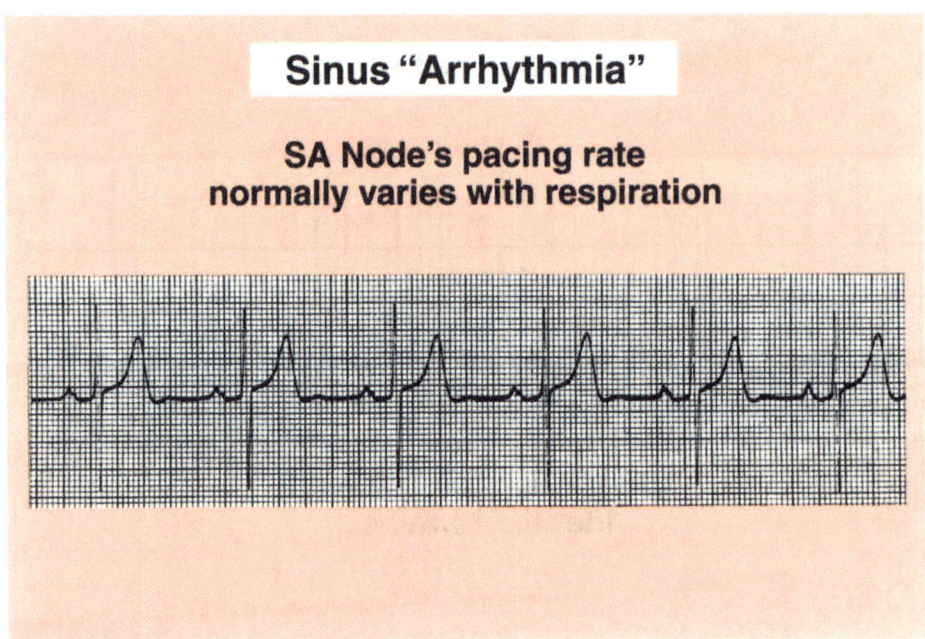

A normal physiological mechanism, **Sinus Arrhythmia**, sounds pathological
("arrhythmia" = abnormal rhythm), but it functions in all humans at all times.
The autonomic nervous system causes barely detectable rate changes in Sinus
pacing that relate to the phases of respiration. This is not a true arrhythmia.

Note: Sinus Arrhythmia is a normal, but extremely minimal, increase
in heart rate during inspiration, and an extremely minimal decrease in
heart rate during expiration.

Sinus Arrhythmia represents normal, minimal variations
in the SA Node's pacing rate in association with the
phases of _____.   respiration

Note: The slight increase in the heart rate is due to inspiration-activated
sympathetic stimulation of the SA Node. The slight decrease in pacing
rate is due to expiration-activated *parasympathetic* inhibition of the SA
Node. Perhaps you knew that already, since Sinus pacing is regulated
by both divisions of the Autonomic Nervous System.

Note: This variability of Sinus Rhythm is normal. In fact, if the
heart rate variability is reduced, this is pathological and is a valuable
indicator of increased mortality, particularly after infarction. Parameters
of "Heart Rate Variability" are being established for determining
patient prognosis in many types of heart disease.

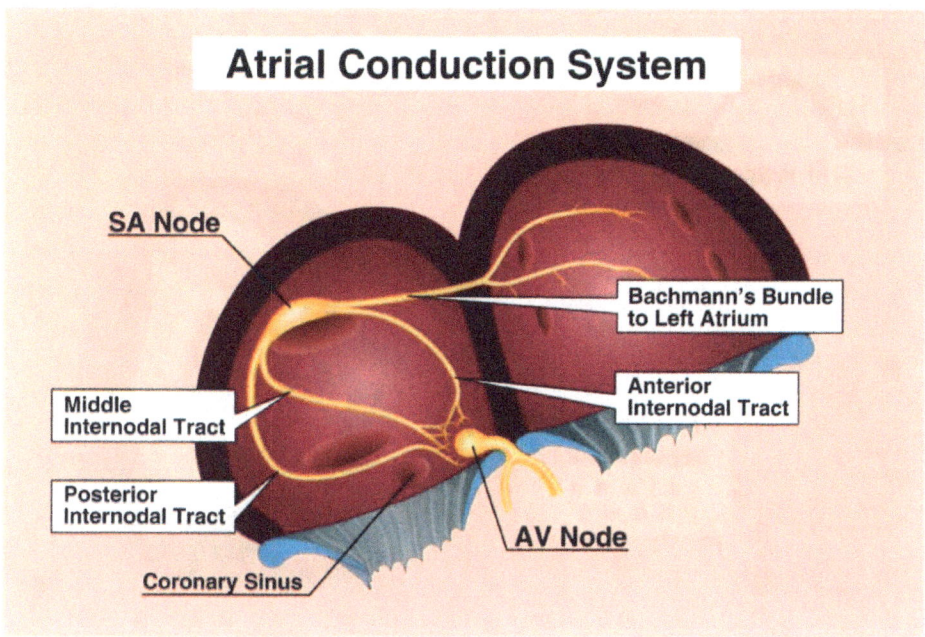

Atrial Conduction System

The atrial conduction system consists of three specialized *internodal tracts* in the right atrium (the *Anterior,* the *Middle,* and the *Posterior*), and one conduction tract known as *Bachmann's Bundle* that innervates the left atrium.

Three conduction pathways in the right atrium course from the SA Node to the AV Node (thus the term "Internodal"). They are the Anterior, the Middle, and the _____ Internodal Tracts.

Posterior

Bachmann's Bundle originates in the SA Node and distributes depolarization to the left _____.

atrium

Depolarization passing rapidly through the atrial conduction system does not record on EKG; however, depolarization of the atrial myocardium produces a ___ wave on EKG.

P

Note: Just as ventricular automaticity foci are within the ventricular Purkinje fibers, similarly, atrial automaticity foci are within the specialized atrial conduction system. Because there is a concentration of merging atrial conduction tracts in the immediate region of the AV Node near the *coronary sinus,* * considerable automaticity activity originates in that area.

* The heart's own venous drainage (i.e., from the myocardium) empties into the right atrium via the coronary sinus.

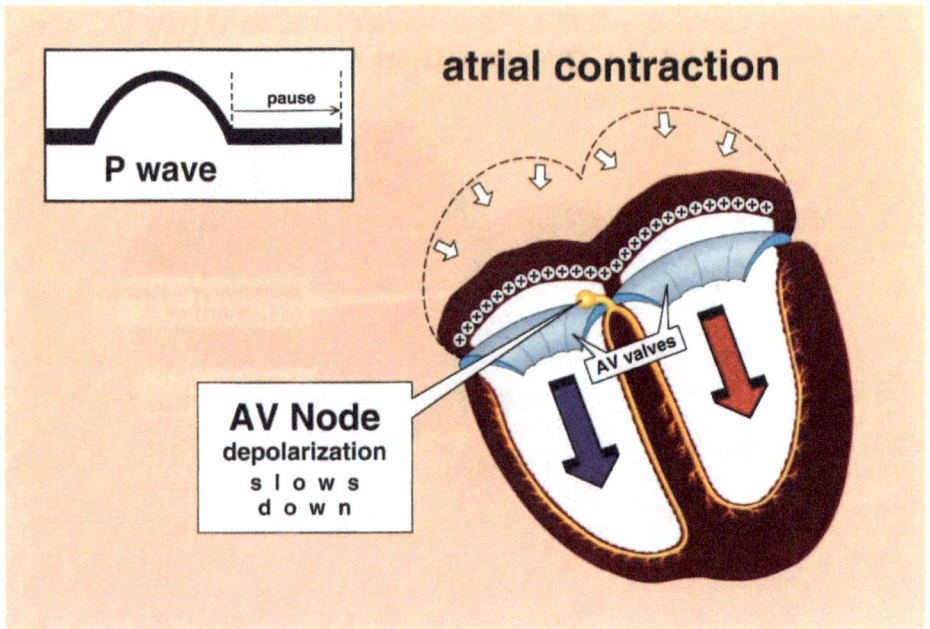

When the depolarization stimulus (passing down from the atria) reaches the AV
Node, the stimulus s l o w s in the AV Node, producing a pause on EKG.

Atrial depolarization eventually reaches the AV Node,
but conduction of depolarization slows within the
AV Node, recording a _____ on EKG.   pause

This pause (during which blood from the atria passes into the
ventricles) is represented by the horizontal piece of baseline
between the P wave and the _____ complex.   QRS

Note: The AV Node is named for its position between the Atria and
the Ventricles (thus "AV"). The proximal end of the AV Node has no
automaticity foci. However, the remainder of the AV Node, an area
known as the AV Junction, does have automaticity foci. These foci
are essential for backup pacing should there be a total failure of all
pacemaking activity from above (SA Node as well as atrial foci), or
(this is important) if a complete conduction block of the proximal end
of the AV Node occurs, preventing all (SA Node or atrial foci) pacing
stimuli from being conducted to the ventricles.

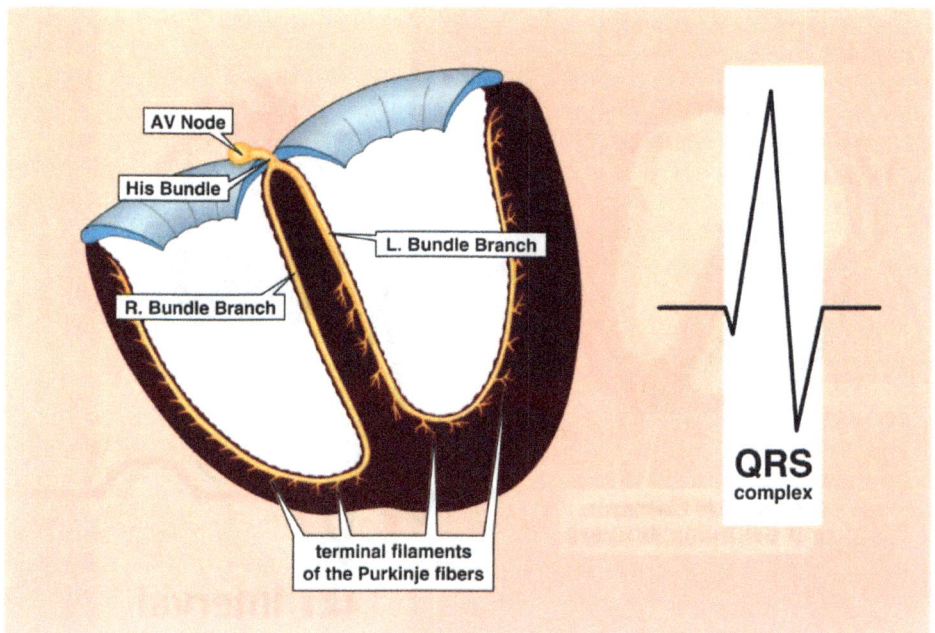

After passing (s l o w l y) through the AV Node, depolarization proceeds <u>rapidly</u> through the His Bundle, Bundle Branches and their subdivisions, and through the terminal Purkinje filaments to distribute depolarization to the ventricles. Ventricular depolarization produces a QRS complex on EKG.

Note: The His Bundle and the Bundle Branches are "bundles" of rapidly conducting Purkinje fibers. Depolarization passing through the Purkinje fibers of the ventricular conduction system is too weak to record on EKG; this is a form of "concealed" conduction.

After c r e e p i n g through the AV Node, depolarization shifts gears and races through the His _____, and...   Bundle

... through the Right and Left Bundle Branches and their subdivisions to rapidly transmit depolarization via the terminal Purkinje filaments to the *endocardial* surface of the _____ myocardium.   ventricular

When the ventricular myocardium depolarizes, it produces a _____ complex on EKG.   QRS

Note: The Purkinje fibers of the ventricular conduction system contain automaticity foci (you knew that already).

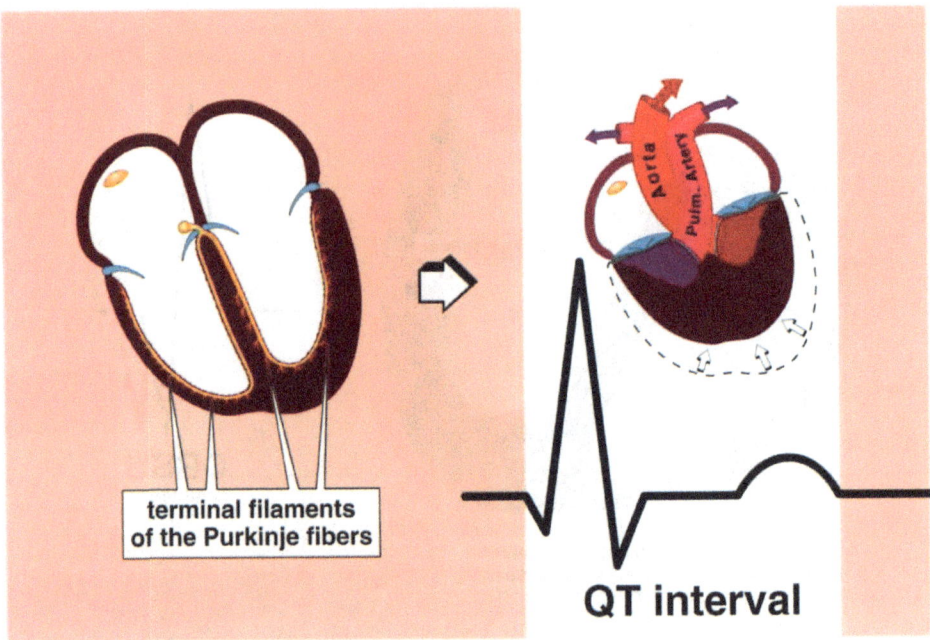

terminal filaments
of the Purkinje fibers

QT interval

The Purkinje fibers of the ventricular conduction system rapidly conduct
depolarization away from the AV Node to the endocardial surface of the ventricles;
when the ventricles depolarize, it produces a QRS complex on EKG.

Note: Ventricular depolarization begins midway down the
interventricular septum, where the Left Bundle Branch produces
fine terminal filaments. The Right Bundle Branch does not produce
terminal filaments in the septum. So left-to-right depolarization of
the septum occurs immediately before the rest of the ventricular
myocardium depolarizes. (Examine the illustration.)

Ventricular depolarization initiates ventricular contraction,
which persists (through both phases of repolarization) to
the end of the __ wave.   T

Ventricular contraction begins and ends during the ___ interval.   QT

Note: Repolarization of the Purkinje fibers takes longer than
ventricular repolarization. That is, the end of the T wave marks the
end of ventricular repolarization; however, repolarization of the
Purkinje fibers terminates a little later — beyond the end of the
T wave. The final phase of Purkinje repolarization may record
a small hump, the **U wave** (following the T wave), on EKG.

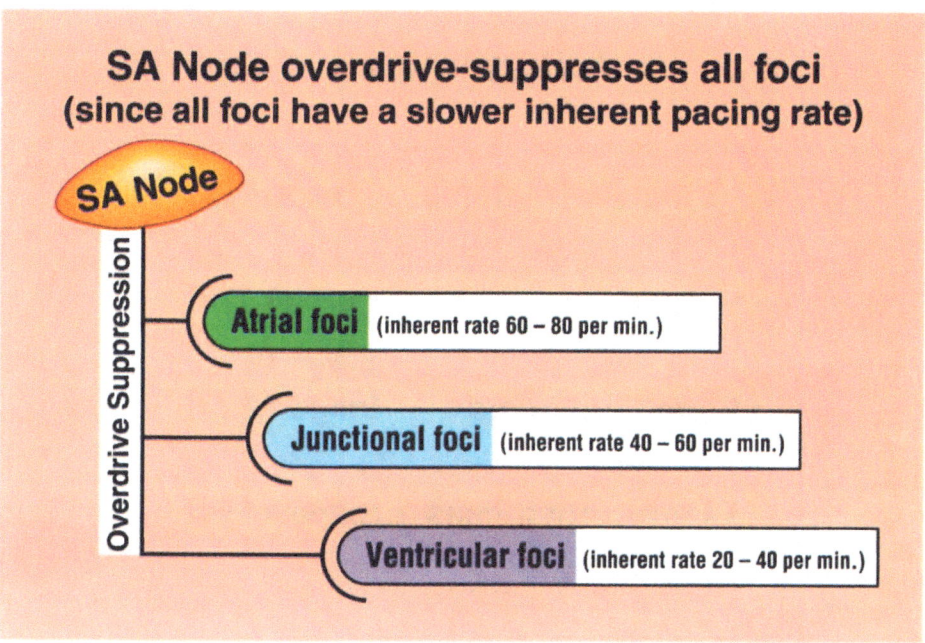

There are three levels of automaticity foci (atrial, Junctional, and ventricular) that can provide backup pacemaker responsibility if pacing activity fails. The foci of each level have a characteristic inherent rate *range*, giving the SA Node a failsafe hierarchy of three levels of backup pacing.

Each level of automaticity foci has a consistent range of _____ rate.   inherent

Note: The SA Node and all automaticity foci are centers of automaticity ("automaticity centers"), which means that they can generate regular pacing stimuli.

Overdrive suppression allows the automaticity center with the fastest rate to be the _____ pacemaker (no competition).   dominant

Should the highest pacemaking center fail, an automaticity focus from the next highest level (no longer overdrive-suppressed) emerges ("escapes") to actively pace at its inherent rate, and it then becomes the dominant pacemaker by overdrive-suppressing all automaticity _____ below it.   foci

Note: A very "irritable" automaticity focus may suddenly pace rapidly.

Arrhythmias

The arrhythmias can be divided into a few general categories, according to the arrhythmia's mechanism of origin. The best students, I've noticed, apply index tabs to the pages that begin each arrhythmia category (see above); try it – you will find it very helpful!

Note: Although arrhythmia literally means "without rhythm," generally it describes any rhythm disturbance, that is, any variance from a Normal Sinus Rhythm. Some authors prefer the term "dysrhythmia" rather than arrhythmia.

Note: The illustration is a simplified arrhythmia classification that is categorized according to the mechanism of origin, so the arrhythmias will be easy for you to understand.

Note: The underlying mechanisms that are basic to the heart's function are very satisfying to learn. But more importantly, conceptual understanding of the basic mechanisms facilitates and perpetuates your knowledge. Don't memorize patterns; your knowledge will be vital to others! Lasting knowledge results from understanding.

Irregular Rhythms
(Atrial)

• Wandering Pacemaker

• Multifocal Atrial Tachycardia

• Atrial Fibrillation

The **irregular rhythms** presented in this section are usually caused by multiple, active automaticity sites.

Rhythms that lack a constant duration between paced cycles are said to be _____.   irregular

Note: The term "irregularly irregular" is an old designation that describes an irregular and chaotic rhythm that has no predictable recurring pattern.

Note: In some hearts with structural pathology or hypoxia, malfunctioning automaticity foci may suffer from *entrance block,* whereby any incoming depolarization is blocked, "protecting" them from passive depolarization by any other source. Such "protection" is not healthy. By being insensitive to passive depolarization, they cannot be overdrive-suppressed, *while their own* automaticity is still conducted to surrounding tissue. When an automaticity focus has entrance block, it is said to be **parasystolic** (the focus paces, but can't be overdrive-suppressed).

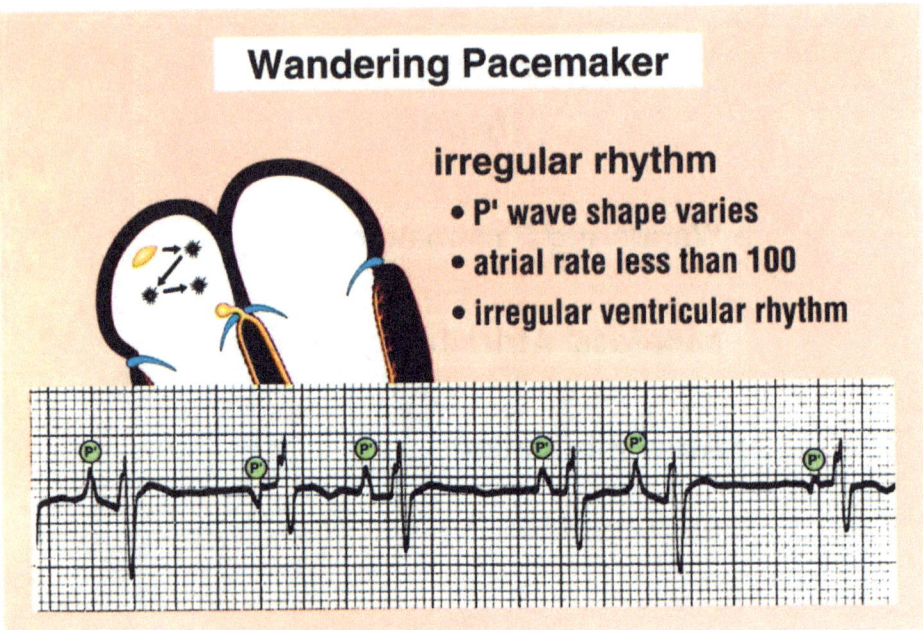

Wandering Pacemaker is an irregular rhythm produced by the pacemaker activity wandering from the SA Node to nearby atrial automaticity foci. This produces cycle length variation as well as variation in the shape of the P' waves. The overall rate, however, is within the normal range.

Note: The P' (pronounced "P prime") wave represents atrial depolarization by an automaticity focus, as opposed to normal Sinus-paced P waves.

Note: Each automaticity focus has a specific inherent rate at which it paces. In a given lead, each atrial automaticity focus produces its own morphological signature, that is, it produces a P' wave of a distinctive shape related to the anatomical location of that focus within the atria.

Wandering Pacemaker is an irregular rhythm (normal rate range); the pacemaking activity wanders from the SA Node to _____ foci...   atrial

... so the cycle lengths vary, and __ wave morphology   P'
(shape) varies as the pacemaking center moves.

Note: Should the rate accelerate into a tachycardia (greater than 100 per minute), it becomes *Multifocal Atrial Tachycardia*. Next page...

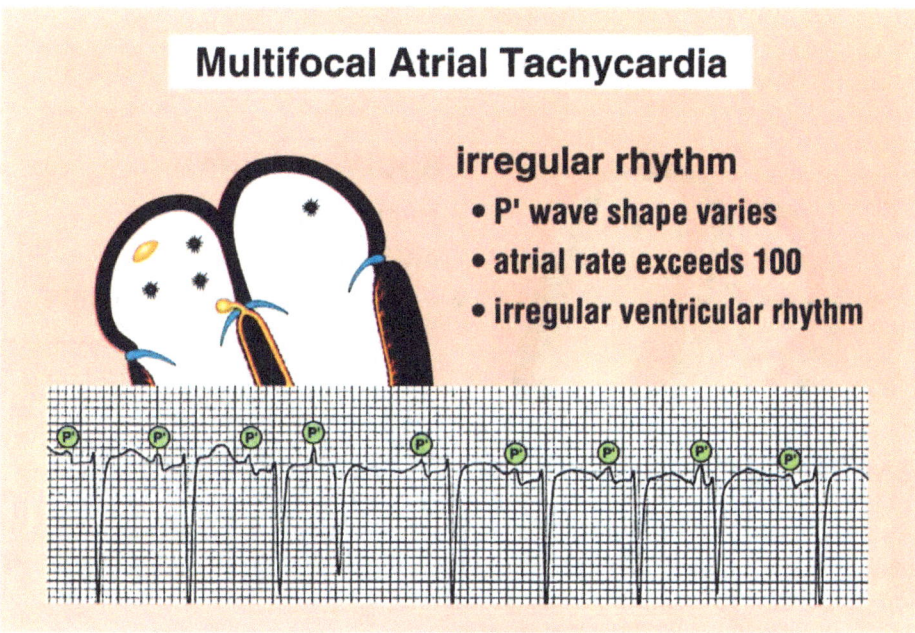

Multifocal Atrial Tachycardia (MAT) is a rhythm of patients with Chronic Obstructive Pulmonary Disease (COPD). The heart rate is over 100 per minute with P' waves of various shapes, since three or more atrial foci are involved.

In MAT, we can recognize each P' wave from a particular _____ focus by its morphological signature, i.e., P' waves from the same focus look the same in a given lead.   atrial

Note: MAT is an arrhythmia of patients who are very ill* with COPD. The atrial automaticity foci are also ill, showing early signs of parasystole (entrance block) by developing a resistance to overdrive suppression. That is why no single focus achieves pacemaking dominance, so they all pace together.

Because of the multifocal origin of MAT, each individual atrial focus paces at its own inherent _____, but the total, combined   rate
pacing of multiple unsuppressed foci produces a rapid, irregular rhythm…

… and in a given lead, each focus produces P' waves with a specific morphological signature, i.e., __ waves of a distinct shape (note that   P'
some P' waves are identical, since they're from the same focus). And remember, this is a tachycardia.

* MAT is sometimes associated with digitalis toxicity in patients with heart disease.

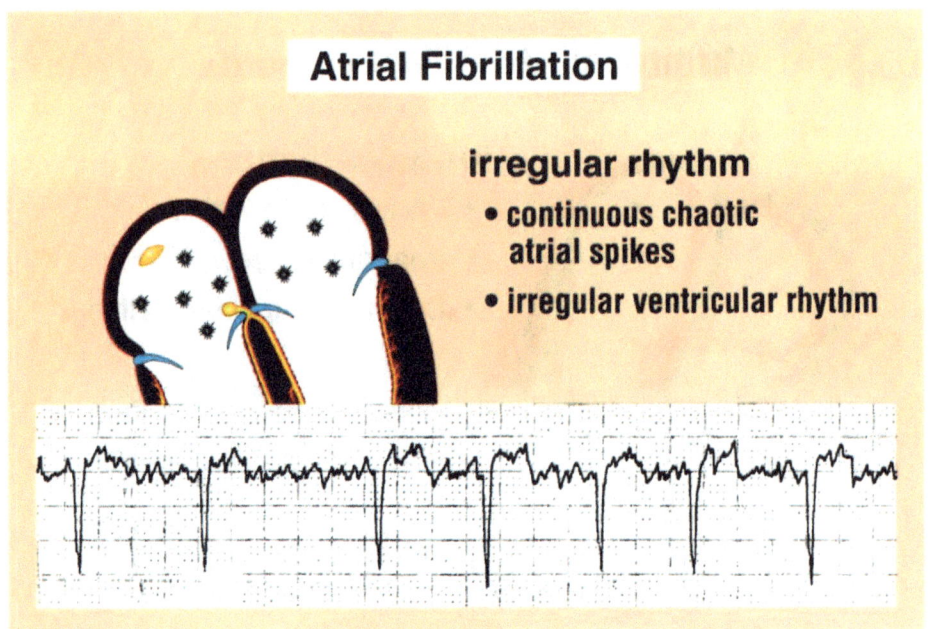

Atrial Fibrillation is caused by the continuous rapid-firing of multiple atrial automaticity foci. No single impulse depolarizes the atria completely, and only an occasional, random atrial depolarization reaches the AV Node to be conducted to the ventricles; this produces an irregular ventricular (QRS) rhythm.

Note: Atrial Fibrillation is NOT an arrhythmia of healthy, young individuals. It is the result of multiple "irritable" atrial foci, suffering from entrance block, pacing rapidly. These multiple atrial foci are *parasystolic*, so they're all insensitive to overdrive suppression; therefore, they all pace at once. What chaos!

During Atrial Fibrillation, no single impulse completely depolarizes both _____, so there are no P waves,   atria
just a rapid series of tiny, erratic spikes on EKG.

Only the occasional atrial impulse gets through the AV Node to initiate a _____ complex. The *irregular ventricular response* may result in   QRS
either a slow or rapid ventricular rate, but it is <u>always</u> irregular.

Note: You must determine and document the general ventricular rate in Atrial Fibrillation (QRS's per six second strip times 10).

Practice Tracing

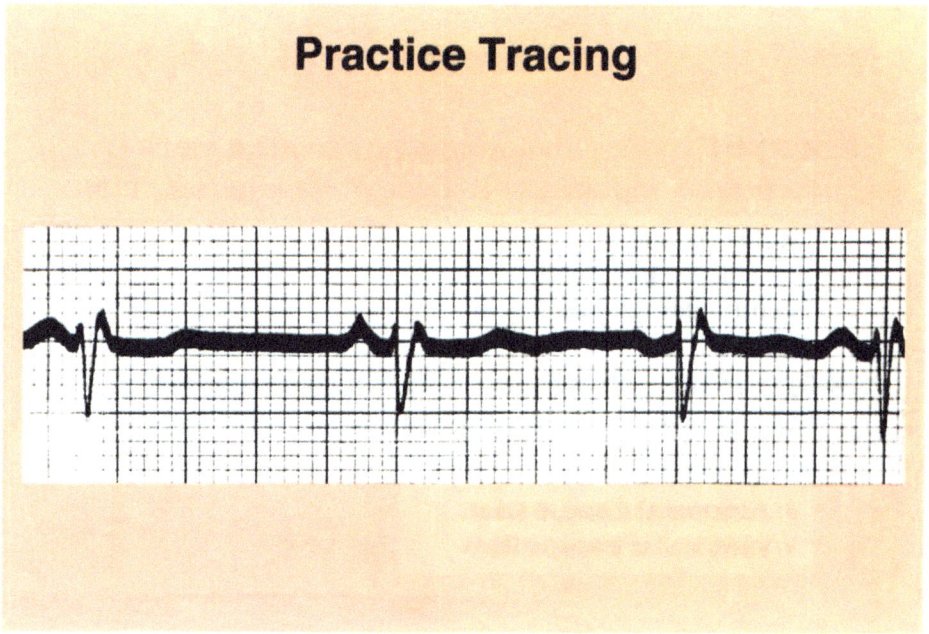

This tracing was monitored from a patient with an irregular pulse.

This practice tracing has an irregular rhythm in which
we see discernible ___ waves, so we know that it is not   P'
Atrial Fibrillation.

The "P" waves are not identical, and the rate does not
gradually increase and gradually decrease, so we
immediately know that this is not _____ Arrhythmia.   Sinus

The rate is less than 100 (which rules out MAT), the
rhythm is irregular, and the P' waves are of different
shapes. This is most likely _____ Pacemaker.   Wandering

Easy, isn't it!

Note: Just to solidify your knowledge of these irregular rhythms,
study the simplified review and tracings of *Irregular Rhythms* on
page 336.

Escape

Escape Rhythm - an automaticity focus escapes overdrive suppression to <u>pace</u> at its inherent rate:

- Atrial Escape Rhythm
- Junctional Escape Rhythm
- Ventricular Escape Rhythm

Escape Beat - an automaticity focus <u>transiently</u> escapes overdrive suppression to emit <u>one beat</u>:

- Atrial Escape Beat
- Junctional Escape Beat
- Ventricular Escape Beat

"Escape" describes the response of an automaticity focus to a pause in the pacemaking activity.

The SA Node's regular pacing overdrive-suppresses all automaticity foci, but a brief pause in SA Node pacing permits an automaticity _____ to escape overdrive suppression.

focus

If SA Node pacing ceases entirely, an automaticity focus will escape to pace at its inherent _____, thereby producing an *Escape Rhythm*. We will, however, need to identify the focus (atrial, Junctional, or ventricular) that escapes to actively pace.

rate

If the pause in pacing is brief (only one cycle missed), an automaticity focus may _____ to emit a single *Escape Beat* before the normal Sinus rhythm returns. So, we will need to identify that focus (atrial, Junctional, or ventricular).

escape

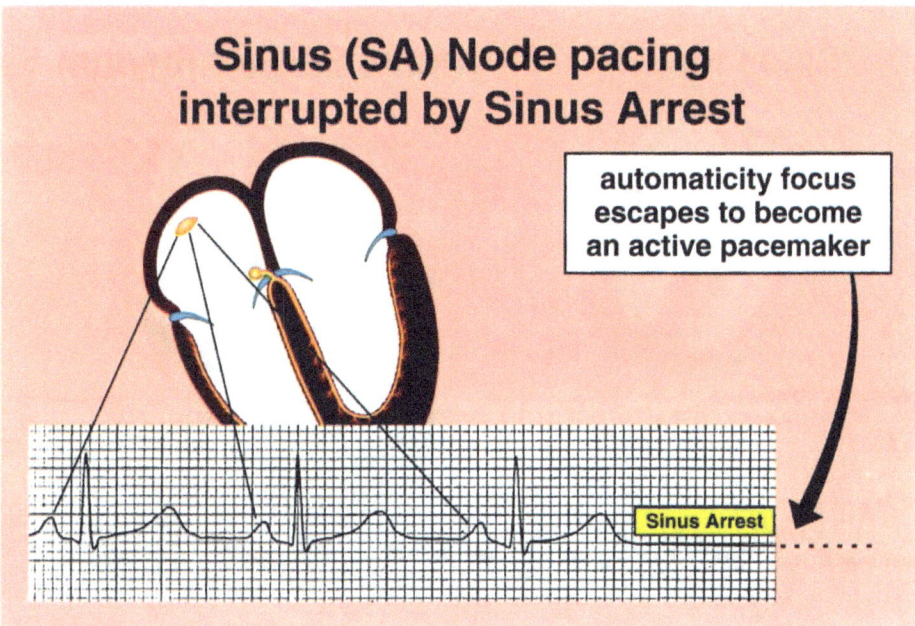

Sinus (SA) Node pacing interrupted by Sinus Arrest

automaticity focus escapes to become an active pacemaker

Sinus Arrest

Sinus Arrest occurs when a very sick SA Node ceases pacemaking completely. But the heart's efficient, failsafe mechanism provides three separate levels of automaticity foci for backup pacemaking. Divine Design.

Note: With Sinus Arrest, the SA Node ceases pacing; then, absent overdrive suppression by the SA Node, an automaticity focus (with the fastest inherent pacing rate) escapes to become an active pacemaker. And since it has the fastest inherent rate, it overdrive-suppresses all foci below, to become the dominant pacemaker.

Note: *An automaticity focus is overdrive-suppressed if it is regularly depolarized by a pacing rate faster than its own inherent pacing rate.* But if an automaticity focus is not overdrive-suppressed – regardless of the cause – it escapes to initiate its own pacemaking activity.

Note: *Each specific focus has its own individual, inherent rate of pacing.* However, the inherent pacing rates of all foci of a given level (for example, the inherent rates of all Junctional foci) are within a rate range.

Note: With a Sinus Arrest, the SA Node ceases pacing, so absent overdrive suppression from above, an automaticity focus escapes to produce an Escape Rhythm. However with Sinus Block, the SA Node misses one pacing cycle, producing only a transient pause. So an automaticity focus escapes to emit an Escape Beat, which actually represents the first beat of the attempt by the focus to pace, but the return of SA Node pacing overdrive-suppresses it again.

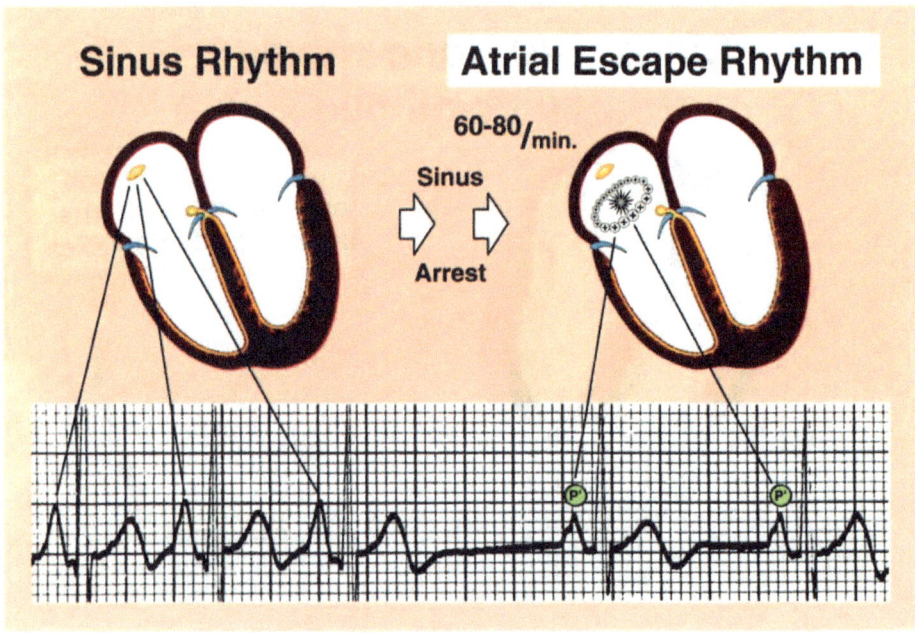

With Sinus Arrest an atrial focus quickly escapes overdrive suppression to become
the dominant pacemaker at its inherent rate. This is an **Atrial Escape Rhythm**.

With a Sinus Arrest, an automaticity focus in the highest
level of foci, the _____, escapes overdrive suppression   atria
to become an active pacemaker in its inherent rate range
of 60 to 80 per minute.

An Atrial Escape Rhythm originates in an atrial automaticity
focus, so the P' waves are not identical to the previous P waves
that were produced by the ___ _____. (See illustration.)   SA Node

Note: The active atrial automaticity focus overdrive-suppresses
all lower, slower foci to become the dominant pacemaker. It also
paces at its inherent rate, which differs from (i.e., is slower than)
the previous Sinus rate. (See illustration.)

When an atrial focus assumes pacing responsibility in the
absence of a Sinus Rhythm, this is an Atrial _____ Rhythm.   Escape

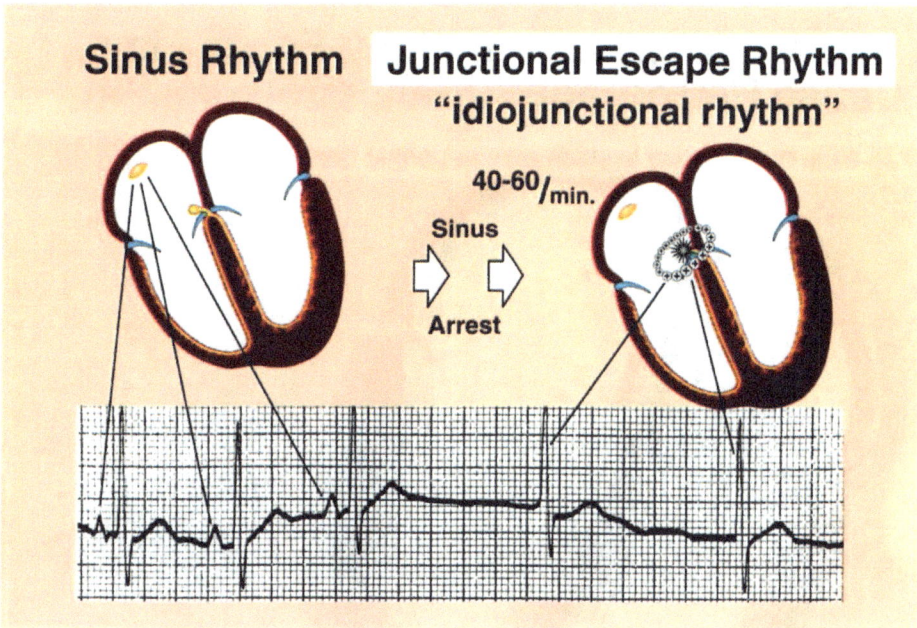

Sinus Rhythm | Junctional Escape Rhythm
"idiojunctional rhythm"

40-60/min.

Sinus

Arrest

Absent regular pacing stimuli from above, an automaticity focus in the AV Junction may escape overdrive suppression to become an active pacemaker producing a **Junctional Escape Rhythm** in its inherent rate range: 40 to 60 per minute.

Note: A Junctional focus escapes the influence of overdrive suppression if there is a Sinus Arrest, and the atrial foci also fail to function properly...

... or if there is a complete conduction block in the proximal end of the AV Node. In either case, the Junctional focus is not regularly stimulated by pacing depolarizations from above.

When a Junctional focus is not overdrive-suppressed, it actively paces, producing a Junctional Escape Rhythm, and it becomes the dominant pacemaker of the ventricles at a rate ranging from 40 to ___ per minute (it's also called an "idiojunctional rhythm").*   60

A Junctional Escape Rhythm usually conducts mainly to the ventricles, producing a series of lone ____ complexes.   QRS
But see the next page for an interesting exception.

* Sometimes the inherent Junctional pacing rate may accelerate beyond its usual range to produce an *Accelerated Idiojunctional Rhythm.*

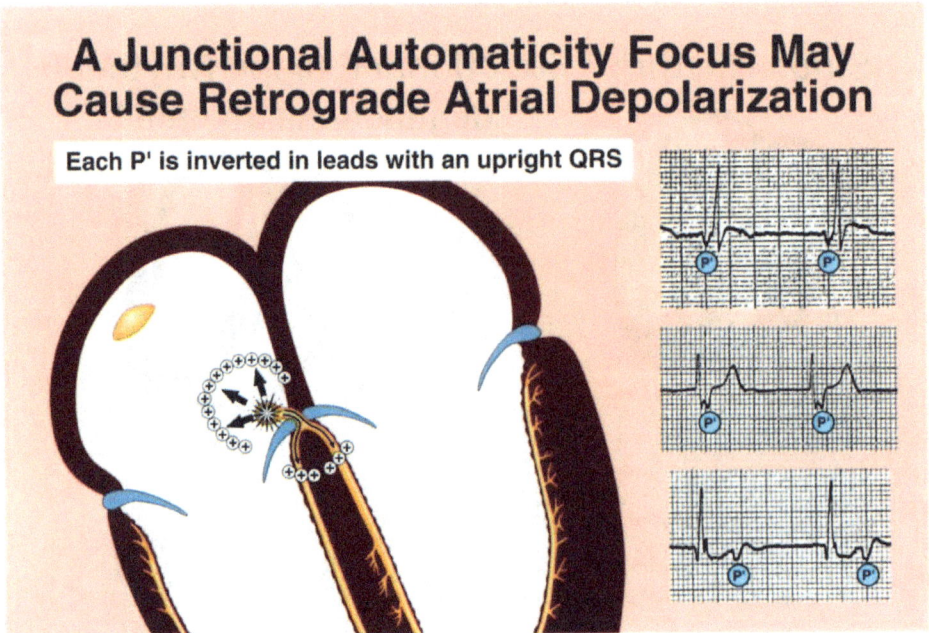

A Junctional Automaticity Focus May Cause Retrograde Atrial Depolarization

Each P' is inverted in leads with an upright QRS

Because each Junctional automaticity focus is located within the AV Node, each pacing stimulus originating there will conduct to the ventricles as expected, but the paced stimuli may also (unexpectedly) depolarize the atria from below ("retrograde"), producing *inverted* P' waves in EKG leads with an upright QRS.

Note: The illustration shows that atrial depolarization and ventricular depolarization proceed in <u>opposite</u> directions from a pacing Junctional focus. Also, most EKG leads produce an upright QRS.

With a Junctional Escape Rhythm, every paced stimulus will depolarize the ventricles, but the pacing may also depolarize the atria from below in a *retrograde* fashion, producing
_____ P' waves in EKG leads with an upright QRS.   inverted

Note: The AV Node conducts very slowly, so depolarization from a Junctional focus may delay <u>either</u> ventricular depolarization or retrograde atrial depolarization (if present)…

… as a result, if there is retrograde atrial depolarization from a Junctional focus, it may record on EKG with one of these three patterns:

- retrograde (inverted) P' wave immediately before each QRS
- retrograde (inverted) P' wave after each QRS
- retrograde (inverted) P' wave buried within each QRS (not shown)

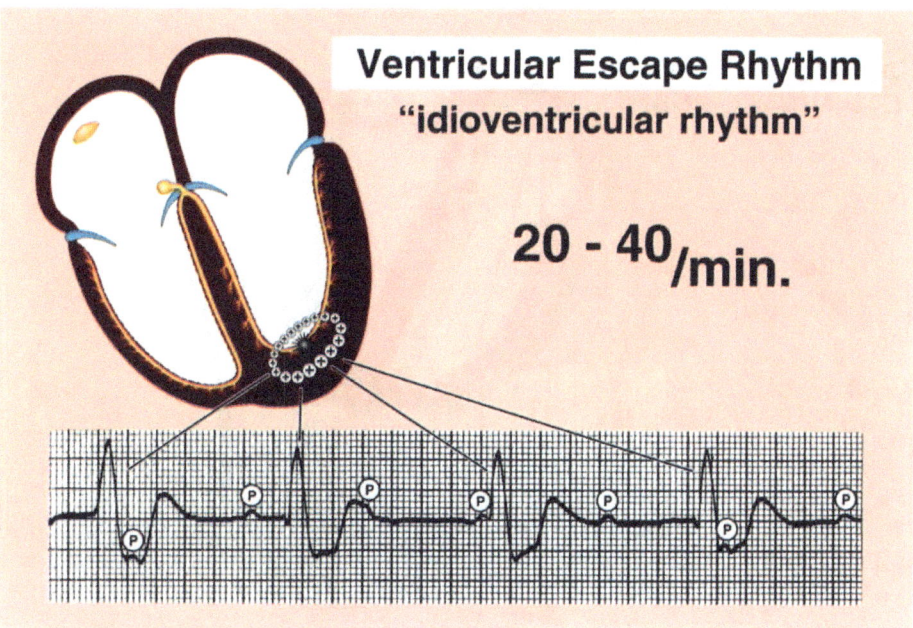

A **Ventricular Escape Rhythm** occurs when a ventricular automaticity focus is not regularly stimulated by paced depolarizations from above, so it escapes overdrive suppression to emerge as the ventricular pacemaker with an inherent rate in the range of 20 to 40 per minute* (so it is also called an "idioventricular rhythm"). Notice the enormous ventricular complexes.

Note: Ventricular Escape Rhythm usually results from one of two mechanisms:

- With complete conduction block high in the ventricular conduction system (but below the AV Node), the ventricular foci are not stimulated by atrial depolarizations from above (see P waves in illustration), so a ventricular focus escapes to pace the ventricles at its inherent rate.

- Total failure of the SA Node and all automaticity foci above the ventricles is a rare and grave condition called *"downward displacement of the pacemaker"*. In extremis, a ventricular focus escapes to become the active ventricular pacemaker in a final, futile attempt to sustain life.

Note: Pacing from a ventricular focus is often so slow that blood flow to the brain is significantly reduced to the point of unconsciousness (syncope). This is **Stokes-Adams Syndrome**. This unconscious patient's airway must be monitored and maintained… constantly. Airway!

* Should this accelerate above the inherent rate range, it becomes an *Accelerated Idioventricular Rhythm*.

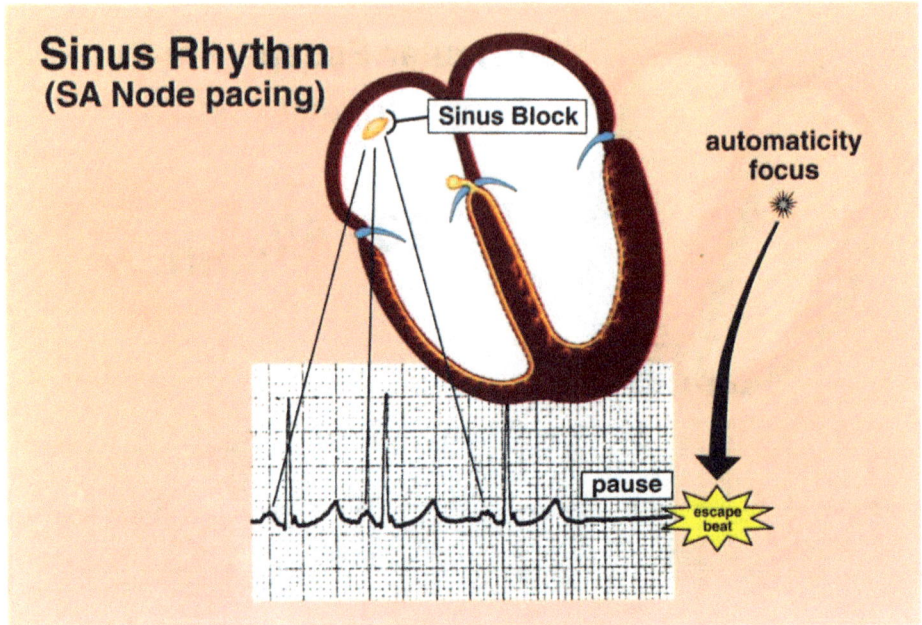

During a Sinus Rhythm, a transient *Sinus Block* makes the SA Node miss a pacing stimulus (one missed cycle), producing a pause in pacing. So an atrial automaticity focus escapes overdrive suppression to emit an **Escape Beat**.

With a transient Sinus Block, an unhealthy SA Node misses one pacing stimulus. This missed cycle produces a _____ during which the heart is electrically silent.

pause

If this pause is long enough (see NOTE below), then an automaticity focus will "escape" _____ suppression.

overdrive

Note: If there is a "sufficient" pause — longer than the inherent (pacing) cycle length of an automaticity focus — that focus will "escape" the SA Node's overdrive suppression to emit a stimulus.*

If the SA Node misses only one cycle, it will then resume pacing, and the SA Node's overdrive suppression of all automaticity _____ resumes as well.

foci

* If you don't understand the Note, don't worry. Just be aware of the escape mechanism.

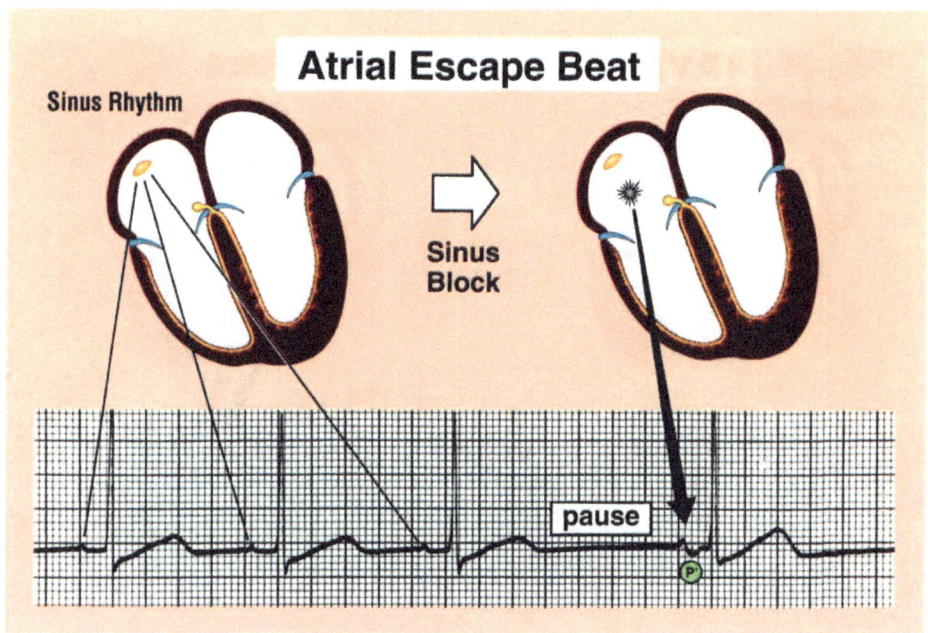

A transient Sinus Block of one pacemaking stimulus (SA Node misses one cycle) is a sufficient pause for an atrial automaticity focus to escape overdrive suppression and emit an **Atrial Escape Beat**. Notice that the P' wave differs from the Sinus-generated P waves.

A transient Sinus Block can prevent the ___ _____ from discharging one pacemaking stimulus, thus producing a pause of electrical silence for one pacing cycle.

SA Node

This pause, resulting from one missed SA Node pacing cycle, is sufficient enough to remove the overdrive suppression of an atrial automaticity _____ and...

focus

... the atrial focus escapes to emit a single stimulus; this is an Atrial Escape Beat (on EKG, a pause followed by a P' that differs from the P waves). Then the SA Node quickly resumes pacing, so the atrial focus is _____-suppressed again.

overdrive

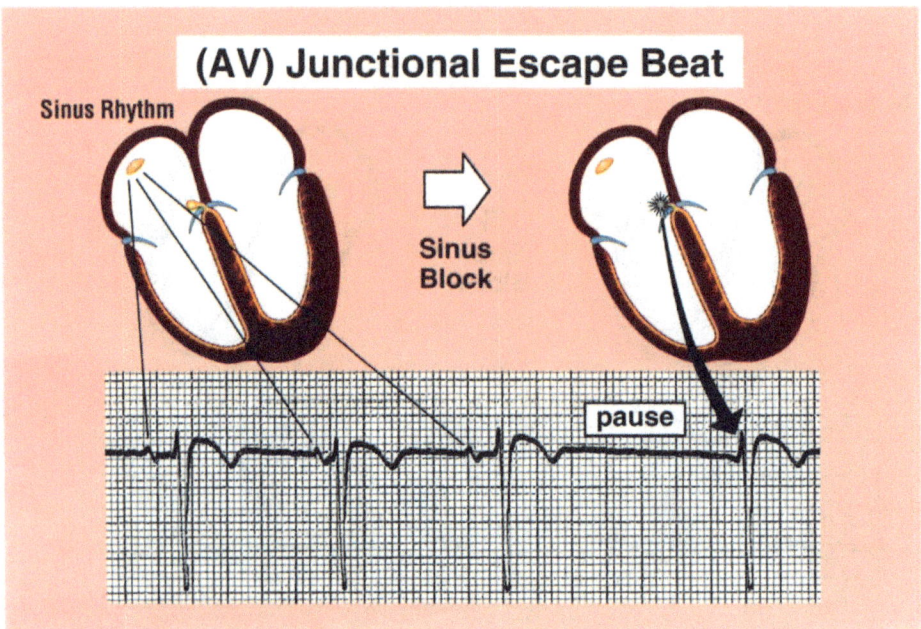

An unhealthy SA Node that suffers a transient Sinus Block misses one pacing
cycle. This pause can induce a Junctional automaticity focus to escape overdrive
suppression and emit a **Junctional Escape Beat**.

If the SA Node suffers a transient Sinus Block, it misses
one pacing cycle, so a sufficient _____ results and…   pause

… absent any atrial focal response, a Junctional automaticity
focus will escape overdrive _____ to emit a   suppression
Junctional Escape Beat.

The depolarization stimulus emitted by the Junctional focus passes
down the ventricular conduction _____ to depolarize the   system
ventricles in a normal fashion, so a normal QRS complex results.
Then the SA Node resumes pacemaking, overdrive-suppressing the
Junctional focus.

Note: A single Junctional Escape Beat may produce retrograde atrial
depolarization that records an inverted P' immediately before the QRS
or an inverted P' after the QRS.

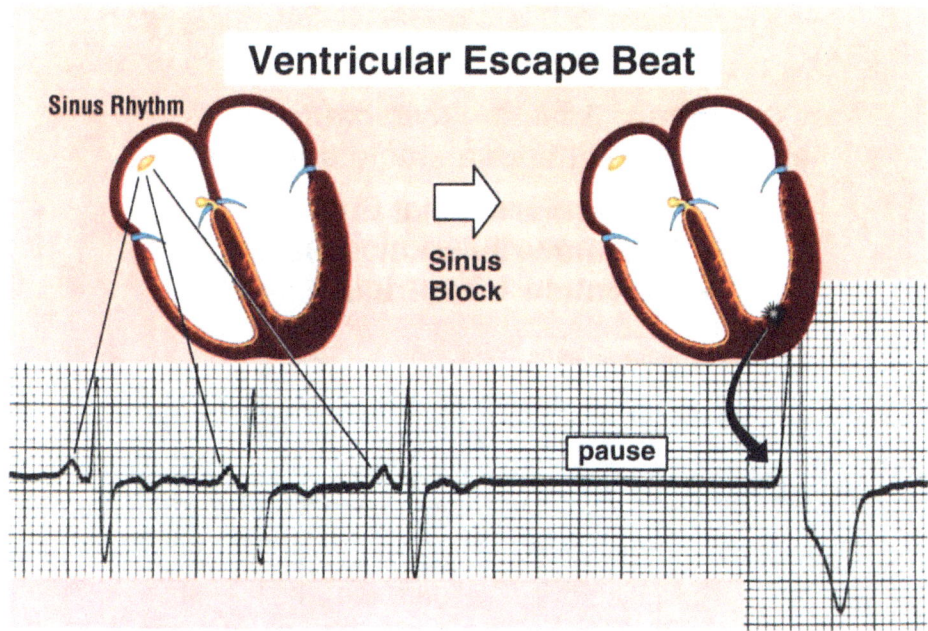

A **Ventricular Escape Beat** originates in a ventricular automaticity focus that is no longer overdrive-suppressed by regular pacing stimuli from above. A ventricular focus typically produces this enormous ventricular (QRS) complex.

A ventricular automaticity _____ can escape overdrive suppression when it is not stimulated by pacemaking activity from above for at least one – maybe two cycles.   focus

It seems a little unusual that the SA Node as well as all of the atrial foci and all the Junctional _____ would fail simultaneously. How then, is it that Ventricular Escape Beats are not so rare? Here's how…   foci

Note: Cardiac parasympathetic innervation inhibits the SA Node <u>and also</u> inhibits the atrial and Junctional foci (see illustration, page 58), but <u>not</u> the ventricular foci. Therefore, a burst of excessive parasympathetic activity depresses the SA Node (producing a pause) and also depresses the atrial and Junctional foci, which leaves only the ventricular foci to respond to the pause. So a ventricular automaticity focus escapes overdrive suppression and discharges, depolarizing the ventricles, producing an enormous ventricular complex. Such a burst of excessive parasympathetic activity is usually transient, so the SA Node resumes its pacemaking activity.

Note: Please study the organized review of *Escape* on page 337, with a focus on understanding.

Premature Beats

Premature Beat - an irritable focus spontaneously fires a single stimulus:

- **Premature Atrial Beat**
- **Premature Junctional Beat**
- **Premature Ventricular Beat**

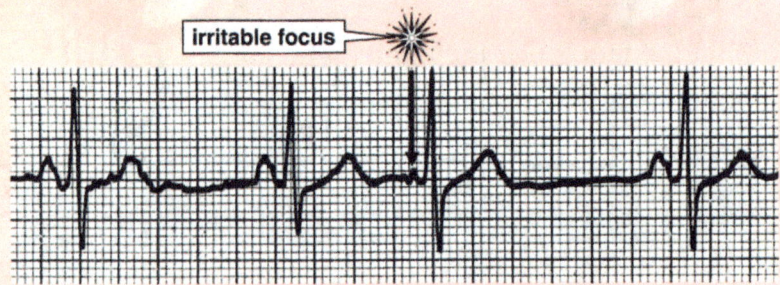

irritable focus

A *premature beat* (premature stimulus) originates in an <u>irritable</u> automaticity focus that fires spontaneously, producing a beat (on EKG we see evidence of a depolarization) earlier than expected in the rhythm.

Note: Those things that make *you* irritable can do the same to an atrial or Junctional automaticity focus. Quickly peek at the next page and you'll see.

A premature beat, like a premature baby, appears earlier than _____.   expected

When we see a premature beat, we recognize that it was fired by an irritable automaticity _____, so we need   focus to identify the focus (atrial, Junctional, or ventricular).

Note: <u>Ventricular</u> automaticity foci are the world's most sensitive O_2 sensors. When they sense low O_2, they become irritable… and they react!

Note: Premature beats can cause peculiarities in the rhythm that may mimic more serious problems such as pathological conduction blocks. While some premature beats are not serious, others are a dire warning – we'll explore them all. You should be cautious and know the difference – lives will depend on it! *Understanding* the basics provides answers, and understanding facilitates rapid judgement.

Atrial and Junctional foci become irritable because of:

- **adrenaline (epinephrine) released by adrenal glands**

- **increased sympathetic stimulation***

- **presence of caffeine, amphetamines, cocaine,**
   or other β_1 receptor stimulants

- **excess digitalis, some toxins, occasionally ethanol**

- **hyperthyroidism**
   (direct stimulation plus heart oversensitive
   to adrenergic stimulants)

- **stretch**
... and to some extent, low O_2

*** decreasing or blocking parasympathetic**
effects may accomplish this.

atrial focus

Junctional focus

An *automaticity focus in the atria or in the AV Junction* may become **irritable** and spontaneously fire an impulse or even suddenly pace very fast. The cause of irritability in atrial and Junctional foci is usually adrenergic substances (page 57).

Should an atrial or Junctional automaticity focus become irritable,* it may fire a spontaneous impulse that depolarizes the surrounding tissue, so we can recognize it on _____ as a premature beat.   EKG

But a *very* _____ atrial or Junctional focus may fire   irritable
a series of rapid pacing impulses to become the dominant
pacemaker, overdrive-suppressing all automaticity centers.

Note: Conditions/substances that can make an atrial focus (usually) or Junctional focus (occasionally) irritable:

- an excess of epinephrine or norepinephrine, the natural substances that activate the adrenergic receptors (of foci).

- adrenergic chemicals that mimic this effect.

- substances or conditions that increase the release of epinephrine or norepinephrine.

* Recalling an irritable person who suddenly yelled at you (too much adrenaline, or maybe too much coffee), you will remember that upper level foci can also become "irritable" (same causes) and spontaneously fire a stimulus.

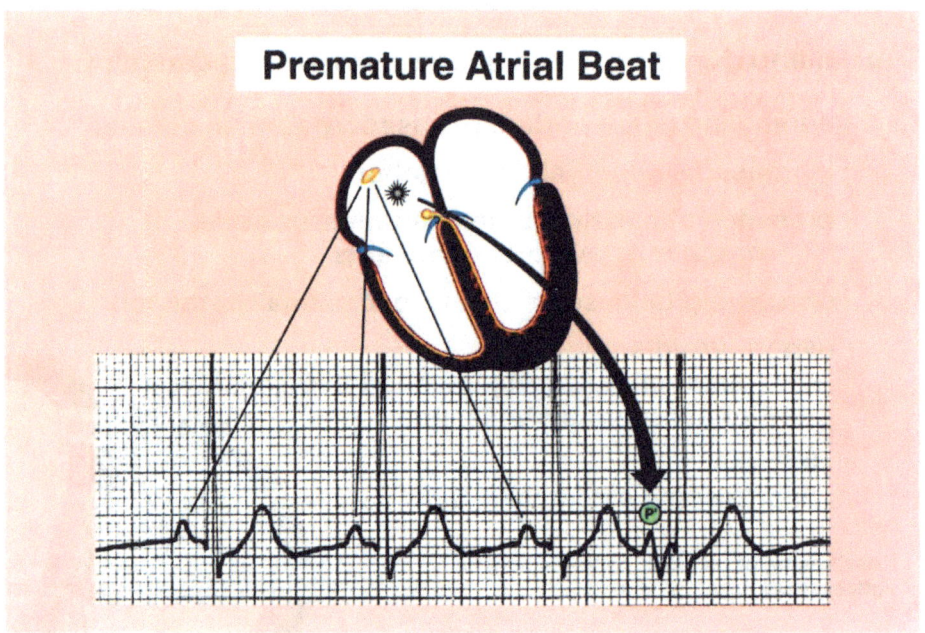

Premature Atrial Beat

A **Premature Atrial Beat** (PAB) originates suddenly in an *irritable* (see previous page) atrial automaticity focus, and it produces a P' wave earlier than expected. On EKG, P' is atrial depolarization by an automaticity focus.

A Premature Atrial Beat (PAB) originates in an irritable atrial automaticity focus that spontaneously fires a depolarization stimulus earlier than the normal ___ wave on EKG.   P

But because an atrial focus is the origin of this premature atrial depolarization (not the SA Node), the stimulus produces a premature and unusually shaped P' wave* that does not look like a normal (Sinus-generated) P _____.   wave

Note: On EKG, a PAB records as a P'. The P' may be difficult to detect when it's hiding on the peak of a T wave; the giveaway is a too-tall T... taller than the other T waves in the same lead.

Note: Each PAB depolarizes the SA Node; the effect of this... (next page)

---

* Atrial depolarization from a focus near the SA Node produces a generally upright P' wave, whereas a focus in the lower atrium depolarizes the atria in a "bottom-upwards" (retrograde) fashion to record an inverted P' wave in most leads.

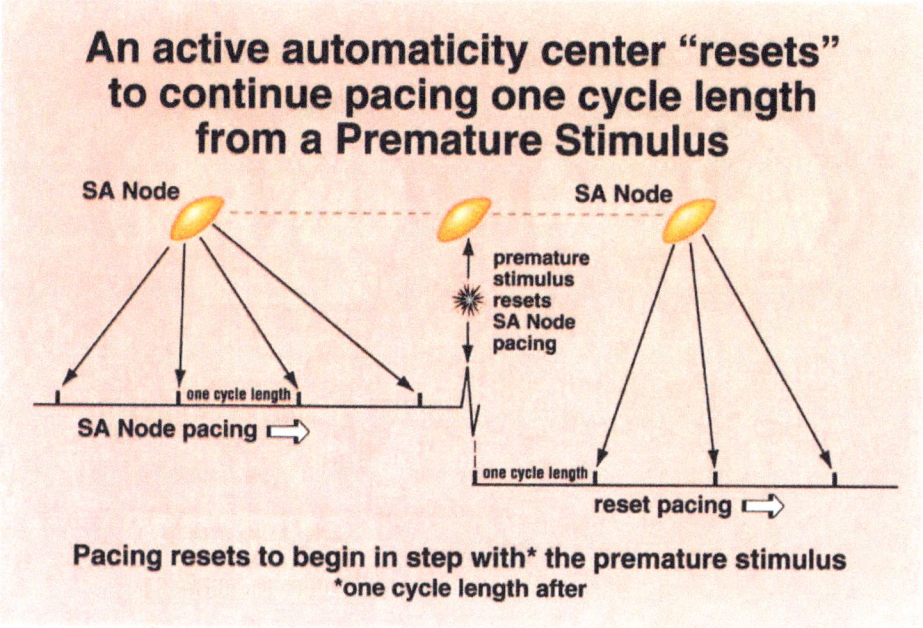

An active automaticity center "resets" to continue pacing one cycle length from a Premature Stimulus

SA Node

SA Node

SA Node

premature
stimulus
resets
SA Node
pacing

one cycle length

SA Node pacing

one cycle length

reset pacing

Pacing resets to begin in step with* the premature stimulus
*one cycle length after

All centers of automaticity **reset**, a characteristic of automaticity. A center of automaticity *resets* its rhythm when it is depolarized by a premature stimulus, so its pacemaking activity *resets* in step with the premature beat. Observing the illustration from left to right, helps clarify the concept.

Resetting occurs when the dominant automaticity center (usually the SA Node) is depolarized by a _____ beat, then...   premature

... its pacemaking activity *resets* in step with the premature stimulus, so that the next pacing stimulus that it generates is one cycle length from the premature _____.   beat
(stimulus)

If the SA Node is depolarized by a premature beat, the SA Node pacemaking is *reset,* so that regular pacing resumes one cycle length from the _____ stimulus.   premature

Note: In order to reset, the dominant (active) center of automaticity must be depolarized by the premature beat. When there is a premature stimulus that does not reach the dominant pacing center, its pacing is not *reset.*

PAB resets SA Node Pacing

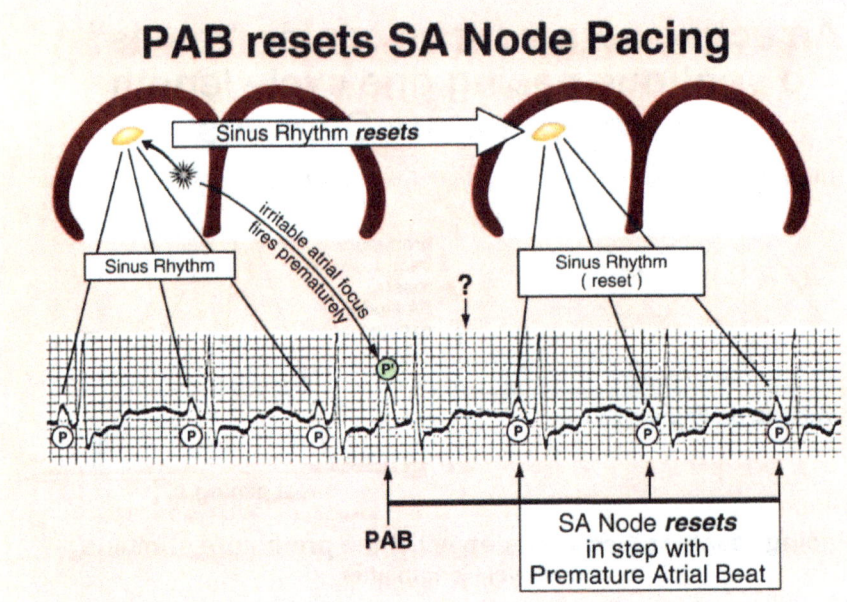

A Premature Atrial Beat from an irritable atrial automaticity focus produces a too-early depolarization of the atria that depolarizes the SA Node as well. So the SA Node *resets* its rhythm in step with the Premature Atrial Beat (P').

Note: The P' on EKG is the funny-looking atrial depolarization wave produced by an automaticity focus. It appears different from all SA Node-generated P waves in the same EKG lead, but a normal QRS follows.

If a Regular Sinus Rhythm produced by the SA _____ is interrupted   Node
by a spontaneous Premature Atrial Beat (from an atrial automaticity focus), the SA Node, which lies within the atria, is depolarized as well so...

... the SA Node *resets*, making the P' the first beat of its (*reset*)
_____. The "?" in the illustration marks where the P wave   rhythm
would have occurred, if the SA Node weren't *reset*.

Note: The *reset* <u>rhythm</u> of the SA Node resumes the same rate (same cycle length) as before the premature stimulus, but it continues one cycle length from (i.e., in step with) the P'. The pacing <u>rate</u> of the SA Node before and after the PAB remains the same.

Note: In reality, the first cycle after a PAB is a little lengthened due to a transient (baroreceptor) parasympathetic effect on the SA Node, which resumes pacing during systole. (Understanding the mechanism is not important.)

Premature Atrial Beat with aberrant ventricular conduction

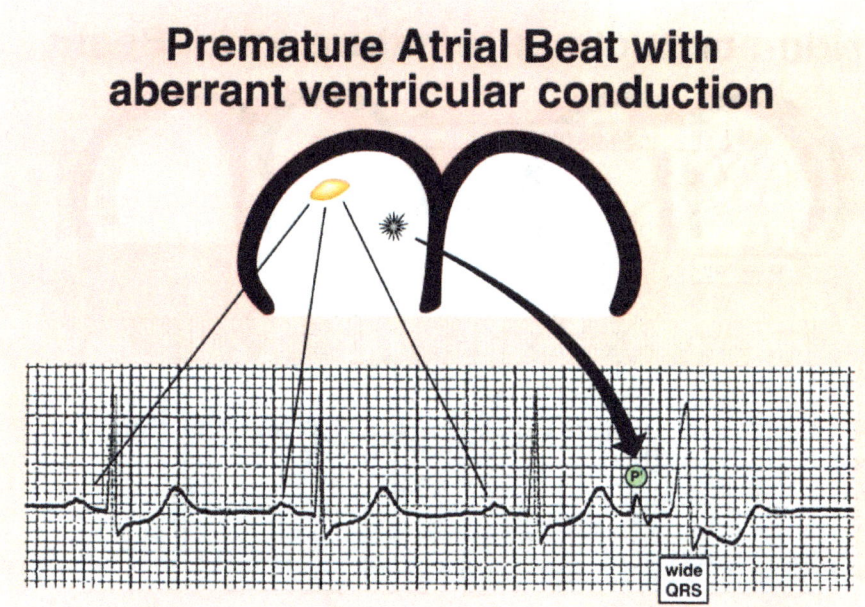

The ventricular conduction system is usually receptive to being depolarized by a Premature Atrial Beat, but one Bundle Branch may not have completely repolarized (that is, it's still a little refractory) when the other is receptive. This **"aberrant ventricular conduction"** produces a slightly widened QRS for that premature cycle only.

<mark>Note:</mark> When a Premature Atrial Beat (P') is conducted to the ventricles, the ventricles are also depolarized earlier than usual.

Sometimes a Premature Atrial Beat can produce aberrant ventricular conduction, because one of the Bundle Branches is not completely _____, and therefore is temporarily   repolarized refractory to depolarization.

So, depolarization of one ventricle is immediate, while depolarization of the other ventricle is slightly _____.   delayed

The non-simultaneous depolarization of the ventricles records as a slightly _____ QRS complex after the P' on the EKG.   widened Normal ventricular conduction resumes with normal cycles.

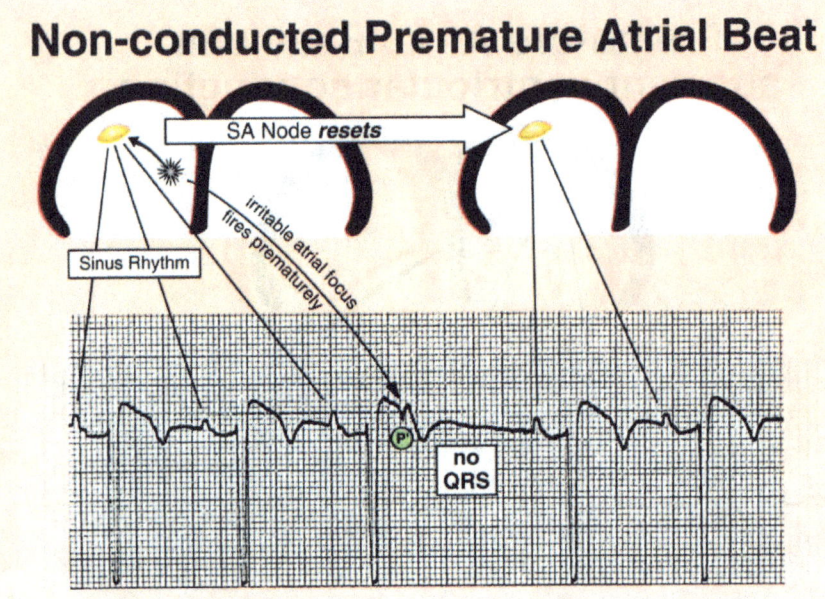

Non-conducted Premature Atrial Beat

At times, the AV Node is completely unreceptive to a premature atrial depolarization stimulus because it reaches the AV Node prematurely, that is, while the AV Node is still in the refractory period of its repolarization. This results in a *"non-conducted"* (to the ventricles) Premature Atrial Beat.

A Premature Atrial Beat may be unable to depolarize
the AV Node if it (the AV Node) is not fully repolarized
and still _____ to an extra-stimulus.   refractory

On EKG, this records as a too-early, unusual ___ wave   P'
that has no ventricular (QRS-T) response.

Note: Warning! Although a "non-conducted" PAB (on EKG,
a premature P' without a QRS response) does not depolarize
the ventricles, it <u>does</u> depolarize the SA Node, which *resets*
its pacemaking one cycle length after the premature stimulus.
The combination of *reset* pacing plus the missing QRS-T creates
a harmless, but dangerous-looking, span of empty baseline…
which has the sinister appearance of a "some-kind-of-block."
And one day you will have the satisfaction of correcting someone
who guessed the wrong diagnosis.

Atrial Bigeminy

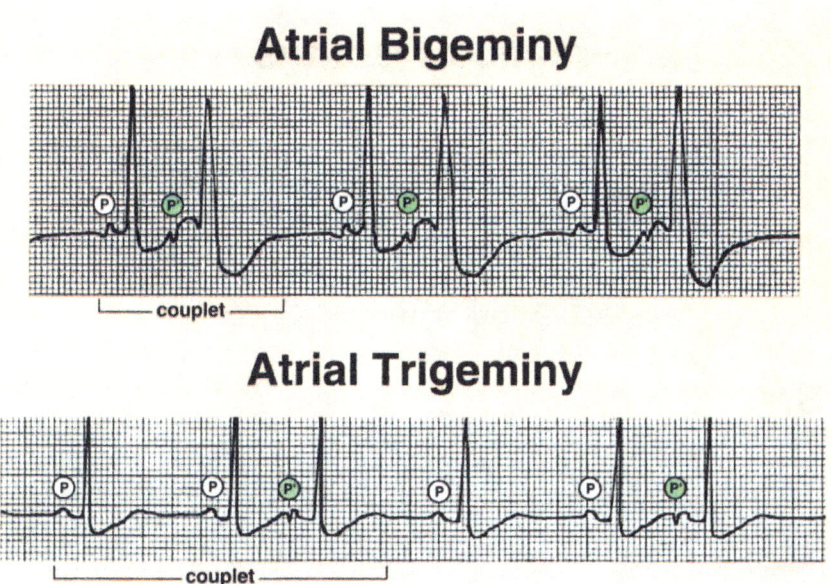

couplet

Atrial Trigeminy

couplet

Occasionally, an irritable automaticity focus fires a Premature Atrial Beat (P') that couples to the end of a normal cycle, and repeats this process by coupling a PAB to the end of each successive normal cycle. This is **Atrial Bigeminy**.

Note: The cycle containing the premature beat together with the cycle or cycles to which it couples, is called a "couplet."

When an irritable atrial focus repeatedly couples a PAB to the end of each (otherwise normal) cycle, this is a run of _____ Bigeminy.*   Atrial

Sometimes, an irritable atrial focus may prematurely fire after two normal cycles; when this couplet _____ continuously,   repeats it is a run of **Atrial Trigeminy**.

Note: With both Atrial Bigeminy and Atrial Trigeminy, each premature stimulus (from the irritable atrial focus) depolarizes the SA Node and *resets* it, producing a span of clear baseline between the couplets. So a series ("run") of couplet groups called "group beating" is often seen with Atrial Bigeminy, Atrial Trigeminy, etc. Just look for the premature (P') beat in each couplet. It's that simple! This is mentioned because group beating may occur with a type of AV conduction block to be discussed later (page 180).

* As you may have noticed, there is a slightly widened (aberrant) QRS after each P' in the upper tracing. Aberrant ventricular conduction can occur after any premature atrial (or Junctional) beat.

Practice Tracings

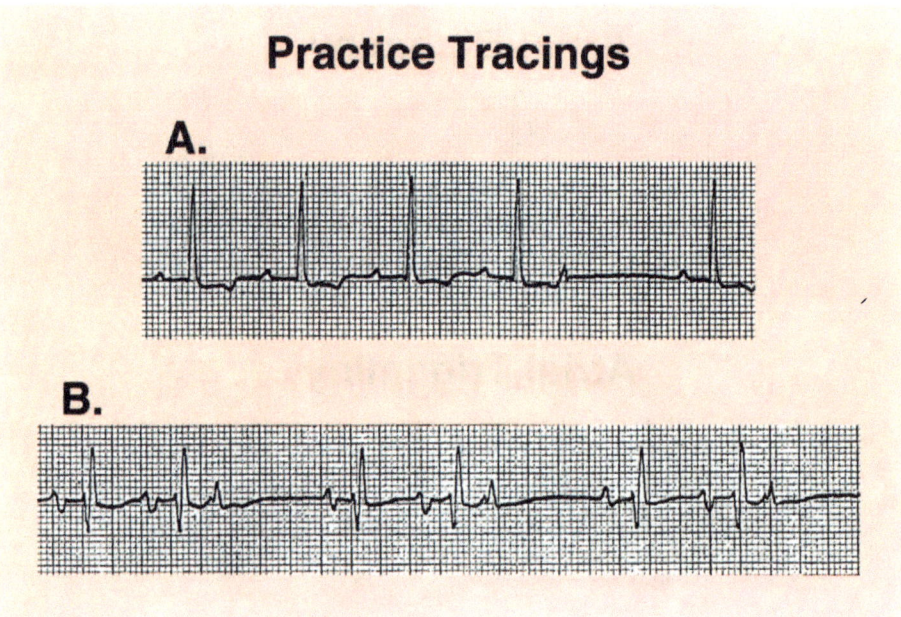

Can you determine what is occurring on each of these practice EKG tracings?

Tracing A:

This tracing is from a medical student who had a few cups of coffee in order to study late. She went to the Emergency Room because her pulse seemed irregular.

The intern on duty thought that the tracing showed "intermittent complete AV Block" and was about to call the attending physician (at 4:00 am) to schedule an emergency artificial pacemaker implantation. Explain the EKG strip to the intern, using only what you have learned so far (before he wakes the attending physician and discovers the real meaning of "irritable").

Tracing B:

This transmitted telemetry tracing is from a known drug abuser who took a large quantity of amphetamines before his emergency ride to the hospital.

Someone in the ambulance suggested what sounded like "Winky bok block," when the telemetry was transmitted. Utilizing only what you have read and understand so far in this book, you will recognize things that you have just learned. Notice that in each grouping only two of the P waves are identical. Carefully analyze what you see, so you can explain it to others.

Note: Carefully examine each tracing and contemplate its subtle information. The answers will appear as you continue reading… somewhere.

Premature Junctional Beat

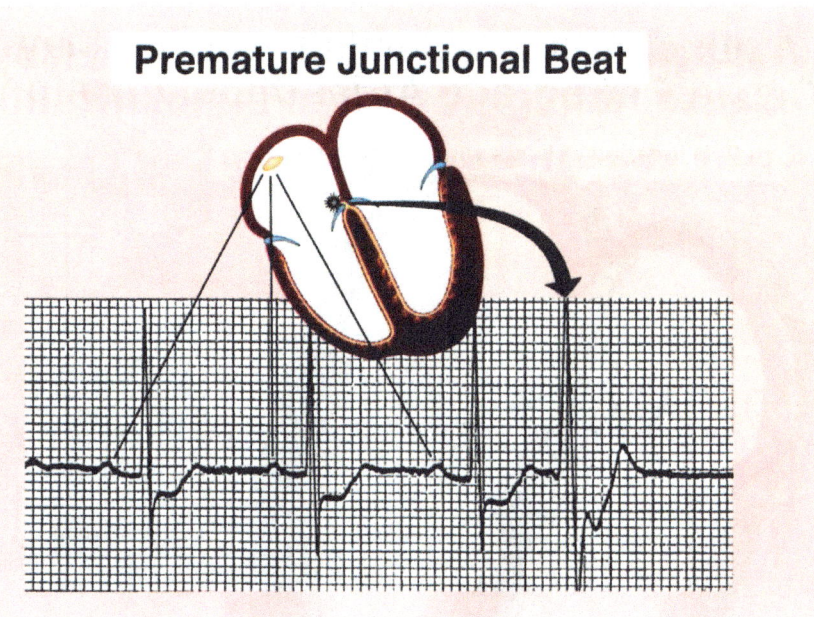

A **Premature Junctional Beat** (PJB) occurs when an *irritable* automaticity focus in the AV Junction suddenly fires a premature stimulus that is conducted to, and depolarizes, the ventricles (and sometimes the atria, in retrograde fashion).

When an irritable focus (see page 123) in the AV Junction spontaneously fires a stimulus, this produces a Premature _____ Beat on EKG.   Junctional

Note: After heart tissue depolarizes, it immediately repolarizes, and during repolarization that tissue is refractory to another stimulus (premature stimulus). As the ventricles repolarize, one Bundle Branch may repolarize slower than the other. So the too-early depolarization from a PJB may conduct through one Bundle Branch, but the impulse is temporarily delayed in the other, still refractory, Bundle Branch (usually the Right). So, instead of depolarizing simultaneously, one ventricle depolarizes punctually and the other is delayed, producing a slightly widened QRS complex typical of a Premature Junctional Beat with *aberrant ventricular conduction.*

If you see a premature QRS complex that is slightly widened, you should consider that it may be due to a Premature Junctional (or Premature Atrial) Beat with _____ ventricular conduction.   aberrant

Previous page answers: A. Non-conducted PAB. B. Atrial Trigeminy with non-conducted PAB.

A Junctional Automaticity Focus May Cause Retrograde Atrial Depolarization

Each P' is inverted in leads with an upright QRS

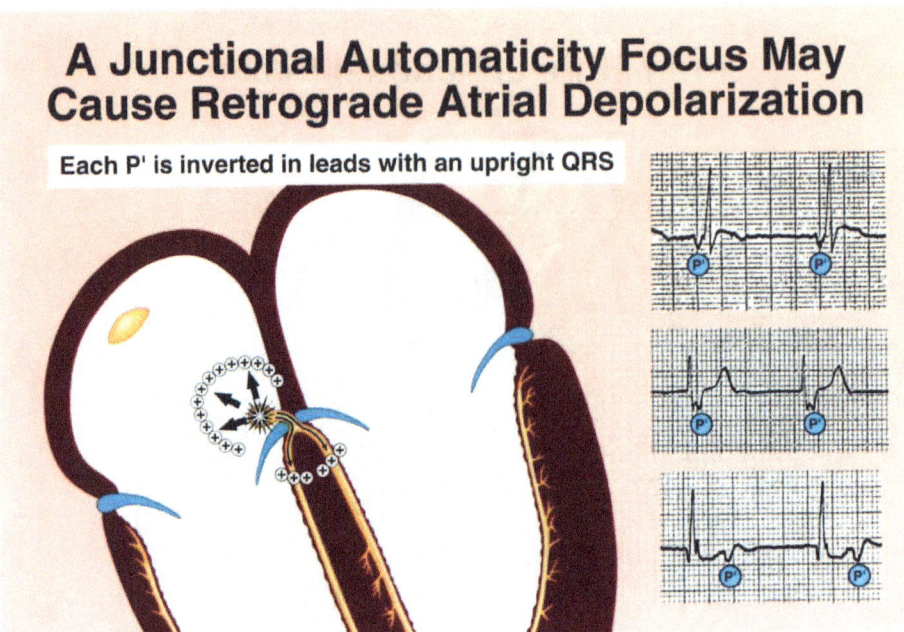

A Premature Junctional Beat originates in an irritable Junctional focus within the AV Node. We expect such a premature stimulus to conduct to the ventricles, but it may also depolarize the atria in a bottom-up "retrograde" fashion that records as an *inverted* P' wave in EKG leads with an upright QRS.

Since atrial and ventricular depolarization move in opposite directions from the Junctional focus, the premature P' wave is _____ i.e., opposite the upright QRS.

inverted

If a PJB produces retrograde atrial depolarization, it may record an inverted P' wave immediately before the premature _____ complex.

QRS

Sometimes an inverted ___ wave associated with a PJB follows the QRS. Occasionally the P' disappears within the QRS when atrial and ventricular depolarization occur simultaneously (not shown in illustration).

P'

Note: Retrograde atrial depolarization from a PJB usually depolarizes the SA Node as well. So the SA Node pacing is *reset* in step with the retrograde *atrial* depolarization.

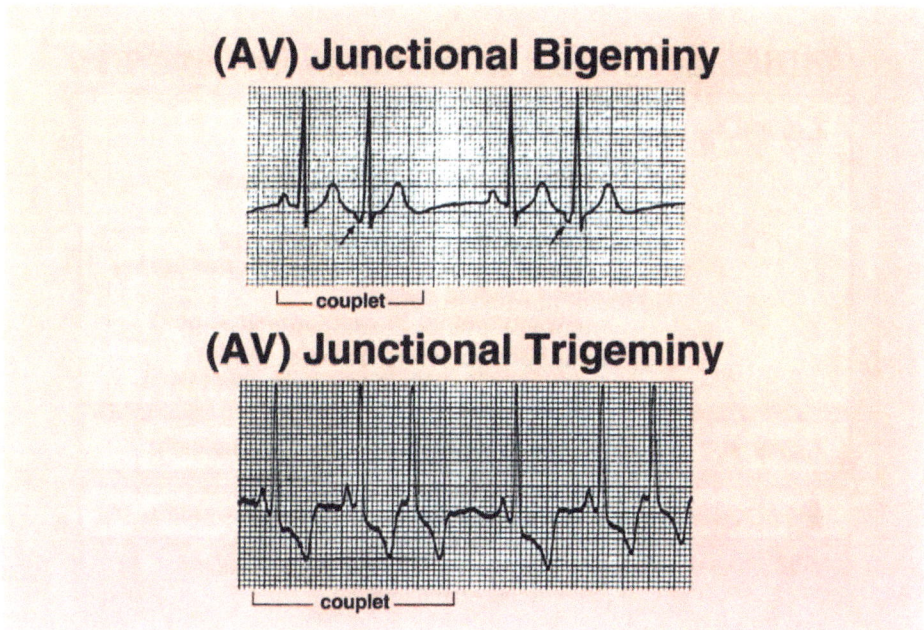

(AV) Junctional Bigeminy

couplet

(AV) Junctional Trigeminy

couplet

An irritable focus in the AV Junction may initiate a Premature Junctional Beat after each normal (SA Node-generated) cycle. This is **Junctional Bigeminy**. When a PJB is coupled with two consecutive, normal cycles in a repeating series of these couplets, this is **Junctional Trigeminy**.

An irritable Junctional automaticity focus may fire a premature stimulus coupled to the end of each normal (SA Node paced) cycle to produce Junctional _____.   Bigeminy

An irritable Junctional focus may fire a stimulus after two consecutive, normal Sinus-generated cycles. A repeating series of these couplets is _____ Trigeminy.   Junctional

Note: Don't forget that on EKG you may see an inverted (retrograde) P' wave (arrows in upper tracing) with every PJB in either Junctional Bigeminy or Junctional Trigeminy. Also, the SA Node will reset its pacing with each retrograde atrial depolarization; this can produce alarming (but innocent) gaps of empty baseline between couplets.

A <u>ventricular</u> focus can be made irritable by:

Low O$_2$	**Airway obstruction**
	Absence of air
	    (near-drowning or suffocation)
	Air with poor O2 content
	Minimal blood oxygenation in lungs
	    (pulmonary embolus or pneumothorax)
	Reduced cardiac output
	    (hypovolemic or cardiogenic shock)
	Poor to absent coronary blood supply
	    (coronary insufficiency or infarction)

Low K$^+$	**Reduced serum potassium ("hypokalemia")**
Pathology	**Mitral Valve Prolapse, stretch, myocarditis, etc.**

... and to a lesser degree, epinephrine-like substances
(β_1 adrenergic stimulants).

A *ventricular focus* may become **irritable** from under-oxygenation ("hypoxia") due to various circumstances and conditions. Hypokalemia, QT-prolonging medications, mitral valve prolapse, cardiac pathology, and stretch, can do the same.

Poor oxygenation (hypoxia) can make a ventricular automaticity
_____ become irritable and fire a spontaneous impulse,   focus
producing a premature ventricular beat on EKG.

A very irritable ventricular focus may be so excessively
provoked by hypoxia or "ischemia" (diminished blood supply)
that it suddenly fires a series of rapid impulses,
overdrive-suppressing the _____ Sinus rhythm...   normal

... so it becomes the heart's dominant pacemaker.

Note: If you study the illustration for a moment, you will quickly realize that there are numorous mechanisms that can reduce the oxygen supply to these sensitive ventricular automaticity foci. In a clinical setting, most (but not all) "deadly" ventricular tachycardias are due to coronary insufficiency or infarction. Know the other causes of ventricular focal irritability (see illustration).

Note: Cocaine is known to make atrial and Junctional foci irritable, but it has more dangerous effects. Cocaine causes coronary spasm, making ventricular foci hypoxic *and* very irritable; dangerous ventricular arrhythmias may ensue.

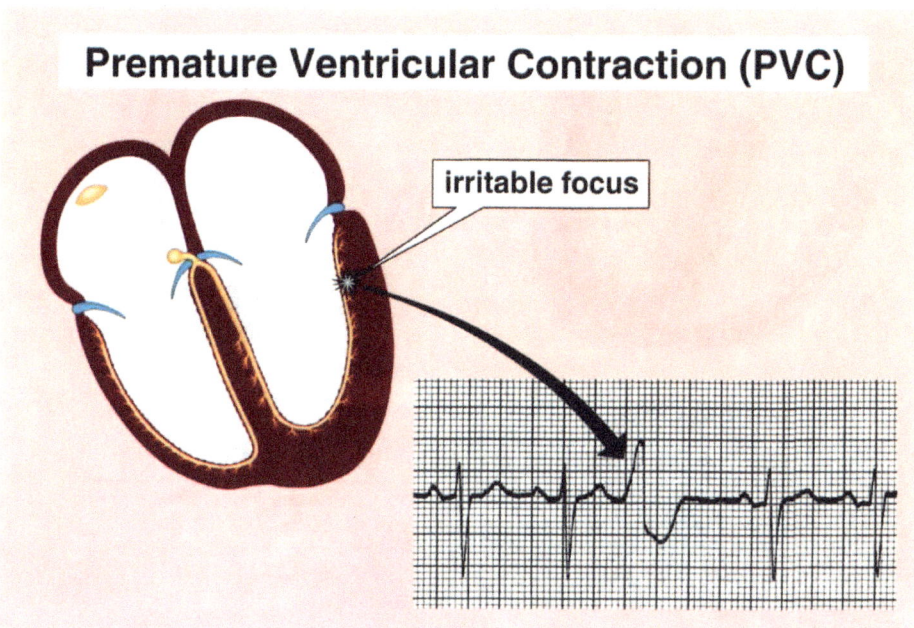

Premature Ventricular Contraction (PVC)

irritable focus

A premature ventricular beat called a **Premature Ventricular Contraction** (PVC) originates suddenly in an *irritable* ventricular automaticity focus and produces a giant ventricular complex on EKG.

An irritable (quickly review the previous page, please) ventricular focus may suddenly fire a stimulus and produce a _____ Ventricular Complex* (PVC) on EKG.   Premature

Note: PVC's occur early in the cycle. Easily recognized by their great width and enormous amplitude (height and depth), they are usually opposite the polarity of the normal QRS's (e.g., if QRS's are upward, PVC's are mainly downward).

The most likely reason for a ventricular automaticity focus to become irritable is under-_____ (hypoxia).   oxygenation

Note: PVC denotes a ventricular "contraction." When you see a PVC, remember that this represents a (premature) ventricular contraction, and an associated premature pulse beat, albeit weaker than normal (the prematurely stimulated ventricles are not completely filled).

* PVC may stand for Premature Ventricular "Contraction" or "Complex." This issue remains unresolved.

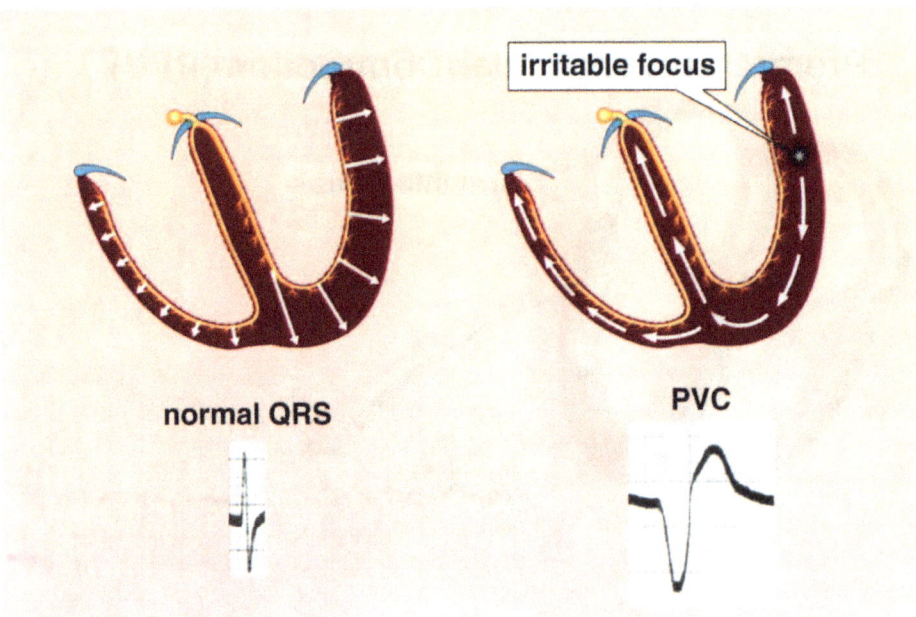

irritable focus

normal QRS   **PVC**

The PVC originates in an automaticity focus within the ventricular conduction
system, usually in a ventricular wall. Thus, one area of the ventricular wall begins to
depolarize before the rest of the ventricle, long before the other ventricle depolarizes.

Note: After a normal, Sinus-generated depolarization stimulus has
passed through the AV Node, the stimulus is quickly transmitted to the
entire endocardial lining of both ventricles at once. This simultaneous
depolarization of both ventricles produces a slender QRS complex.

Note: When an irritable ventricular automaticity focus suddenly
fires an impulse, that ventricular region depolarizes before the rest
of the ventricle, and then the depolarization wave creeps to the other
ventricle, which then depolarizes… producing an enormously wide
ventricular complex.

Note: Normally, ventricular depolarization passes through the entire
thickness of both ventricles at once. Left ventricular depolarization in
the leftward direction tends to be counterbalanced by the simultaneous
right ventricular depolarization in the opposite direction. This
minimizes the QRS amplitude. But depolarization originating in a
remote ventricular focus (as with a PVC), gradually spreads without
simultaneous opposition from the other side, and in its slow course,
produces (unopposed) deflections of immense amplitude.

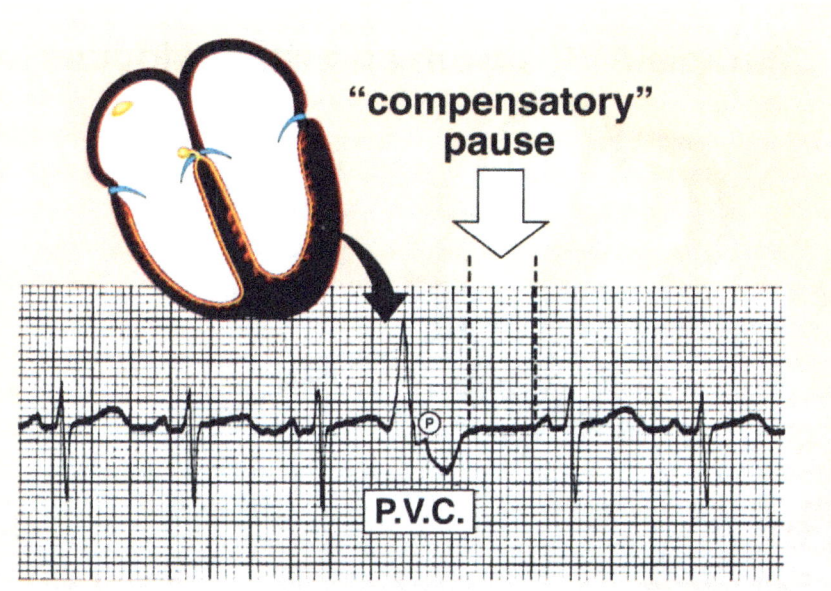

The PVC is an enormous ventricular complex that is much wider, taller, and deeper than a normal QRS. There is a pause after the PVC, but it is <u>not</u> caused by resetting of the SA Node; in fact, sometimes you can see the punctual, but ineffective, P wave within the PVC (see P in the illustration).

The PVC is a gigantic ventricular complex that jumps out
at you from the EKG, warning you that there is a ventricular
focus that is irritable, usually because of _____.   hypoxia

PVC's depolarize only the _____, not the SA Node,   ventricles
so the SA Node discharges on schedule. In fact, by measuring
P-P cycles, you can often locate the punctual P wave within a PVC.

But that timely P wave occurs while the ventricles are still
refractory (from the PVC) and not fully _____.   repolarized
When this normal stimulus arrives, they can't depolarize...

... so there is a _____ as the ventricles finish repolarizing,   pause*
making them receptive to the next Sinus-generated cycle.

Note: *Interpolated PVC's* are rare, but are somehow sandwiched
between the beats of a normal rhythm, producing no pause and no
rhythm disturbance.

* The pause, sometimes called a "compensatory" pause, doesn't "compensate" for anything.

Multiple PVC's from an irritable focus

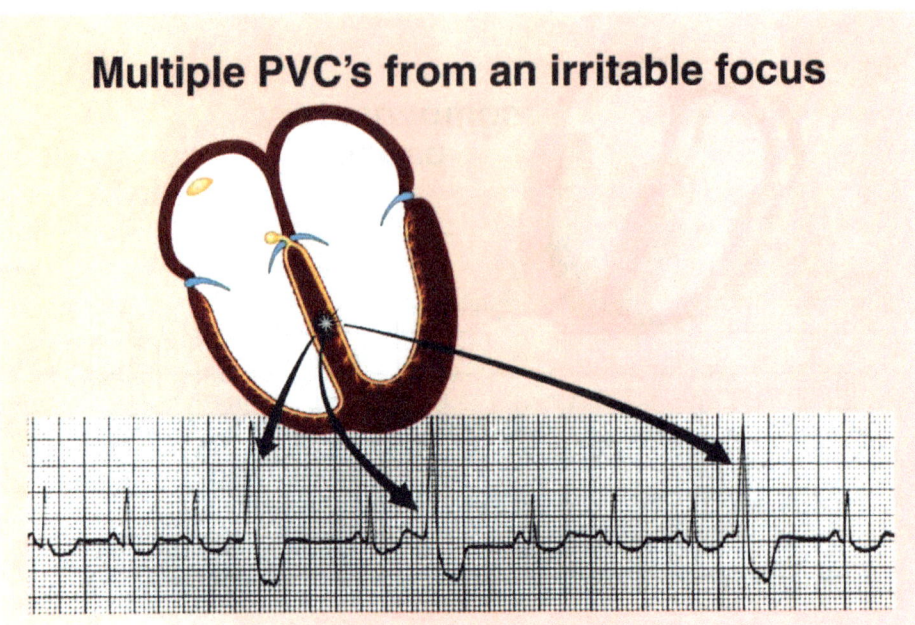

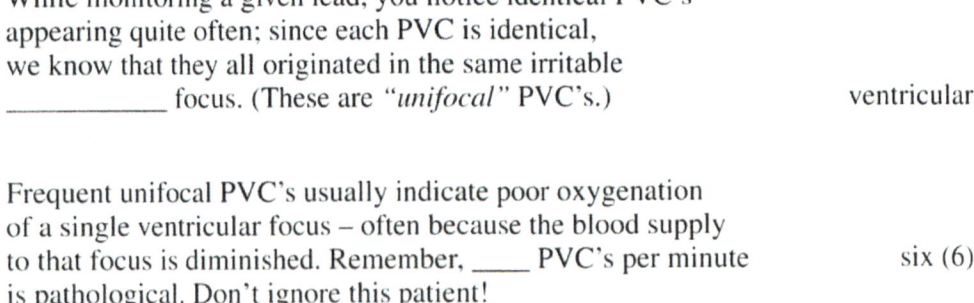

Numerous PVC's may emanate from the same ventricular focus, warning that the focus is very irritable, usually because of its poor state of oxygenation. Six or more PVC's per minute is considered pathological.

While monitoring a given lead, you notice identical PVC's
appearing quite often; since each PVC is identical,
we know that they all originated in the same irritable
_____ focus. (These are *"unifocal"* PVC's.)   ventricular

Frequent unifocal PVC's usually indicate poor oxygenation
of a single ventricular focus – often because the blood supply
to that focus is diminished. Remember, _____ PVC's per minute   six (6)
is pathological. Don't ignore this patient!

Note: There are situations when the coronary blood flow is adequate, but the blood is poorly oxygenated (e.g., drowning, pneumothorax, pulmonary embolus, tracheal obstruction, etc.). When a highly irritable ventricular focus is warning you with multiple PVC's... you must respond! Low serum potassium, as well as certain medications, can also irritate a ventricular focus. In addition, adrenergic stimulants like epinephrine can aggravate the situation.

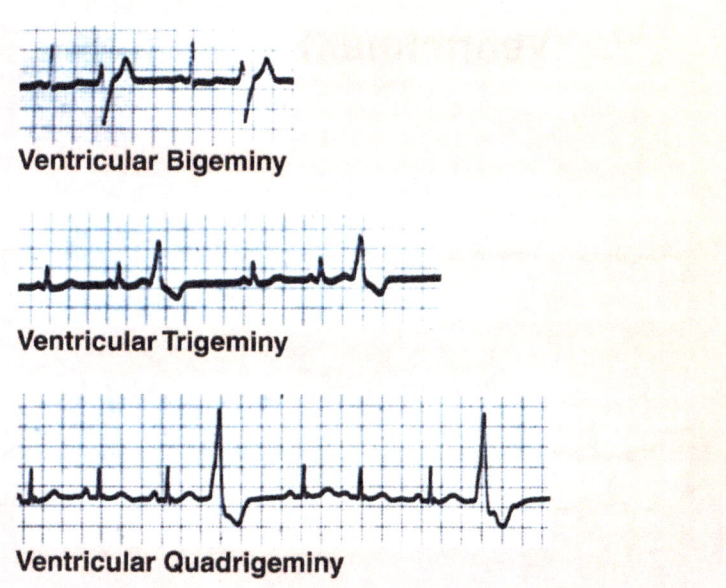

Ventricular Bigeminy

Ventricular Trigeminy

Ventricular Quadrigeminy

A very irritable ventricular automaticity focus may fire a stimulus that couples to one or more normal cycles to produce **Ventricular Bigeminy**, or **Ventricular Trigeminy**, etc.

Note: By convention, 6 PVC's per minute is considered pathological. A continuous run of any of these couplet patterns quickly exceeds that criterion and usually indicates that a very irritable focus is hypoxic and calling for help.

When a PVC becomes coupled to a normal cycle,
and the pattern continues with every cycle in succession,
we identify this as Ventricular _____.   Bigeminy

If you see a repetitive pattern of a PVC coupling with every
two normal cycles, this is a run of Ventricular _____.   Trigeminy

Note: Ventricular automaticity foci are the heart's hypoxia early warning system. Respond!

Ventricular Parasystole

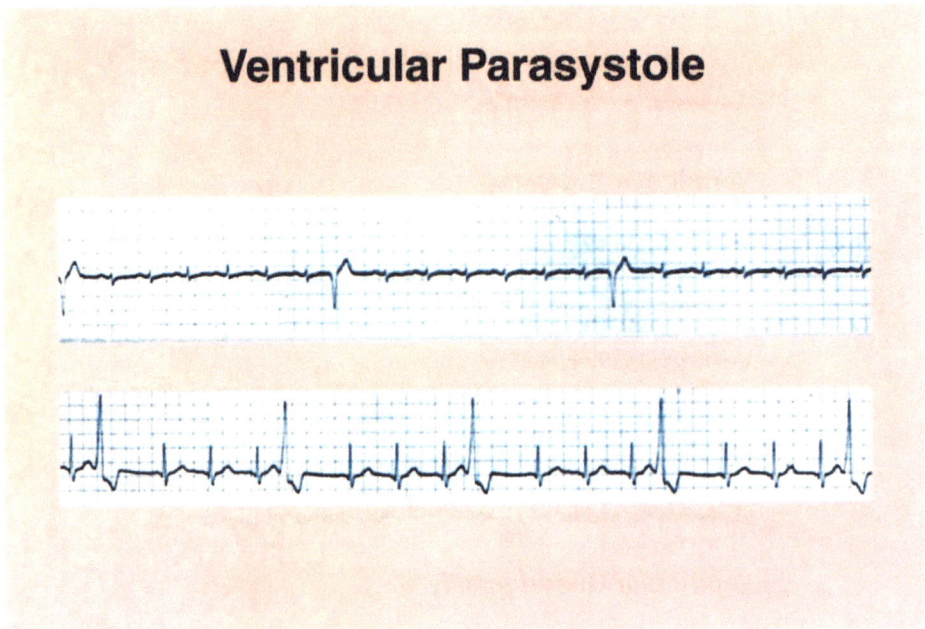

Ventricular Parasystole is produced by a ventricular automaticity focus that suffers from entrance block (but is *not* irritable). The parasystolic focus is not vulnerable to overdrive suppression, so it paces at its inherent rate, and the ventricular complexes that it generates poke through the dominant Sinus Rhythm.

Note: A solitary ventricular focus suffering from entrance block is "parasystolic", that is, it can't be overdrive-suppressed yet it can deliver pacing stimuli at its inherent rate.

Note: A parasystolic ventricular focus suffers from entrance block, insulating it from depolarization by outside sources. Absent overdrive suppression, it paces at its inherent rate. The result is a dual rhythm with pacing from two sources, the SA Node and the ventricular focus.

When you see PVC's that appear to be coupled to a long series of normal cycles, you should suspect Ventricular _____.   Parasystole

Note: Because this represents two unrelated, independent rhythms (from two different pacing locations), the interval between the normal cycle and the large ventricular complex is not always consistent. Occasionally a large ventricular complex may fail to appear because the ventricular focus happens to discharge during the refractory period of the (Sinus-paced) ventricles.

A very irritable ventricular focus can emit consecutive stimuli

one PVC   **run of 3 PVC's (VT)**

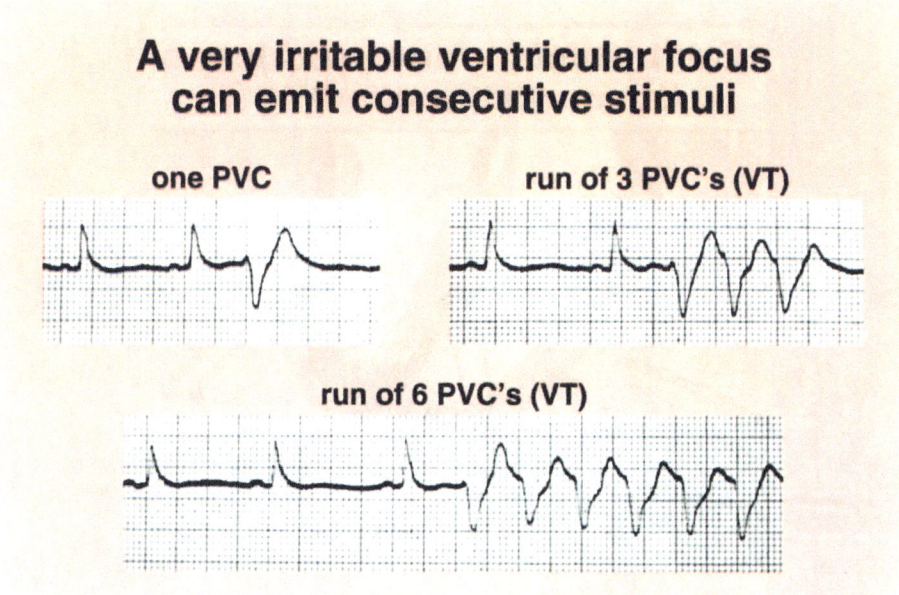

run of 6 PVC's (VT)

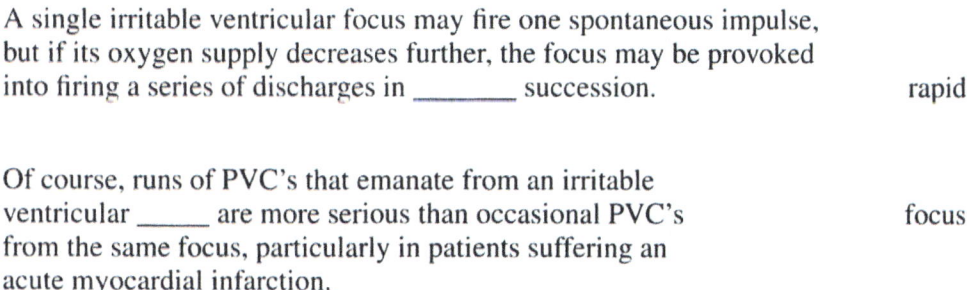

An irritable ventricular automaticity focus may fire once or, if extremely irritable (under-oxygenated), it may fire a rapid series of impulses to produce a *run* of PVC's.

A single irritable ventricular focus may fire one spontaneous impulse, but if its oxygen supply decreases further, the focus may be provoked into firing a series of discharges in _____ succession.   rapid

Of course, runs of PVC's that emanate from an irritable ventricular _____ are more serious than occasional PVC's   focus
from the same focus, particularly in patients suffering an acute myocardial infarction.

Note: A *run* of three or more PVC's in rapid succession is really a *run* of **Ventricular Tachycardia** (VT). Two of the examples in the above illustration are VT. If a run of VT lasts longer than 30 seconds, it is called "sustained" VT.

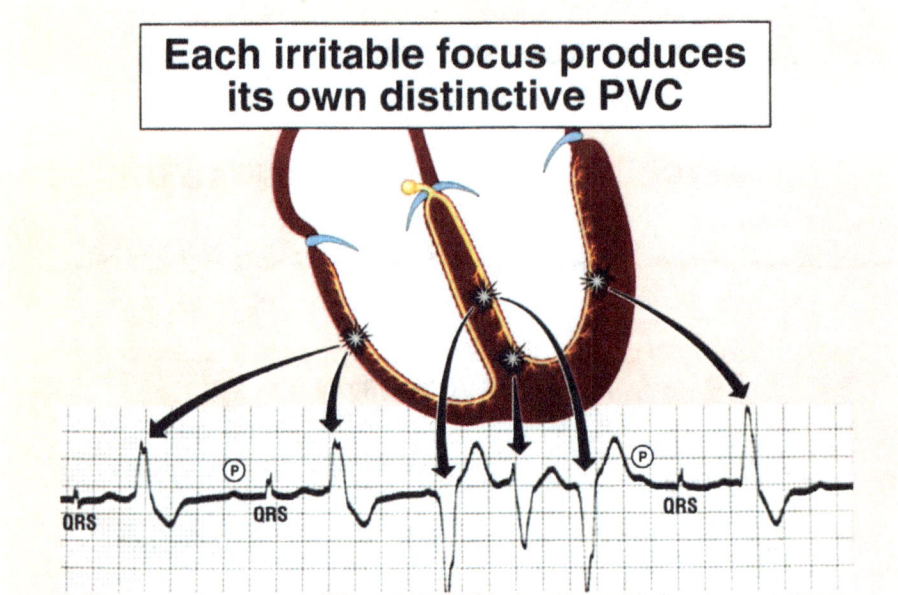

Each irritable focus produces its own distinctive PVC

Severe cardiac hypoxia can cause **Multifocal PVC's** – a desperation measure produced by multiple, exceptionally irritable (hypoxic), ventricular foci. Each focus produces its own unique, identifiable PVC every time it fires.

In a given lead, PVC's originating in a specific ventricular focus all appear the _____.   same

Note: Severe cardiac hypoxia can cause numerous *multifocal* PVC's to appear. This is indeed dangerous and requires immediate intervention. Because a single irritable ventricular focus can suddenly fire a series of rapid discharges to produce a dangerous tachy-arrhythmia (e.g., Ventricular Tachycardia), the presence of numerous multifocal PVC's means that a number of extremely irritable foci are discharging, and trouble is imminent. The chance of developing a dangerous or even deadly arrhythmia (e.g., Ventricular Fibrillation) under these dire circumstances is obviously enhanced. With infarction patients, this is an alarm of crisis proportions!

Mitral Valve Prolapse
(Barlow syndrome)

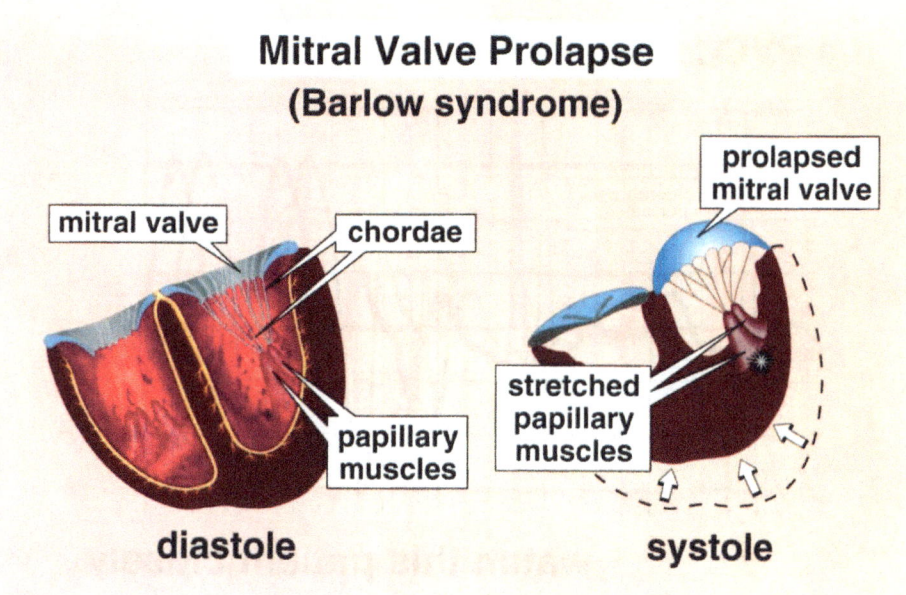

mitral valve

chordae

prolapsed
mitral valve

stretched
papillary
muscles

papillary
muscles

diastole   **systole**

Mitral Valve Prolapse (MVP) causes PVC's, including runs of VT and multifocal
PVC's, yet it is considered a benign condition. With MVP the mitral valve is "floppy"
and billows into the left atrium during ventricular systole.

First described by Dr. J. B. Barlow in 1968 (MVP is also
called "Barlow Syndrome"), this is quite common; 6% to 17% of
females, and about 1.5% of males. Females with MVP typically have
a slender body with a slight chest deformity, experience "dizzy" spells,
and are anxiety prone. They first experience symptoms after age 20.

During ventricular systole, the billowing valves pull on the
chordae that tether them to the papillary muscles in the left
ventricle. In the author's opinion, this traction on the papillary
muscles causes localized stretch and ischemia, irritating adjacent
ventricular automaticity _____.   foci

MVP patients usually have a mid-systolic click with a
decrescendo murmur on auscultation.

If a PVC falls on a T wave...

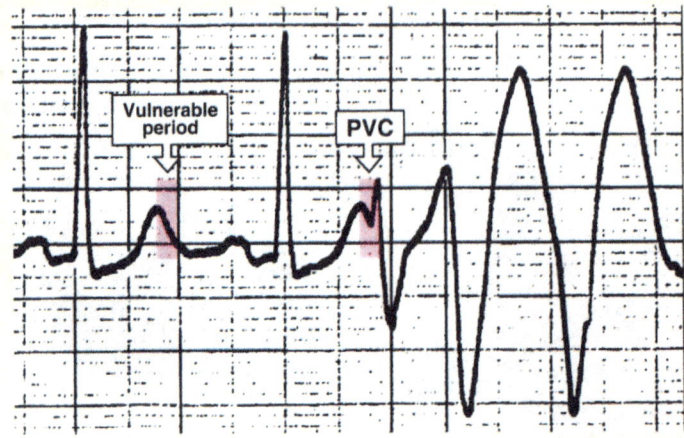

watch this patient closely.

If a PVC falls on a T wave ("**R on T phenomenon**"), particularly in situations of hypoxia or low serum potassium, it occurs during a "vulnerable period" and dangerous arrhythmias may result. Notice how a PVC hits the second T wave directly in its vulnerable period (ouch!)... and see what happens!

PVC's are, of course, premature and usually occur
just after the ___ wave of a normal cycle.   T

When a PVC falls on the peak of a T wave or on the initial part
of its downslope, it catches the ventricles during a vulnerable period,
particularly in the presence of _____ (often caused by cardiac   hypoxia
ischemia from a narrowed coronary artery) or in the presence
of low potassium.

Note: Repolarization of Purkinje fibers (along with their vulnerable
period) extends beyond the T wave, so a PVC falling just after the
T wave may, in fact, occur during the vulnerable period of ventricular foci.
Ischemia can extend Purkinje repolarization even further.

Note: This well known warning sign, "R on T" is often noted after the
fact, during the review of an EKG strip from a patient who suffered a
dangerous or deadly arrhythmia. By being cautious and vigilant, you
can respond quickly.

Practice Tracing

The discerning eye of a coronary care nurse detected a beat that appeared a little too
early on the EKG strip taken from a patient's monitor. Let's determine the location
of the irritable focus that produced the premature beat.

The last QRS complex in the strip catches your eye because
it occurs prematurely, and it is not preceded by a ___ wave.   P

The last QRS complex looks the same as the other QRS's, so we know
that, although premature, the last QRS resulted from depolarization
that passed (in a normal fashion) down the ventricular conduction
system. Therefore, it is <u>not</u> from a _____ focus.   ventricular

Carefully examining the EKG strip, we don't see a P' (with a little baseline)
before the premature QRS, so we know that the QRS did not emanate
from an atrial focus. Therefore the irritable automaticity focus that
produced the premature QRS must be in the ___ _____.   AV Junction

Note: Sure you understand this, but it probably would be a good
idea to take a minute to review this section, and study the simplified
review of *Premature Beats* on page 337. Then, let's take a break, and
I'll be right here when you return.

Tachy-arrhythmias
rapid rhythms originating in
very irritable automaticity foci

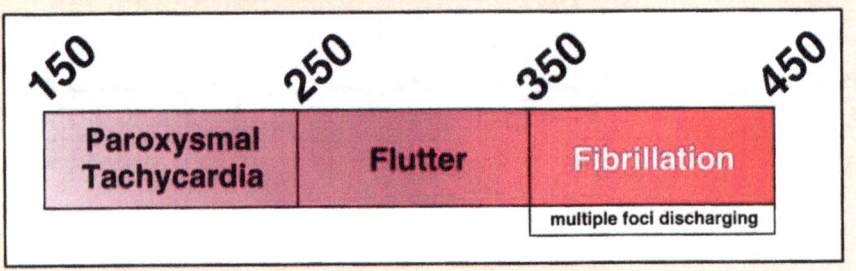

A *"tachy-arrhythmia"* originates in a very irritable focus that paces rapidly. Sometimes more than one active focus is generating pacing stimuli at once.

Note: Tachy-arrhythmia ("rapid arrhythmia"), hyphenated for recognition purposes here, is not usually hyphenated, so henceforth the hyphen will be omitted.

The rate ranges of the tachyarrhythmias are:

Paroxysmal Tachycardia . . . . _____ to _____ /minute.   150 to 250

Flutter. . . . . _____ to _____ /minute.   250 to 350

Fibrillation . . . . _____ to _____ /minute.   350 to 450

Note: A tachyarrhythmia is easily recognized by rate alone, but the specific diagnosis requires that we identify the origin, that is, we must determine the location of the irritable automaticity focus (atrial, Junctional, or ventricular). You already have a solid understanding* of normal conduction in the heart, so we merely need to get up to speed (pun intended) in learning the behavior of very irritable automaticity foci, and how they record on EKG.

* "Understanding is a kind of ecstacy." Carl Sagan (from *Broca's Brain.*)

Paroxysmal (sudden) Tachycardia
a very irritable automaticity focus suddenly paces rapidly:

- **Paroxysmal Atrial Tachycardia**
- **Paroxysmal Junctional Tachycardia**
- **Paroxysmal Ventricular Tachycardia**

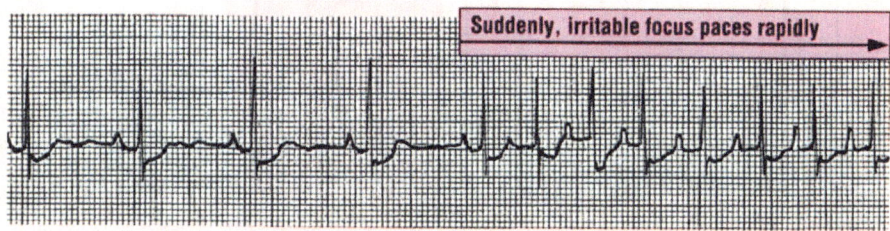

Suddenly, irritable focus paces rapidly

Paroxysmal ("sudden") *tachycardia* ("rapid heart rate") indicates rapid pacing (150 to 250 per minute) by a <u>very</u> irritable automaticity focus. Once we recognize a paroxysmal tachycardia, we need only identify the focus (atrial, Junctional, or ventricular) of its origin.

The medical term for rapid heart rate is _____.   tachycardia

Paroxysmal means _____.   sudden

Note: Paroxysmal tachycardia arises <u>suddenly</u> from a very irritable automaticity focus. Generally speaking, stimulants like epinephrine make higher level foci irritable, whereas more threatening physiological conditions like hypoxia (or low potassium) make ventricular foci irritable. There is some overlap, however. In addition, a single premature stimulus from another focus can provoke an irritable focus into a run of paroxysmal tachycardia.

In contrast, Sinus tachycardia is the SA Node's <u>gradual</u> response to exercise, excitement, etc. Although the SA Node's rate of pacing may eventually become quite rapid, Sinus tachycardia is neither sudden nor does it originate in an automaticity focus, so by definition, it is <u>not</u> a _____ tachycardia.   paroxysmal

Paroxysmal Tachycardia

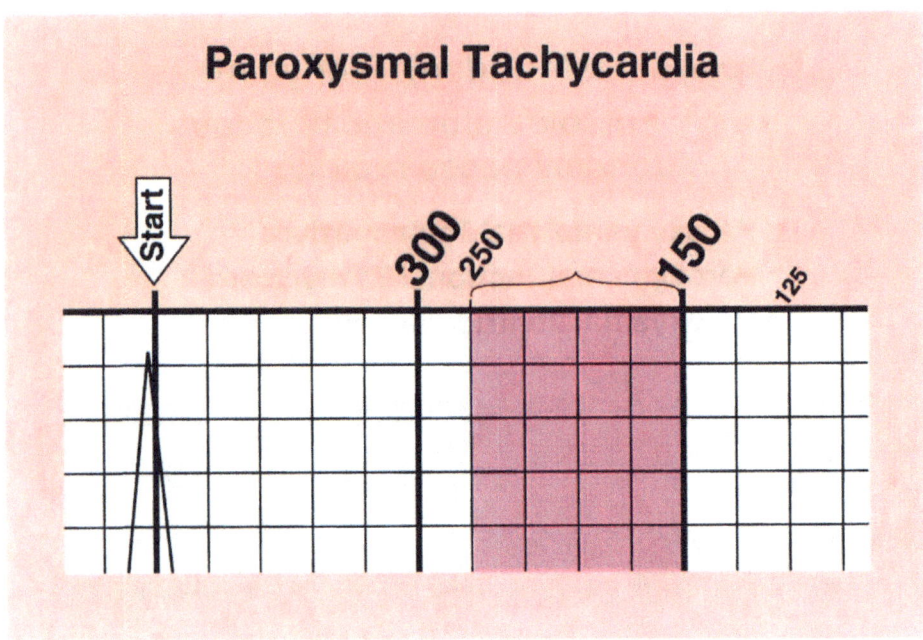

The rate range of the paroxysmal tachycardias is 150* to 250 per minute, so they are easy to recognize. Locating the causative irritable focus (atrial, Junctional, or ventricular) gives us the diagnosis.

When calculating rate, we find an R wave that peaks on a heavy black "start" line. The next three heavy black lines are called "300, 150, _____."

100

The fine line immediately to the right of the heavy black "300" line is the thin "250" line. Therefore, if an R wave falls on the "start" line (see illustration) the next R wave will fall within the shaded area during paroxysmal _____.

tachycardia

You can instantly recognize a paroxysmal tachycardia by noting the rate range of _____ to 250 per minute. Now you have to determine at which of three levels there is a very irritable automaticity focus causing the tachycardia. Easy enough!

150

* Some authors now set the lower rate limit of paroxysmal tachycardia at 125 per minute.

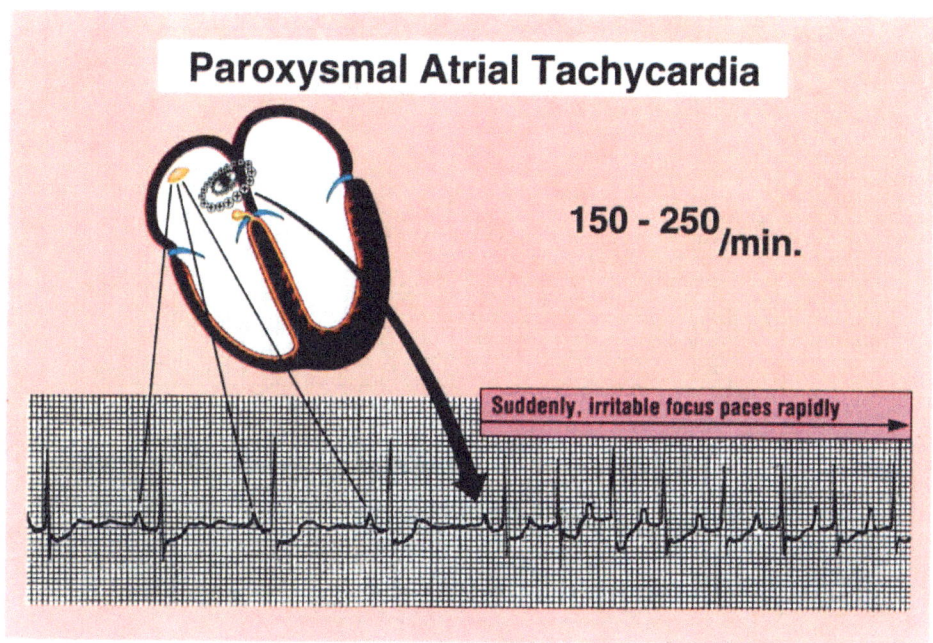

Paroxysmal Atrial Tachycardia

150 - 250 /min.

Suddenly, irritable focus paces rapidly

Paroxysmal Atrial Tachycardia (PAT) is caused by the sudden, rapid firing of a very irritable* atrial automaticity focus. You may see the beginning of this arrhythmia only occasionally, so become familiar with its general appearance.

Paroxysmal Atrial Tachycardia has a rapid heart rate that originates suddenly in a very irritable focus in one of the _____. The rate   atria
range is usually 150 to 250 per minute, so it overdrive-suppresses the SA Node and all other automaticity foci.

Because the origin of this tachyarrhythmia is a very irritable atrial focus, the atrial depolarizations of PAT are ___ waves   P'
that do not look like the Sinus-generated P waves.

Each depolarization impulse from the rapidly-pacing, irritable _____ focus depolarizes the atria and then is conducted   atrial
down the ventricular conduction system to the ventricles, yielding normal-appearing P'-QRS-T cycles.

Note: A premature stimulus from another focus may set off PAT.

* Quickly review page 123.

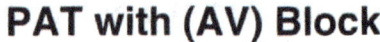

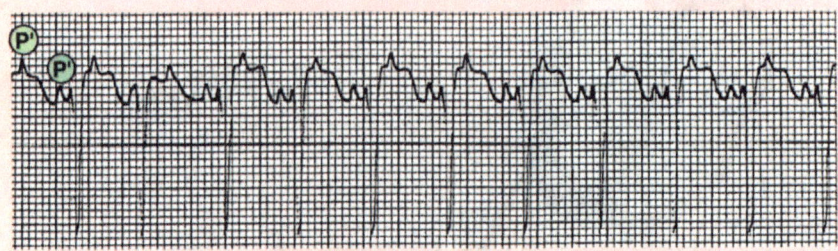

- **rapid rate, spiked P' waves**
- **2:1 ratio of P':QRS**

Suspect digitalis excess or toxicity.

Paroxysmal Atrial Tachycardia with AV block has more than one P' wave spike for every QRS response. Suspect digitalis excess or toxicity; atrial foci are very sensitive to the irritating effects of digitalis preparations.

<mark>Note:</mark> Excess digitalis can provoke an atrial focus into such an irritable state that it suddenly paces rapidly. At the same time, digitalis markedly inhibits the AV Node, so that only every second stimulus conducts to the ventricles (every-other atrial stimulus is blocked in the digitalis-inhibited AV Node).

PAT with block* is a tachyarrhythmia that has two P' waves
for each QRS response on EKG, because the ___ _____ blocks   AV Node
the conduction of every-other atrial stimulus.

PAT with block is usually a sign of _____ excess or toxicity,   digitalis
particularly if the patient has a low serum potassium, so careful
administration of intravenous potassium can help. Also, digitalis
antibodies can be employed to reduce toxicity.

* The "AV" is sometimes omitted, but is always understood.

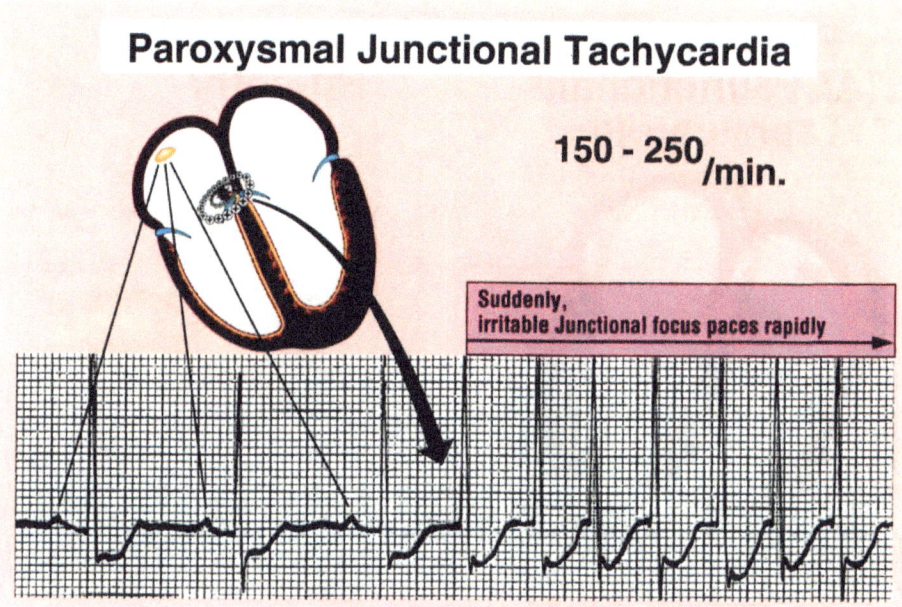

Paroxysmal Junctional Tachycardia

150 - 250/min.

Suddenly,
irritable Junctional focus paces rapidly

Paroxysmal Junctional Tachycardia (PJT) is caused by the sudden rapid pacing of a very irritable automaticity focus in the AV Junction. The Junctional focus may suddenly initiate tachycardia pacing, because of marked irritability induced by stimulants and/or by a well-timed premature beat from another focus.

Paroxysmal Junctional Tachycardia is due to a very irritable* focus
in the AV Junction that paces at the rate of _____ to 250 per minute.   150

Note: A rapidly pacing (irritable) Junctional focus *may* also
depolarize the atria from below in retrograde fashion to record:

- an inverted P' immediately before each upright QRS, or   (see illustration
- an inverted P' after each upright QRS, or   page 132)
- an inverted P' buried within each QRS (difficult to detect).

Note: Each stimulus from a rapidly pacing (irritable) Junctional focus
may occur at a time in the cycle when the Left Bundle Branch has fully
repolarized (i.e., recovered from its refractory period), but the Right
Bundle Branch is still refractory (in some patients, the reverse occurs).
As a result, this *aberrant ventricular conduction* depolarizes the left
ventricle before the right, to produce somewhat widened QRS's during
the tachycardia.

* One more look at page 123, and I'll never bother you again.

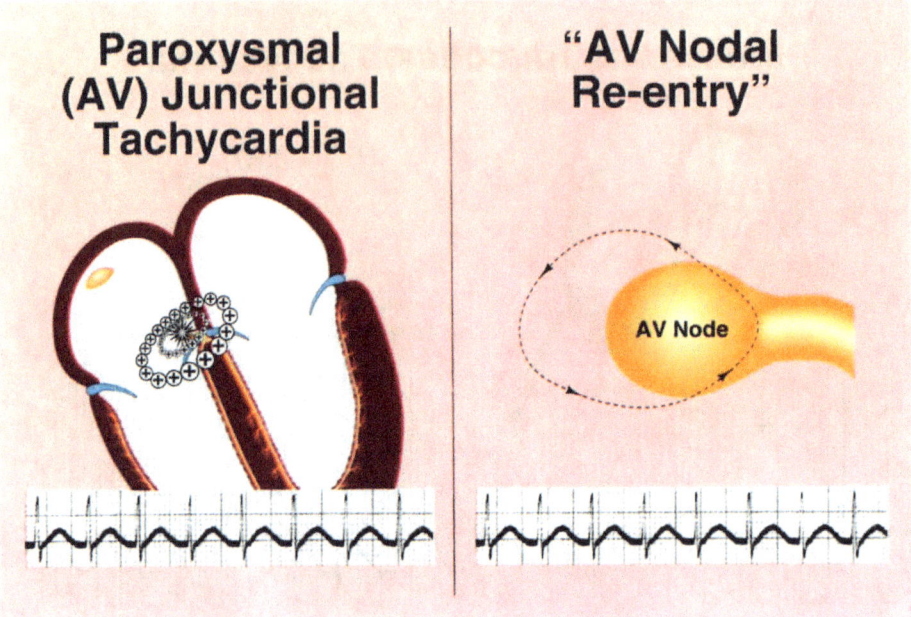

Paroxysmal (AV) Junctional Tachycardia

"AV Nodal Re-entry"

AV Node

Another type of Junctional Tachycardia is *AV Nodal Reentry* Tachycardia* (AVNRT). In theory, a continuous reentry circuit develops (which includes the AV Node and the lower atria) and rapidly paces the atria and ventricles.

Note: A theoretical "reentry circuit" may continuously circle (like perpetual motion) through the AV Junctional region, giving off a depolarization stimulus to the atria and to the ventricles with each pass in the circuit. This is "circus reentry," an aptly named tachycardia that looks suspiciously like PJT.

Note: In AVNRT, each pacing stimulus first records from an origin near the coronary sinus — an area loaded with automaticity foci. Although the putative reentry circuit includes a broad area around the AV Node, only catheter ablation of the focus-laden region can successfully eliminate this tachycardia (very suggestive of focal automaticity origin). Dogmatic loyalty to this theoretical reentry model persists. The jury is still out.

* Pronounced "ree-EN-tree".

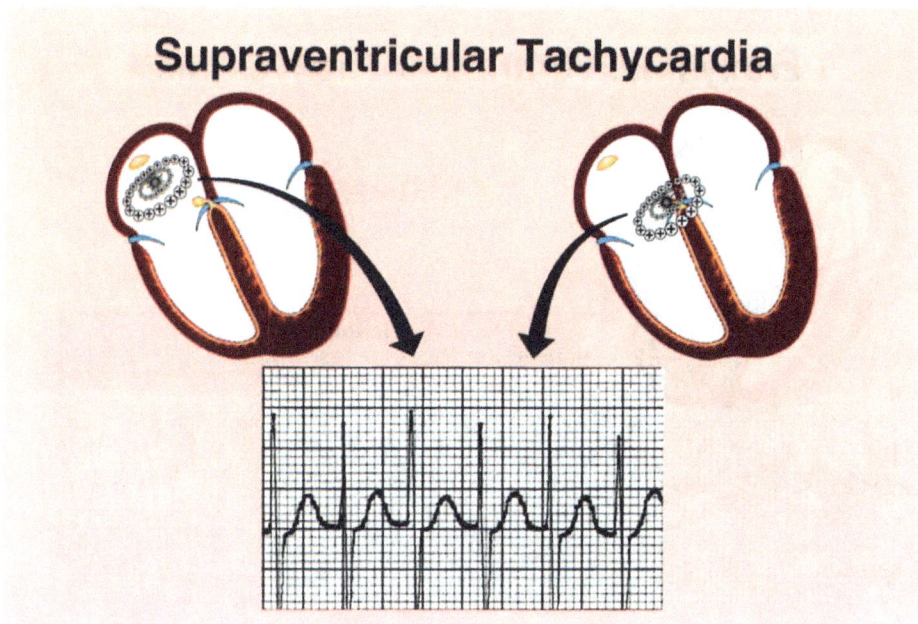

Supraventricular Tachycardia

The very irritable* automaticity foci that produce both Paroxysmal Atrial Tachycardia and Paroxysmal Junctional Tachycardia originate above the ventricles, so these arrhythmias are known as **Paroxysmal Supraventricular Tachycardia**.

Supraventricular tachycardia (the word "paroxysmal" is often omitted) is a general term, which includes both PAT and _____.   PJT

The term "supraventricular" imparts the understanding that all atrial foci and all Junctional foci are above the _____.   ventricles

Note: Paroxysmal Atrial Tachycardia can be so rapid that the P' waves run into the preceding T waves to become indistinguishable. This can make differentiation between PAT and PJT very difficult. But since treatment for both is so similar, the umbrella term Supraventricular Tachycardia (SVT) suffices, and further distinction between the two is unnecessary. Certain conditions may widen the QRS's in SVT, so it may then resemble Ventricular Tachycardia (next page).

* Usually an atrial or Junctional focus is made irritable by adrenergic stimulants, but a focus may be further provoked into tachycardia pacing by a premature stimulus from another irritable focus.

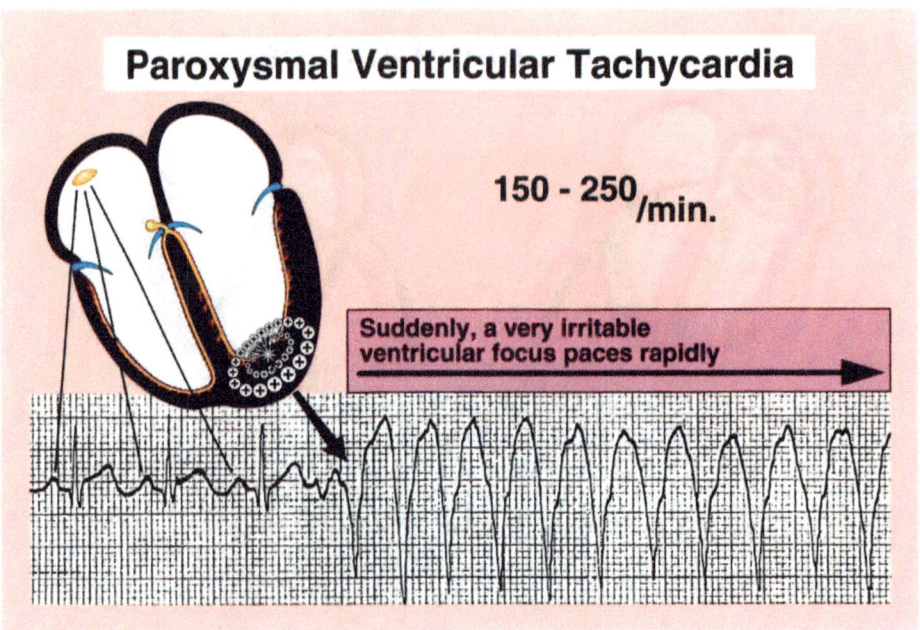

Paroxysmal Ventricular Tachycardia (PVT or VT)* is produced by a very irritable ventricular automaticity focus that suddenly paces in the 150 to 250 per minute range. It has a characteristic pattern of enormous, consecutive PVC-like complexes. Please conscientiously review page 134 now.

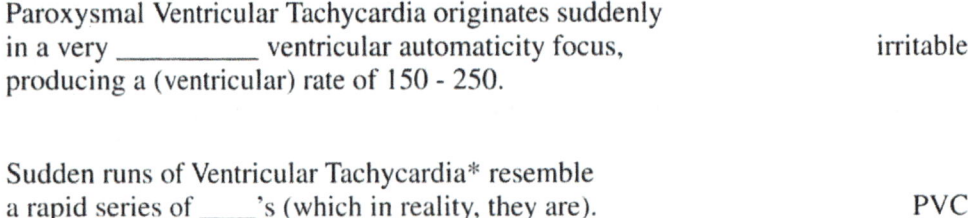

Paroxysmal Ventricular Tachycardia originates suddenly
in a very _____ ventricular automaticity focus,   irritable
producing a (ventricular) rate of 150 - 250.

Sudden runs of Ventricular Tachycardia* resemble
a rapid series of ____'s (which in reality, they are).   PVC

<mark>Note:</mark> During Ventricular Tachycardia, the SA Node still paces the
atria, but the large, dramatic ventricular complexes hide the individual
P waves that can be seen only occasionally. So, there is independent
pacing of the atria and the ventricles… a type of *AV dissociation.*

* The "Paroxysmal" is often left off, so "Ventricular Tachycardia" or "VT"
  are used commonly.

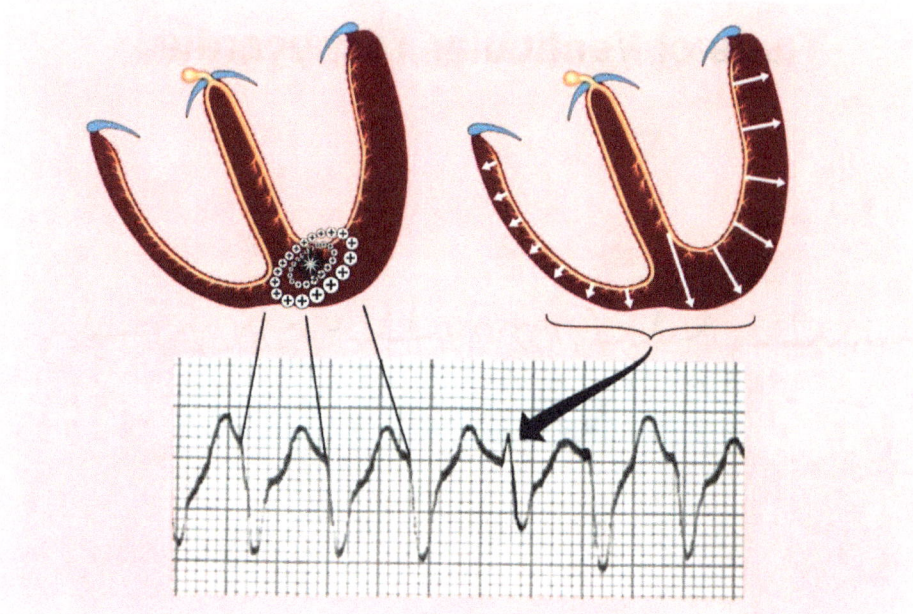

During Ventricular Tachycardia, the SA Node continues to pace the atria (AV dissociation), but an occasional atrial depolarization catches the AV Node in a receptive state, and then this depolarization stimulus conducts to the ventricles.

Occasionally (during VT), one of the regular (Sinus-paced) atrial depolarizations finds the AV _____ receptive to depolarization and…   Node

… that stimulus passes through the AV Node to depolarize the ventricles via the ventricular _____ system.   conduction

Note: On occasion during VT, a (Sinus-paced) depolarization stimulus from the atria finds the entire ventricular conduction system receptive to depolarization and produces a normal-appearing QRS (*capture beat*) in the midst of the ventricular tachycardia. More commonly during VT, an atrial depolarization finds a receptive AV Node, but ventricular depolarization only proceeds so far before it meets ventricular depolarization progressing from the ventricular focus. This produces a *fusion beat,* which is a blending on EKG of a normal QRS with a PVC-like complex (see illustration). The presence of "captures" or "fusions" confirms the diagnosis of Ventricular Tachycardia, because they could not occur during SVT.

Runs of Venticular Tachycardia

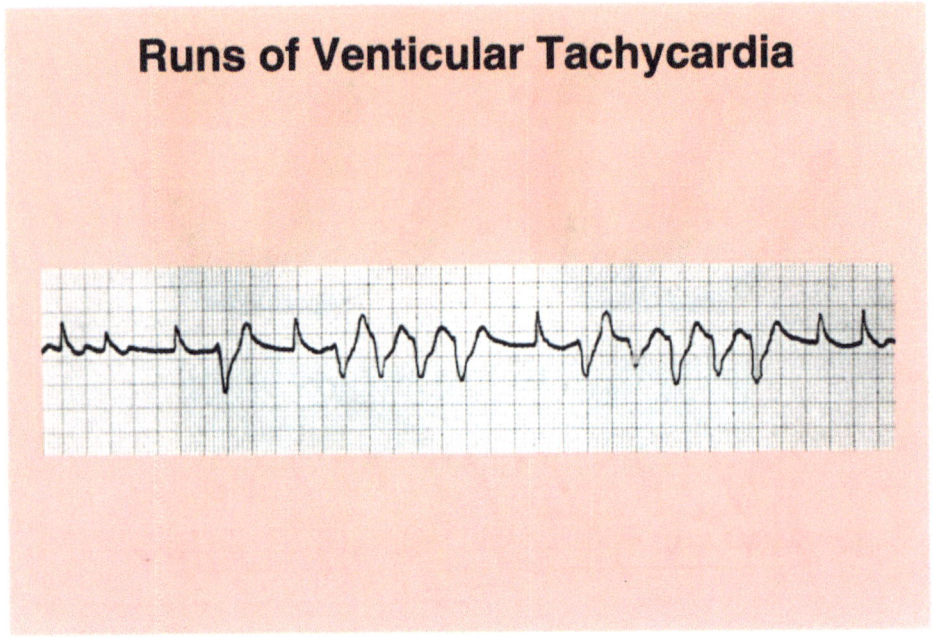

Runs of (Paroxysmal) Ventricular Tachycardia may signify coronary insufficiency (ischemia) or other causes of cardiac hypoxia that make a ventricular automaticity focus very irritable.

Ventricular Tachycardia appears like a run of _____'s.   PVC

Paroxysmal Ventricular Tachycardia often indicates coronary _____, causing poor oxygenation   insufficiency of the heart (and ventricular foci). For other causes of cardiac hypoxia see page 134.

Note: This rapid ventricular rate suddenly erupts from an irritable (hypoxic) ventricular focus. The rapid rate is too fast for the heart to function effectively, particularly in the elderly with compromised coronaries. It should be treated quickly (but cautiously) in patients with a myocardial infarction.

Caution: A rapid (Junctional or atrial) Supraventricular Tachycardia with aberrant conduction can produce a tachycardia with widened QRS's that mimics VT. Also, pre-existing Bundle Branch Block with SVT will widen the QRS complexes to give the same impression. NEVER give medications for SVT to a patient with VT.

Distinguishing
Wide QRS complex SVT from Ventricular Tachycardia

Helpful Clues	Wide QRS Complex SVT	Ventricular Tachycardia
Patient with coronary disease or infarction	uncommon	very common
QRS width (duration)	less than .14 sec.	greater than .14 sec.
AV dissociation showing captures or fusions	rare	yes
Axis: Extreme Right Axis Deviation (R.A.D., see page 231)	rare	yes

A few clues and good judgement can help you distinguish between VT and wide QRS complex SVT (with aberrant ventricular conduction). Begin with the history, and get a 12 lead EKG.

The patient with VT is most likely elderly and suffering from diminished coronary blood _____, reducing the   flow oxygen supply to the ventricular foci.

Signs of AV dissociation (e.g., presence of fusions or captures, or Extreme R.A.D. (-90° to -180°) are characteristic of ___.
VT

Note: If the QRS complex can be measured with accuracy, the QRS in SVT, even if widened by aberrant ventricular conduction, is usually .14 sec. or less in duration. However the ventricular complexes in VT are very wide, .14 sec. or greater. There are many criteria for distinguishing VT from SVT with aberrancy, but probably the most reliable to date are in:

Brugada et al: The differential diagnosis of a regular tachycardia with a wide QRS complex on the 12 lead ECG. *PACE* 1994; Vol.17: 1515-1524.

Torsades de Pointes

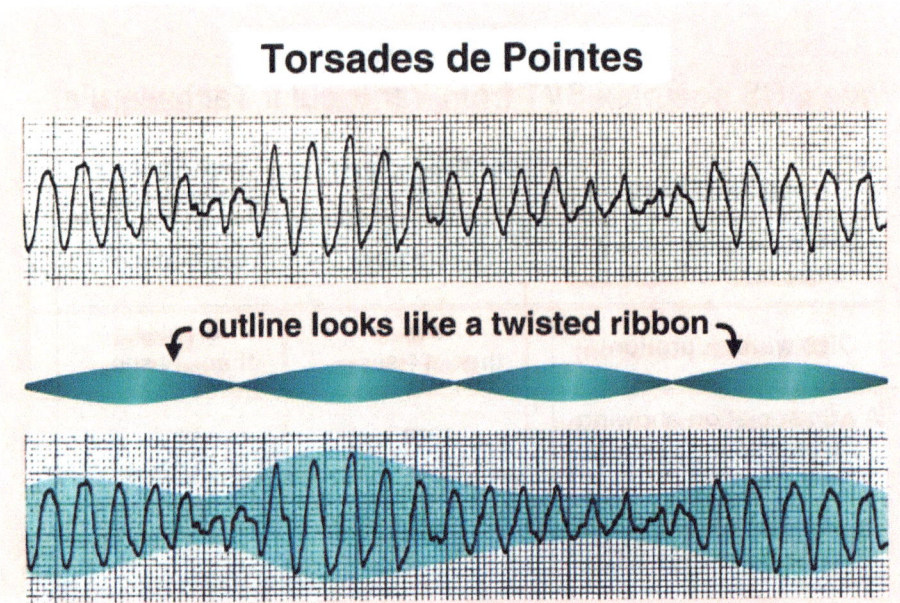

outline looks like a twisted ribbon

Torsades de Pointes is a peculiar form of (very) rapid ventricular rhythm caused by low potassium, medications that block potassium channels, or congenital abnormalities (e.g., Long QT syndrome), all of which lengthen the QT segment. The rate is a variable 250 to 350 per minute, usually in brief episodes.

<mark>Note:</mark> Torsades* de Pointes means "twisting of points," which refers to the series of ventricular complexes that are upward-pointing then downward-pointing in a repeating continuum. In 1966, Dr. F. Dessertenne presented the first scientific description of this arrhythmia. He theorized that it was caused by two competitive, irritable foci in different ventricular areas, pacing at the same rate – an explanation that seems quite plausible.

The rate of this arrhythmia is 250 to _____ per minute, but   350
fortunately it usually occurs only in brief self-terminating
bursts, for at that rate there is no effective ventricular pumping.

<mark>Note:</mark> On EKG, the amplitude of each successive complex gradually increases and then gradually decreases, so when viewed as a whole, the general outline or silhouette of the tracing looks like a series of end-to-end spindle shapes. Some say the tracing outline resembles a twisted ribbon. If unresolved, it can lead to a deadly arrhythmia.

* This is the correct spelling; don't forget the "s" at the end of "Torsades", even though it is
   not pronounced.

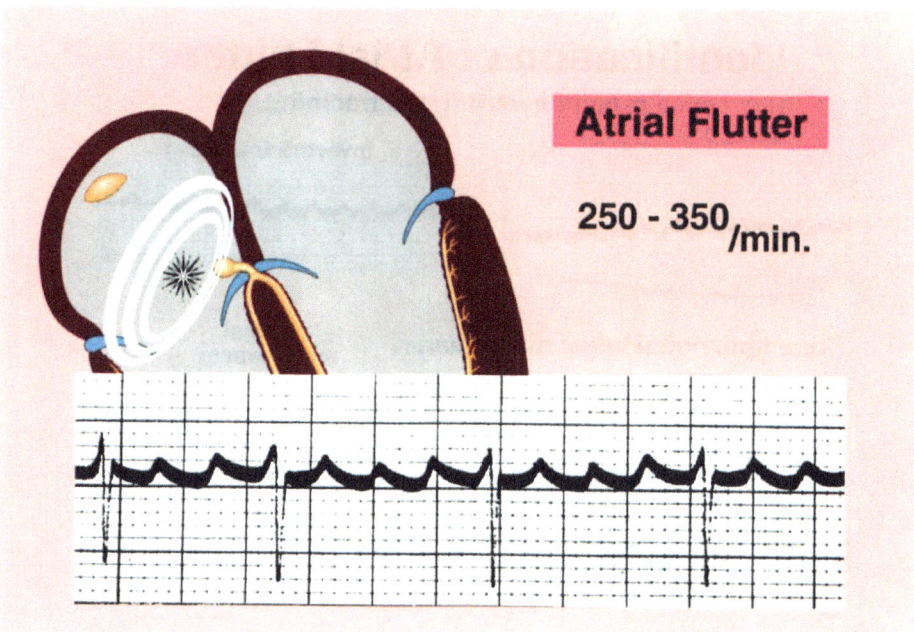

Atrial Flutter originates in an atrial automaticity focus. The rapid succession of identical, back-to-back atrial depolarization waves, "flutter" waves, suggest a reentry origin to some experts (see the last paragraph on the next page).

In atrial flutter an extremely irritable atrial automaticity focus fires at a rate of 250 to 350 per minute, producing a rapid series of _____ depolarizations.   atrial

Note: On EKG, atrial flutter is characterized by consecutive, identical "flutter" waves in rapid back-to-back succession. The baseline appears to vanish between the back-to-back flutter waves, and because the waves are identical, they are described as having the appearance of the teeth of a saw or a "saw tooth" baseline. Turn back to PAT with (AV) block to make sure that you recognize the difference.

Note: The AV Node has a long refractory period, so only one in a series of flutter waves conducts to the ventricles. Therefore, this very rapid series of atrial depolarizations cannot drive the ventricles at the same excessive rate; perhaps only one of two (or commonly, one of three, as above) atrial depolarizations reaches the ventricles in atrial flutter.

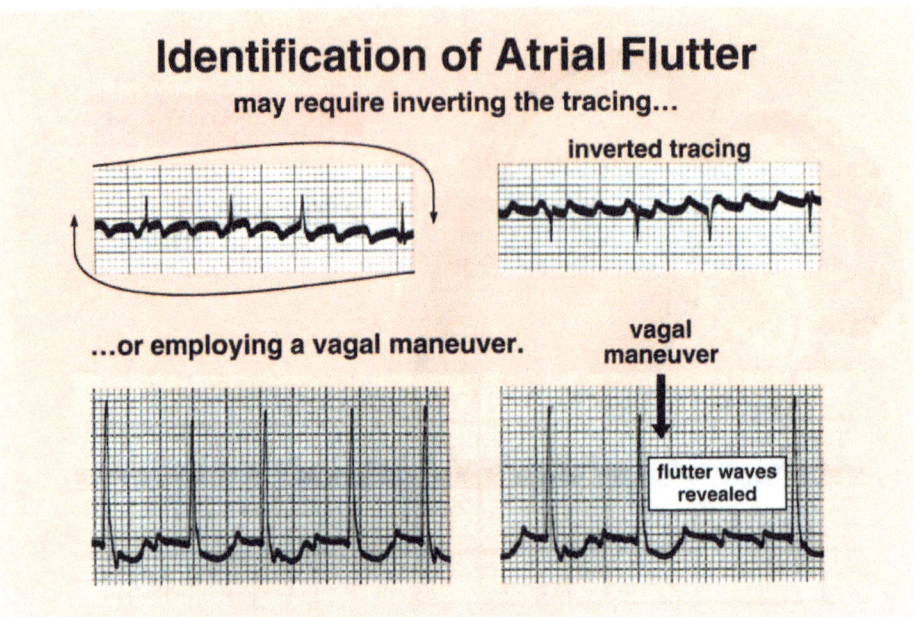

Identification of Atrial Flutter
may require inverting the tracing...

inverted tracing

...or employing a vagal maneuver.

vagal maneuver

flutter waves revealed

Inverting a tracing of suspected atrial flutter can help in its identification. Also, vagal maneuvers can be an effective diagnostic aid (see page 61.)

When in doubt about atrial flutter, inverting the _____ tracing may be helpful.

EKG

Note: With atrial flutter there may be a rapid QRS response rate, particularly in 2:1 ratios (flutter waves:QRS response), masking the flutter waves. Vagal maneuvers increase AV Node refractoriness, allowing fewer flutter waves to be conducted to the ventricles. This produces a longer series of flutter waves that are easier to identify.

Note: The "Maze" surgical procedure cuts (and resutures) the atria into a maze of channels that provides a continuous pathway from the SA Node to the AV Node. This procedure eliminates any possibility of reentry circuits. Yet a study of patients recovering from the maze procedure, revealed that 47% developed atrial flutter (or atrial fibrillation) postoperatively. This raises considerable doubt that the origin of atrial flutter could be reentry.

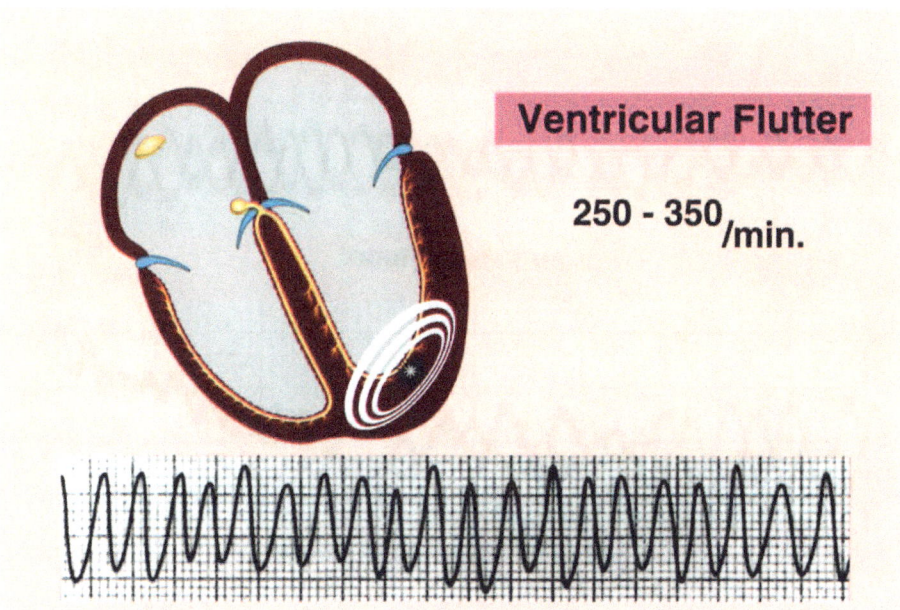

Ventricular Flutter

250 - 350/min.

Ventricular Flutter is produced by a single ventricular automaticity focus firing at an exceptionally rapid rate of 250 to 350 per minute. It produces a rapid series of smooth sine-waves of similar amplitude.

Ventricular flutter is caused by a highly irritable ventricular focus that is desperately discharging at a rate of _____ to _____ per minute.   250
                                                                    350

The ventricular rate in ventricular flutter is so rapid that the _____ hardly have enough time to fill – even partially, so this arrhythmia rapidly deteriorates into a deadly arrhythmia.   ventricles

The smooth _____-wave pattern of ventricular flutter is its distinguishing characteristic.   sine

Note: Ventricular flutter produces a rapid series of smooth sine-waves of similar amplitude, whereas the waves of Torsades de Pointes get progressively larger, then smaller, producing a general outline of connected spindle shapes (page 158). Ventricular Flutter rarely self-resolves and is nearly always a prelude to a deadly arrhythmia... see next page.

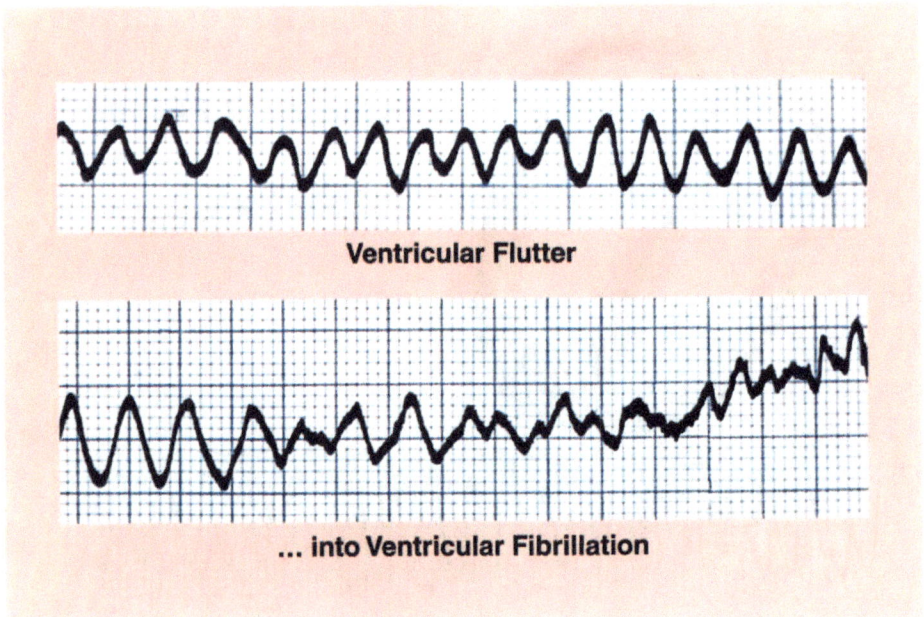

Ventricular Flutter

... into Ventricular Fibrillation

True ventricular flutter almost invariably deteriorates into ventricular fibrillation, which requires immediate Cardio-Pulmonary Resuscitation and defibrillation.

Note: During ventricular flutter, the ventricles are contracting at an alarming rate. The above (separated but continuous) tracing shows ventricular flutter at a rate of about 300 per minute, which is five contractions per second. Blood is a viscous fluid, and the ventricles cannot properly fill (and empty) at a rate of 5 times per second; in fact, they hardly fill at all. For this reason, there is no effective cardiac output. Therefore, the coronary arteries are not receiving blood, and the heart itself has no blood supply. Ventricular Fibrillation ensues, as many profoundly hypoxic ventricular automaticity foci desperately try to compensate... in vain.

Practice Tracing

A monitored patient became very concerned about a sudden pounding in his chest.

By the history and the rate (which you determined by observation),
you identify the rhythm as a paroxysmal _____.   tachycardia
Now, we'll determine the causative irritable automaticity focus.

Because this paroxysmal tachycardia has narrow, normal
looking QRS's, it could <u>not</u> have originated in an irritable
_____ focus; therefore it must be some type of   ventricular
supraventricular tachycardia.

There appear to be P' waves present, so we are probably dealing
with an automaticity focus in the _____. You have already ruled   atria
out a Junctional focus, because any retrograde depolarizations
that it might have produced, would record as <u>inverted</u> P' waves
(which are usually adjacent to the QRS when they precede it).

Note: This is Paroxysmal Atrial Tachycardia (PAT), and because
each P' wave produces a QRS response, it could not be PAT with block.
Quickly review the illustrations for the paroxysmal tachycardias and
flutter before we go on. Take your time.

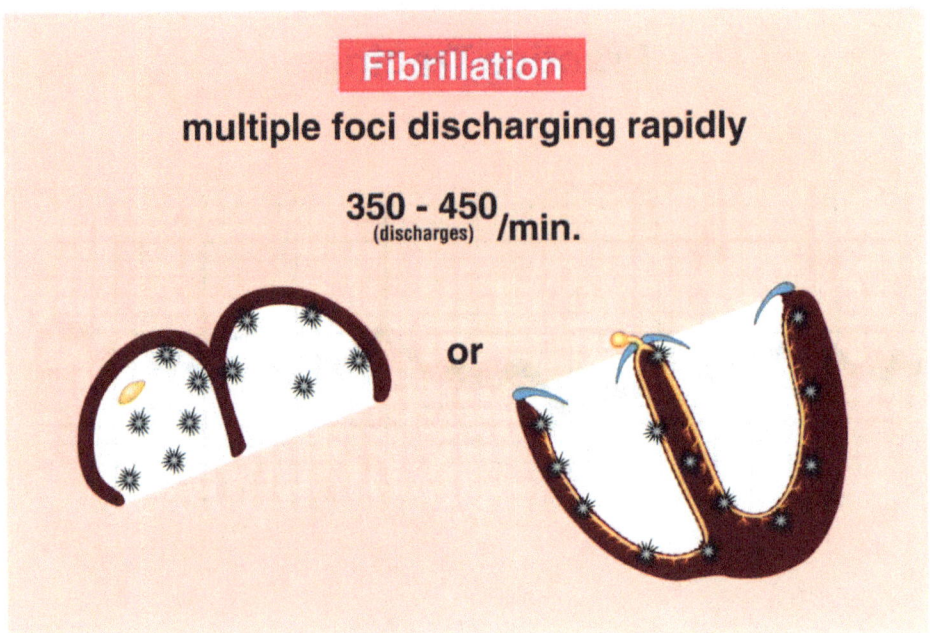

Fibrillation

multiple foci discharging rapidly

350 - 450 (discharges) /min.

or

"Fibrillation" is a totally erratic rhythm caused by continuous, rapid rate discharges from numerous automaticity foci in either the atria or in the ventricles.

Note: Fibrillation is caused by rapid discharges from numerous profoundly irritable automaticity foci in the atria (**Atrial Fibrillation**), or due to numerous profoundly irritable foci in the ventricles rapidly discharging (**Ventricular Fibrillation**). Both types represent a pathological condition: these *irritable* foci all suffer from entrance block, so they are parasystolic. Since they cannot be overdrive-suppressed, they all pace rapidly at once. The resulting rhythm is so erratic and uncoordinated that distinct, complete waves are not distinguishable, thus rates are impossible to determine. The involved chambers merely twitch rapidly.

Note: The "rate" 350 to 450 per minute is not a true rate, since many of the foci discharge simultaneously. The number and the tachy-rate of individual foci is conjectural. The range of "rate" is more relative and hypothetical than real, because fibrillating chambers do not effectively pump at all.

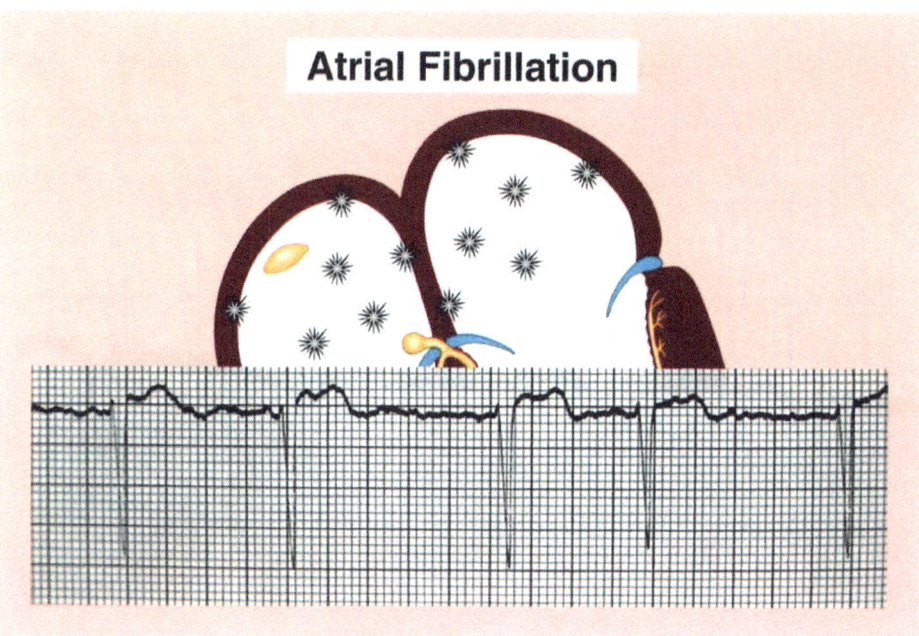

Atrial Fibrillation

Atrial Fibrillation (AF) is caused by many irritable <u>parasystolic</u> atrial foci (with entrance block) firing at rapid rates, producing an exceedingly rapid, erratic atrial rhythm. The atrial "rate" is 350 to 450 per minute. Notice the irregular ventricular response.

Atrial fibrillation occurs when many irritable atrial foci* fire rapidly, but since they are parasystolic, none of them can be overdrive-_____; they all rapidly pace at once to produce   suppressed an excessively rapid series of tiny, erratic spikes on EKG.

==Note:== Because so many atrial foci are rapidly firing, no single depolarization spreads very far. Only a small portion of the atria is depolarized by any one discharge from an atrial focus. Depolarizations from foci near the AV Node conduct to the ventricles, producing a very <u>irregular</u> ventricular rhythm. see rhythm strip, page 351.

==Note:== With a Normal Sinus Rhythm, each pacing impulse that the SA Node generates spreads through the atria like an enlarging, circular wave; much like a pebble dropped into a pool of water. However, the multiple erratic depolarizations of atrial fibrillation are analogous to a rain shower striking the same pool.

* Atrial fibrillation is usually initiated by parasystolic foci in the
  pulmonary vein ostia of the left atrium.

Atrial Fibrillation

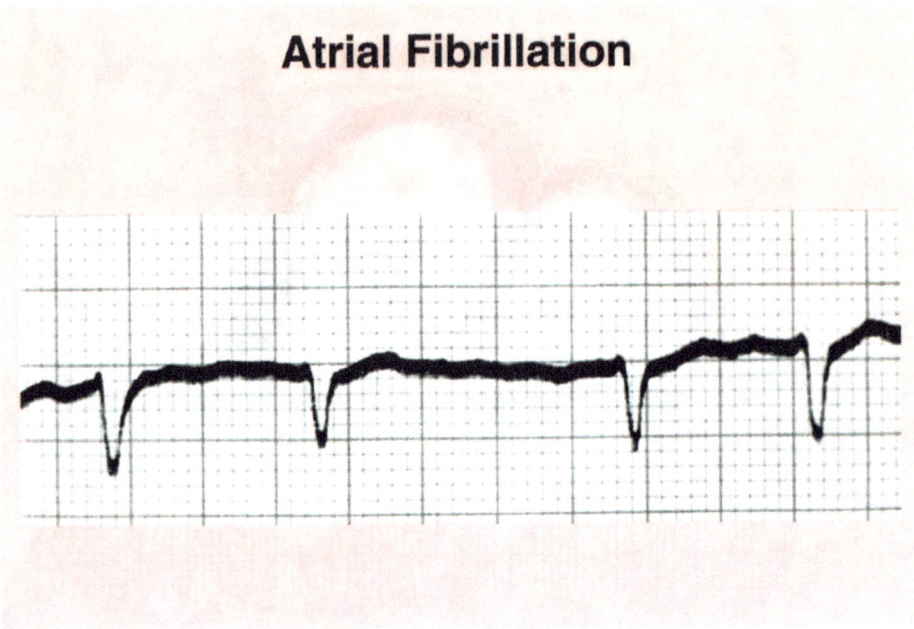

Atrial Fibrillation often appears as a wavy baseline without identifiable
P or P' waves. The QRS response is not regular and may be fast or slow.

Atrial Fibrillation may cause such small, erratic spikes that it
appears like a wavy baseline without visible __ waves   P
(and without distinguishable P' waves either).

Note: Only discharging foci near the AV Node can (occasionally)
stimulate it, but the AV Node sorts out a normal ventricular rate.

The AV Node is irregularly stimulated during atrial fibrillation,
so the _____ (QRS) response is irregular. On EKG,   ventricular
you may see only random QRS's (see illustration), so the pulse
is irregular also.

Note: With Atrial Fibrillation, the ventricular rate depends on the
AV Node's duration of refractoriness after it is stimulated. During AF,
the AV Node usually allows a relatively normal range of ventricular
rate, albeit always *irregular.* Sometimes the AV Node permits an
increased number of depolarization stimuli to pass through, producing a
rapid ventricular rate that may require pharmacological control. Always
determine the ventricular (pulse) rate (QRS's per 6-second strip times
10) and document it. If the ventricular rate is out of a safe range for the
patient, it should be treated appropriately.

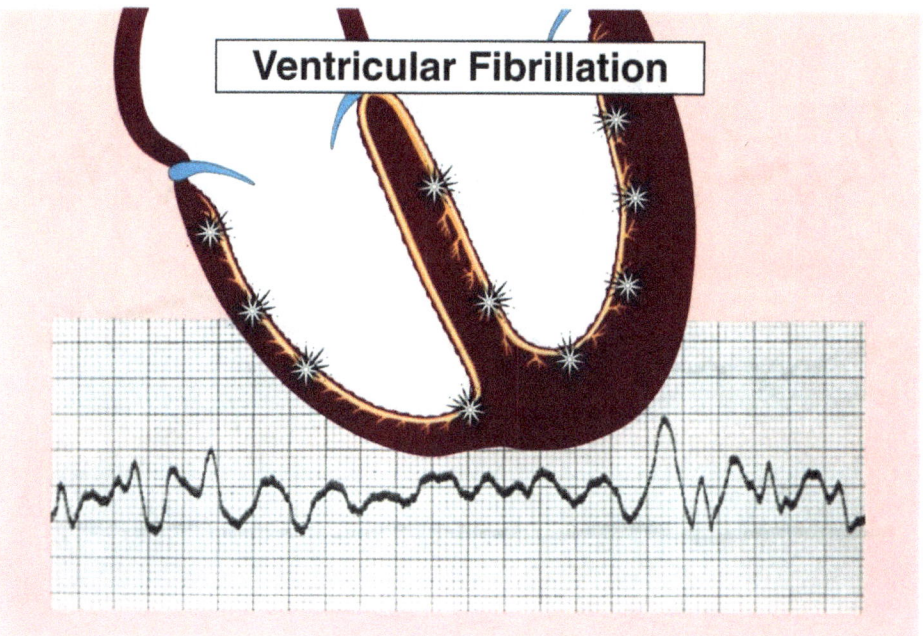

Ventricular Fibrillation (VF) is caused by rapid-rate discharges from many irritable, parasystolic ventricular automaticity foci, producing an erratic, rapid twitching of the ventricles (ventricular "rate" is 350 to 450 per minute).

Ventricular Fibrillation is due to numerous parasystolic ventricular foci pacing rapidly (each of them suffering from entrance block, so they can not be _____-suppressed); this produces an erratic twitching of the ventricles.   overdrive

Because there so many ventricular _____ firing rapidly, each one repeatedly depolarizes only a small area of ventricle. This results in a rapid, ineffective twitching of the ventricles.   foci

This erratic twitching of VF has been called a "bag of worms," for this is the way the ventricles actually appear. On EKG the tracing is totally erratic, without identifiable _____, and the ventricles do not provide mechanical pumping. Emergency!   waves

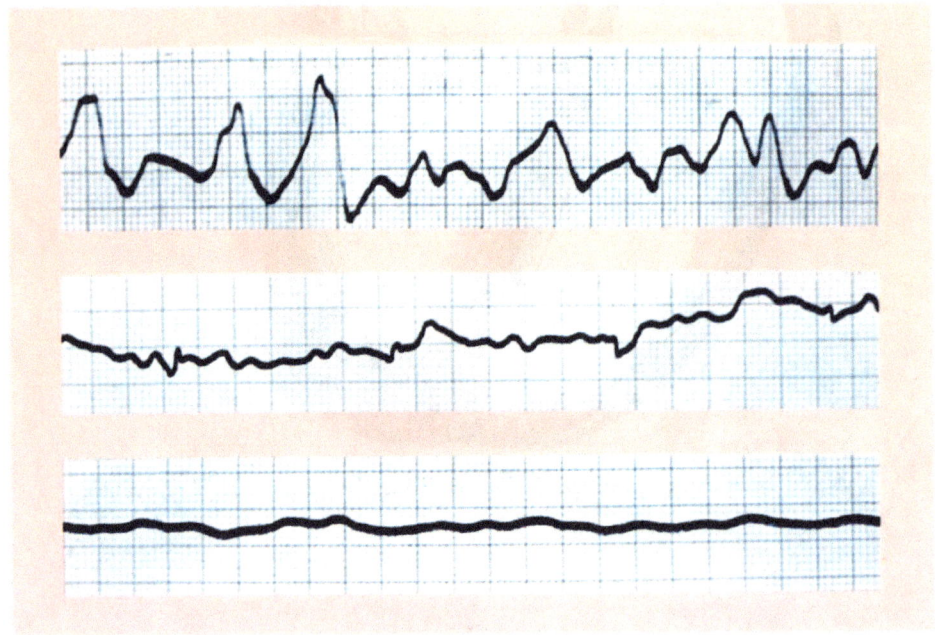

Ventricular Fibrillation is easily recognized by its totally erratic appearance and lack of any identifiable waves on the electrocardiogram.

Note: These three strips are from a continuous tracing of the same patient's dying heart. Notice how the amplitude of the deflections diminishes as the heart dies.

We recognize Ventricular Fibrillation by its completely erratic appearance on the EKG tracing. Even with large deflections, there are no identifiable _____.

waves

There is no predictable pattern with _____ Fibrillation. As you can see, it looks different at every moment, but it is so erratic that it is difficult to miss, thank Goodness!

Ventricular

If you do recognize any repetition of pattern or regularity of deflections, you probably are not dealing with __ __.

VF

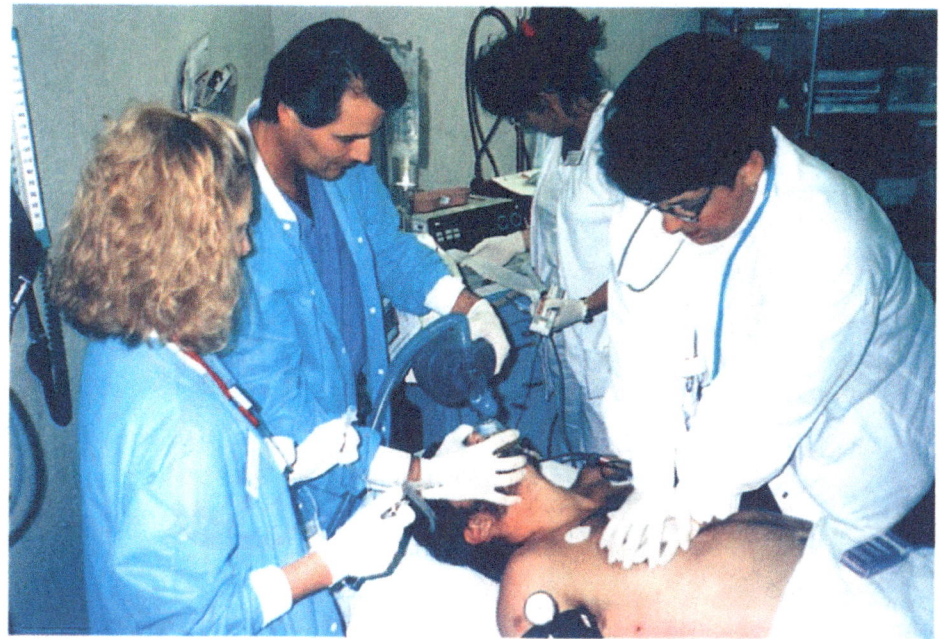

Ventricular Fibrillation is a type of *cardiac arrest,* for there is no pumping action by the heart; this is a dire emergency! VF requires immediate CPR and defibrillation, with some type of electrical defibrillator.

Ventricular Fibrillation is a type of cardiac _____. There is no   arrest
effective cardiac output, because the ventricles are only twitching
erratically. There is no ventricular pumping, so there is no circulation.

Note: VF requires immediate defibrillation. Cardiac Arrest is an
emergency that demands immediate intervention. Cardio-Pulmonary
Resuscitation (cardiac massage and assisted respiration) is carried out
in order to circulate oxygenated blood by external mechanical means.
The technique of CPR was originally taught only to hospital and
ambulance personnel, but it is imperative that every person master
this technique. Only when CPR skills are universally known, can all
victims of cardiac arrest get immediate lifesaving care at any location.

Note: There are two other types of cardiac arrest. *Cardiac Standstill*
("Asystole") occurs when there is no detectable cardiac activity on
EKG. This is a rare circumstance when the SA Node and the escape
mechanisms of all the foci at all levels are unable to assume pacing
responsibility. *Pulseless Electrical Activity* (PEA) is present when a
dying heart produces weak signs of electrical activity on EKG, but
the moribund heart cannot respond mechanically (no detectable pulse).

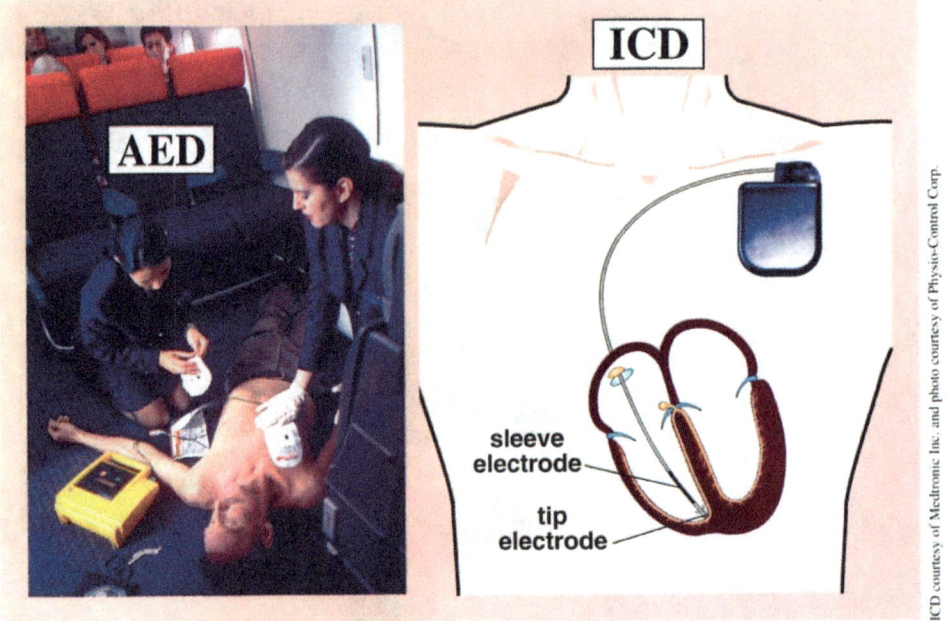

There are now computerized defibrillators that can detect Ventricular Fibrillation and immediately deliver a defibrillating shock. One type, the AED, is a portable unit that can be operated by the public. Another type, the ICD, is a small unit that is implanted under the chest skin to automatically defibrillate appropriate patients as needed.

Note: The *Automated External Defibrillator* (AED) is a small portable unit. When its electrodes are placed on the chest of an unconscious person, it is programmed to identify VF and deliver a defibrillating shock.

Note: The *Implantable Cardioverter Defibrillator* (ICD) is implanted under the chest skin of patients likely to develop Ventricular Fibrillation. Wire leads from the ICD are attached to the heart to detect VF and deliver a defibrillating shock. This mini-computer can also identify other arrhythmias and treat them with timed electrical stimuli, and it can pace if a bradycardia ensues. A technological wonder!

Please review all "fibrillation" illustrations.

Wolff-Parkinson-White Syndrome

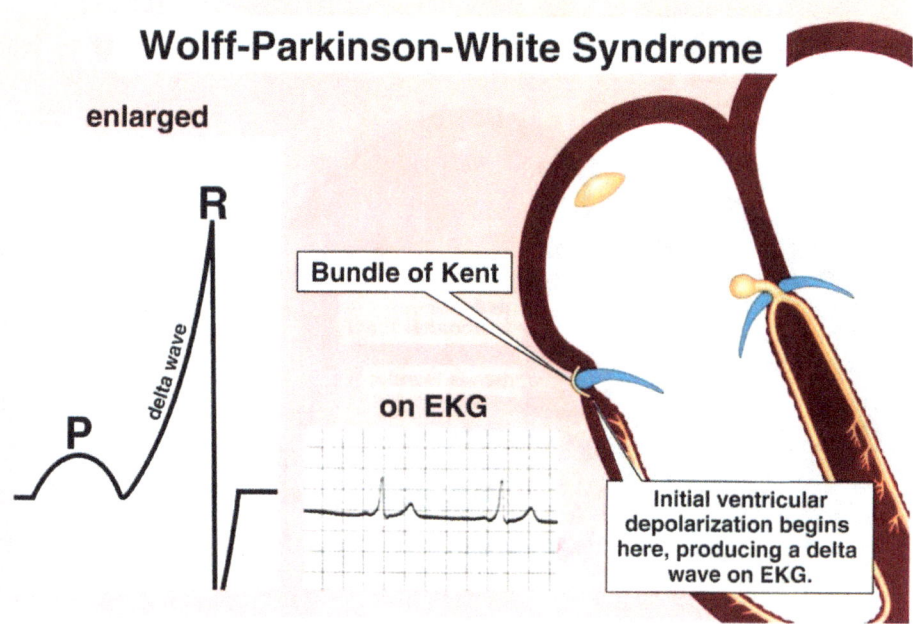

An abnormal, accessory AV conduction pathway, the *bundle of Kent*, can "short circuit" the (usual) delay of ventricular conduction in the AV Node. This prematurely depolarizes ("pre-excites") a portion of the ventricles (producing a delta wave on EKG) just before normal ventricular depolarization begins.

The accessory Bundle of _____ causes ventricular   Kent
pre-excitation in **Wolff-Parkinson-White** *(WPW)* syndrome.

The delta wave creates the illusion of a "shortened" PR interval
and "lengthened" QRS. The delta wave actually records the
depolarization of an area of _____ pre-excitation.   ventricular

Note: WPW syndrome is very important because persons with such an
accessory pathway can have paroxysmal tachycardia by three possible
mechanisms:

- rapid conduction — supraventricular tachycardia (including atrial flutter
  or atrial fibrillation) may be rapidly conducted 1:1 through this accessory
  pathway producing dangerously high ventricular rates.

- some Kent Bundles have been found to contain automaticity foci
  that can initiate a paroxysmal tachycardia.

- re-entry — ventricular depolarization may immediately restimulate
  the atria in a retrograde fashion via the accessory pathway causing
  a theoretical circus re-entry loop.

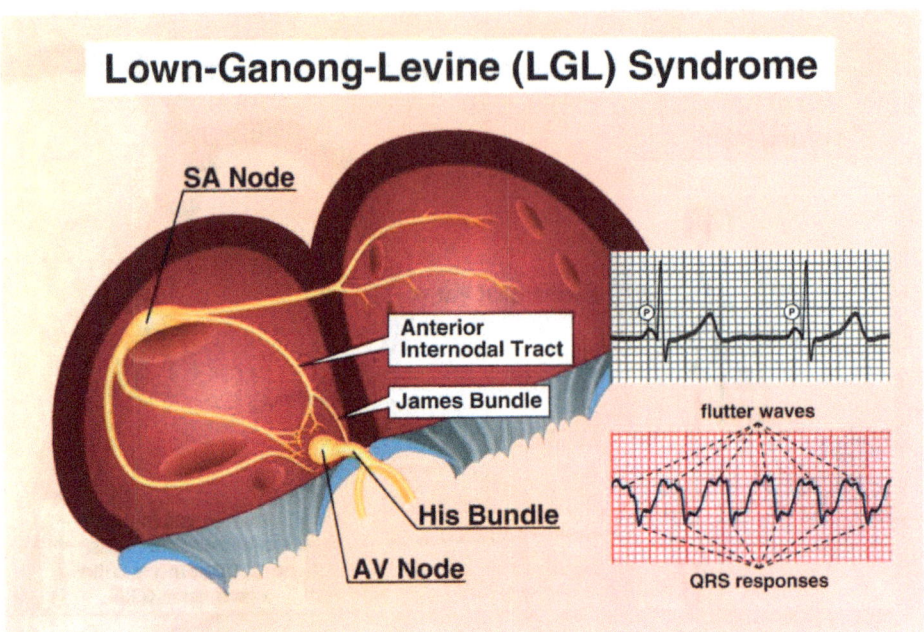

Lown-Ganong-Levine (LGL) Syndrome

In patients with **LGL syndrome,** the AV Node is bypassed by an extension of the Anterior Internodal Tract. Absent the conduction delay in the AV Node, this "James bundle" conducts atrial depolarizations directly to the His Bundle without delay. This can pose a serious problem with rapid atrial arrhythmias like atrial flutter.

Ordinarily the AV Node filters rapid supraventricular rates,
in order to transmit depolarization to the _____ at   ventricles
a physiologically reasonable rate.

Absent the filtering effect of the AV Node, patients with
LGL syndrome can transmit rapid atrial rates directly (1:1)
to the His Bundle, driving the ventricles at very _____ rates.   rapid

With this syndrome, the AV Node is bypassed by the
James tract, so there is no significant PR interval delay;
the P _____ are adjacent to their QRS's on the EKG.   waves

Note: You may now review *Rhythm, Part I* by turning to the
Personal **Q**uick **R**eference Sheets on page 336-338, and relate this
to the simplified methodology that is summarized on page 334.

Before you begin, look at this chapter's summary on pages 334 and 339.

Rhythm, Part II

Blocks

- **Sinus Block**

- **AV Block**

- **Bundle Branch Block**

- **Hemiblock**
  (begins on page 295, Chapter 9)

Blocks retard or prevent the conduction of depolarization; they can occur in the SA Node, the AV Node, or in the larger divisions of the ventricular conduction system. The general public and the media often refer to them as "heart blocks".

Blocks may develop in any of these areas: the SA _____, the AV Node, the His Bundle, the Bundle Branches, or in either of the two subdivisions of the Left Bundle Branch (Hemiblock).

Node

These are blocks of electrical conduction that prevent (or retard) the passage of _____ stimuli.

depolarization

Note: When examining the rhythm on a tracing, *always* check for all the varieties of block, because the same patient can have more than one type of block.

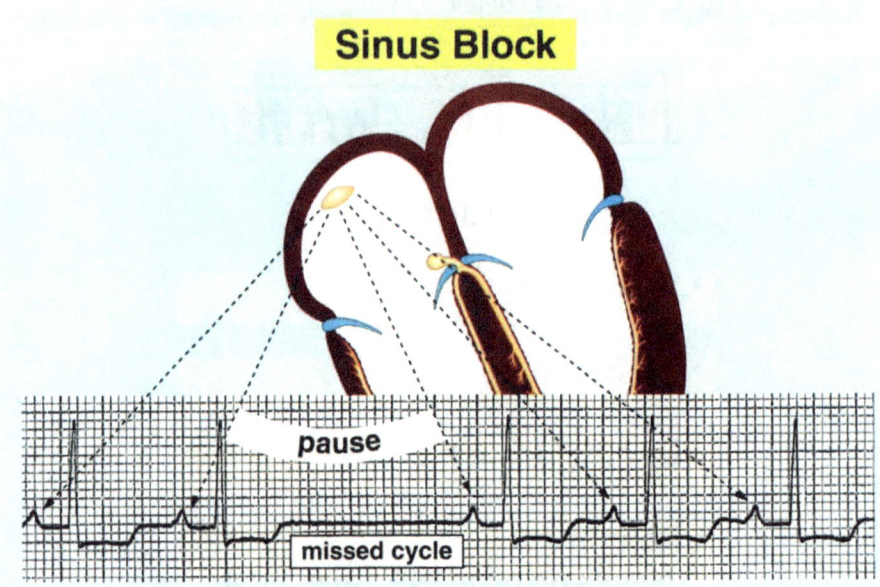

Sinus Block

pause

missed cycle

An unhealthy SA Node (Sinus Node) may temporarily fail to pace for at least one cycle, this is **Sinus Block**, then the SA Node resumes pacing. Notice that the missed cycle has no P wave; a very important feature.

With Sinus Block (also called *"SA Node Block"* or simply *"SA Block"*), an unhealthy SA Node* stops its pacing activity for at least one complete _____, so the block is usually transient.   cycle

After the pause of Sinus Block, pacing resumes at the same rate (and timing) as prior to the block. The SA Node resumes its pacing responsibility in step with its previous rhythm. However, the pause may induce an <u>escape beat</u> from an automaticity _____.
focus

Note: The P waves before and after the pause are identical, since they originate in the SA Node. The SA Node continues to generate atrial depolarizations with the same timing as before the block. However a long pause may elicit an escape beat from an automaticity focus before the SA Node can resume pacing (see pages 119-121).

* Some experts claim that the SA Node does generate a stimulus, but that it is blocked from leaving the SA Node. This is referred to as *Sinus "Exit" Block*.

Sick Sinus Syndrome

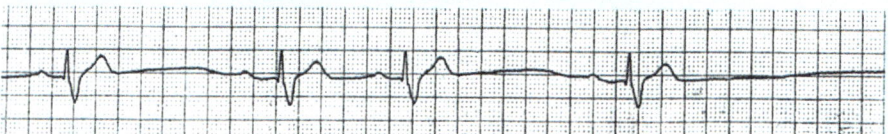

Bradycardia - Tachycardia Syndrome

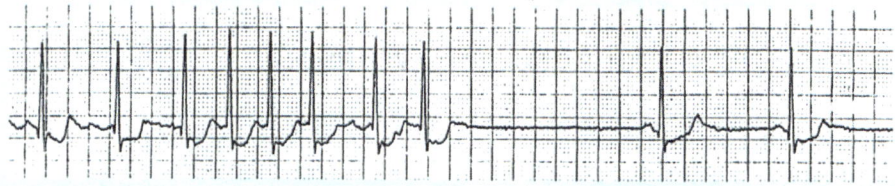

Sick Sinus Syndrome (SSS) is a wastebasket of arrhythmias caused by SA Node dysfunction associated with unresponsive supraventricular (atrial and Junctional) automaticity foci, which are also dysfunctional and can't employ their normal escape mechanism to assume pacing responsibility.

Note: Sick Sinus Syndrome most often occurs in elderly individuals who have heart disease. It is usually characterized by marked Sinus Bradycardia, but without the normal escape mechanisms of atrial and Junctional foci. SSS may also present as recurrent episodes of Sinus Block or Sinus Arrest associated with faulty (or absent) escape mechanisms of all supraventricular foci.

Note: Because of the extensive parasympathetic innervation to the SA Node and all supraventricular (atrial and Junctional) foci, excessive parasympathetic activity depresses the pacing rate of the SA Node, and depresses the atrial and Junctional foci as well. Therefore, young, healthy individuals (e.g., conditioned athletes like marathon runners) who often have parasympathetic hyperactivity at rest, appear to exhibit convincing signs of SSS (*"pseudo" Sick Sinus Syndrome*).

Note: Patients with SSS may develop intermittent episodes of SVT (sometimes even Atrial Flutter or Atrial Fibrillation) mingled with the Sinus Bradycardia. This is **Bradycardia-Tachycardia Syndrome**.

AV Block

1° (first degree) AV Block

2° (second degree) AV Block

3° (third degree) AV Block

AV (<u>A</u>trio-<u>V</u>entricular) **blocks** either retard or eliminate (or both!) conduction from the atria to the ventricles.

Minor AV blocks lengthen the brief pause between atrial depolarization and ventricular _____.

depolarization

Most AV blocks completely block some (or all) supraventricular impulses from reaching the _____.

ventricles

Note: The AV blocks are:

- **first degree (1°) AV block**
  (lengthens the delay between atrial and ventricular depolarization)

- **second degree (2°) AV block** (*Wenckebach* and *Mobitz* types)

- **third degree (3°) AV block** (completely blocks the conduction of atrial stimuli to the ventricles)

Note: Whether "first degree" is written out or the shorthand notation, 1°, is used, both have the same meaning. This book will alternately use both methods for all degrees of AV block, since you will see both in the current literature. Although it is currently popular to omit the "AV" it is always understood.

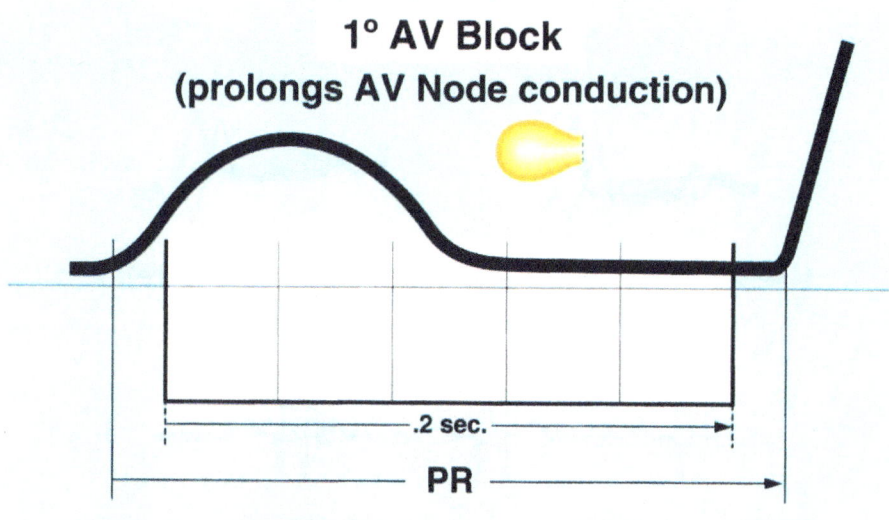

1° AV Block
(prolongs AV Node conduction)

PR interval more than .2 sec. indicates 1° AV block

First degree (1°) AV block retards AV Node conduction, prolonging the *PR interval* more than one large square (.2 sec.) on EKG.

Note: Technically, a "segment" is a portion of baseline, while an "interval" contains at least one wave. So the PR interval includes the P wave and the baseline that follows, up to the point where the QRS complex begins. Therefore, the PR interval is measured from the beginning of the P wave to the beginning of the QRS complex.

The delay caused by 1° AV block prolongs the ___ interval.   PR

The PR interval normally should be less than one large square,
which is less than ___ second.   .2 (2/10)

Note: You must observe (and record) the PR interval for every EKG. Some kind of AV block is present, if the PR interval is longer than one large square anywhere on an EKG.

1° AV Block

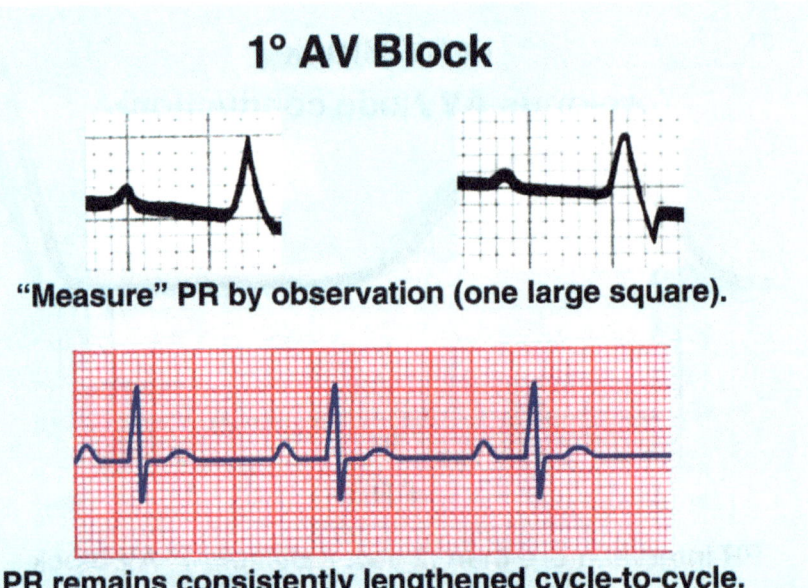

"Measure" PR by observation (one large square).

PR remains consistently lengthened cycle-to-cycle.

A *first degree (1°) AV block* is characterized by a PR interval greater than .2 second (one large square). The PR prolongation is consistent in every cycle.

Once you recognize a prolonged PR _____, you should determine the type of AV block that is present.

interval

Some type of AV block is present if any PR interval is longer than ___ second, anywhere in the tracing.

.2
(two-tenths)

A 1° block* is present when the PR interval is consistently prolonged the same amount in every _____, and the P-QRS-T sequence is normal in every cycle also.

cycle

* Whenever you hear "1° block," understand that it means "1° AV block."

2° AV Blocks

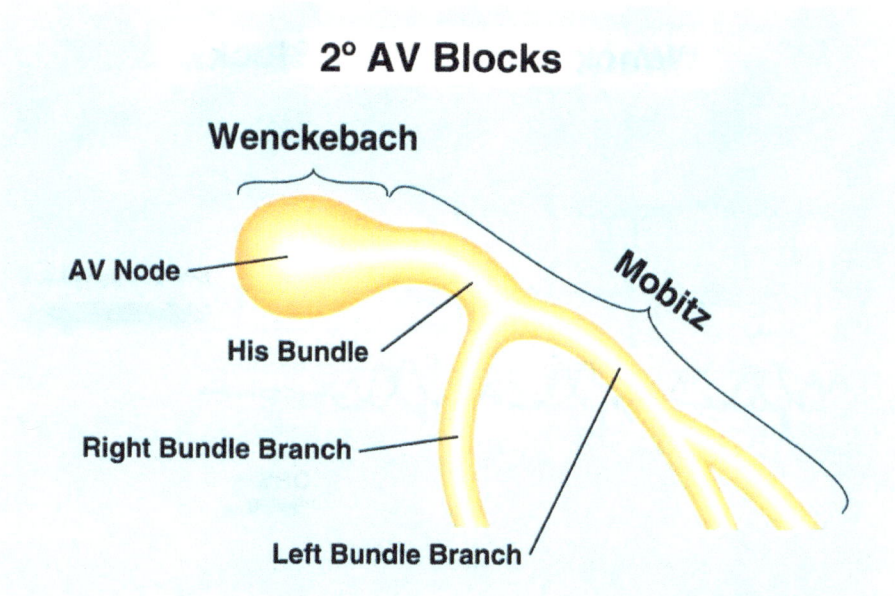

Second degree AV blocks allow some atrial depolarizations (P waves) to conduct to the ventricles (producing a QRS response), while some atrial depolarizations are blocked, leaving lone P waves without an associated QRS. There are two general types of 2° AV block; those that occur in the AV Node, and those that occur below the AV Node.

Note: There are two types of 2° AV blocks:

- 2° blocks of the AV Node are "**Wenckebach***" (formerly called "Type I"). They produce a series of cycles with progressive blocking of AV Node conduction until the final P wave is totally blocked in the AV Node, eliminating the QRS response. Each repeating Wenckebach series has a consistent P:QRS ratio like 3:2, 4:3, 5:4, etc. (one less QRS than P waves in the series).

- 2° blocks of Purkinje fiber bundles (His Bundle or Bundle Branches) are "**Mobitz**" (formerly called "Type II"). They usually produce a series of cycles consisting of one normal P-QRS-T cycle preceded by a series of paced P waves that fail to conduct through the AV Node (no QRS response). Each repeating Mobitz series has a consistent P:QRS ratio, like 3:1, 4:1, 5:1, etc.

Note: Don't be intimidated by these descriptions, once you see the tracings on the next few pages, you will understand immediately.

* Pronounced "WINKY-bok"

"Wenckebach" 2° AV Block

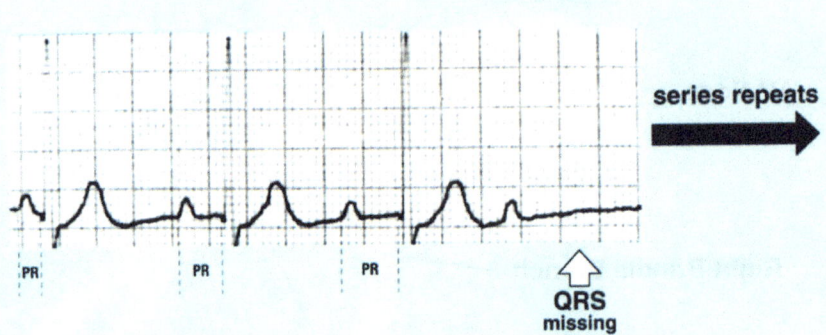

Wenckebach 2° AV block occurs in the AV Node. On EKG, the PR interval gradually lengthens in successive cycles, but the last P wave of the series fails to conduct to the ventricles (the final P lacks a QRS response). This series repeats.

On EKG, Wenckebach (2° AV block) gradually prolongs the PR interval in each successive cycle, until the final P wave of the series fails to produce a _____ response ("dropped QRS").

QRS

Each P wave and its associated QRS get progressively farther apart in successive cycles; the last P wave stimulus (totally blocked in the AV Node) stands alone at the end of the series. This typical Wenckebach pattern ("footprint") consists of anywhere from two to eight or more _____.

cycles

Note: Wenckebach is usually located in the AV Node. Wenckebach is sometimes caused by parasympathetic excess (inhibits the AV Node) or drugs that mimic or induce parasympathetic effects. Carefully examine EKG's for this characteristic, progressive lengthening of the PR in consecutive cycles, ending in a final lone P wave (see page 329). Repeating short series of Wenckebach footprints can produce "group beating" that looks somewhat like couplets of premature beats. Don't be fooled.

"Mobitz" 2° AV Blocks

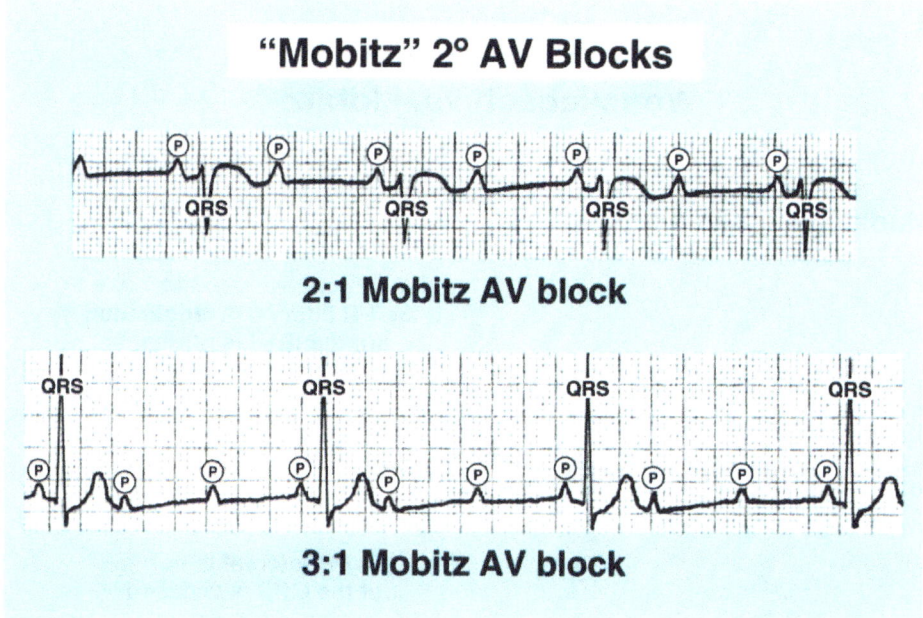

2:1 Mobitz AV block

3:1 Mobitz AV block

Mobitz* 2° (AV) Block totally blocks a number of paced atrial depolarizations (P waves) before conduction to the ventricles is successful. This produces 2:1 (two P waves to one QRS) or 3:1 (three P waves to one QRS) or even higher AV ratios. The series repeats. Mobitz is a serious problem; notice the extremely slow ventricular rates, which may produce loss of consciousness (syncope).

Mobitz (2° AV Block) may appear (<u>at a normal Sinus rate</u>) as two P waves to one _____ response, often referred to as "2:1 AV block" (or simply "2:1 block").   QRS

<mark>Note:</mark> Mobitz sometimes blocks three atrial depolarizations (P waves) producing a single ventricular response (QRS); this is written "3:1 AV block," or just "3:1 block", which describes the mechanism of conduction. Poorer conduction ratios (e.g., 4:1, 5:1, etc.) relate to *increased severity* of the block and are sometimes called *"advanced"* Mobitz block.

<mark>Warning!</mark> With Mobitz, every cycle that is missing its QRS has a regular, <u>punctual</u> P wave — but *never* a premature P' wave (see Note, page 128). This distinction is critical!

* Previously called "Type II" or "Mobitz II."

2:1 AV Block
Wenckebach vs. Mobitz

Most likely Wenckebach... ⇨

**if the PR interval is lengthened,
but the QRS is normal.**

Most likely Mobitz... ⇨

**if the PR interval is normal,
but the QRS is widened.**

Both Wenckebach and Mobitz have missing ("dropped") QRS's, so how can we differentiate between 2:1 Wenckebach and 2:1 Mobitz? Wenckebach is considered innocuous and Mobitz is considered pathological, so we should differentiate.

Note: On EKG, a 2:1 AV block could be a short, two-cycle Wenckebach. For example, if the first cycle is fairly normal but in the second cycle the PR lengthens just enough to prevent conduction through the AV Node, this is 2:1 Wenckebach. But by its appearance alone, most of us would probably interpret (correctly?) a 2:1 block as Mobitz. Perhaps the following will help...

Because Wenckebach commonly originates in the AV _____,   Node
a 2:1 AV block of this origin often has an initial lengthened PR
with no wide QRS pattern* (typical of Bundle Branch Block).

But since Mobitz originates below the AV Node, usually in the
His Bundle, we recognize that it often has a normal PR
with a widened _____ (Bundle Branch Block) pattern.*   QRS

Note: Since differentiating between these two types of 2:1 AV Block is clinically very important, we may need to employ bedside diagnostic techniques to make the distinction (next page).

* The wide QRS pattern, typical of Bundle Branch Block, is soon explained (pages 191-202).

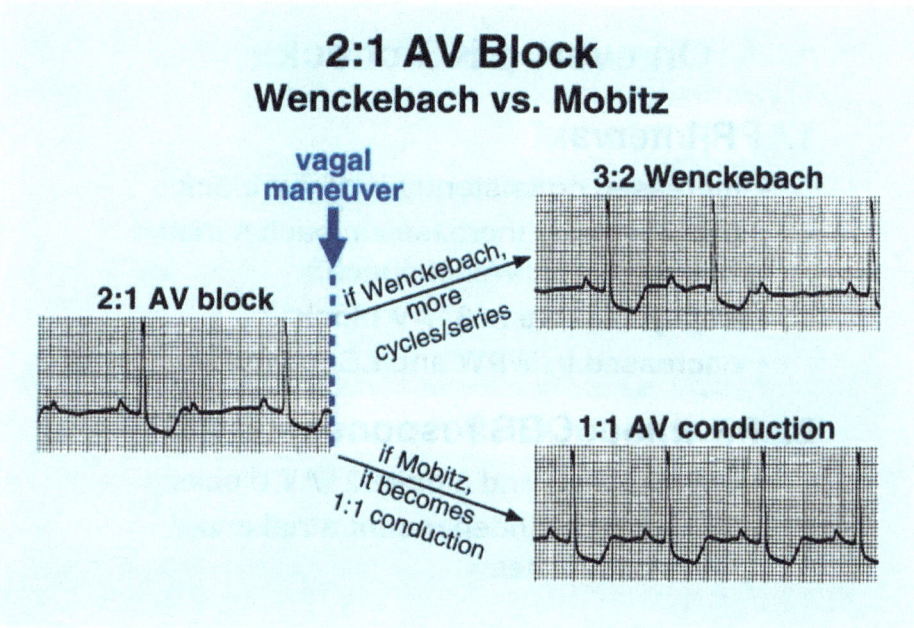

2:1 AV Block
Wenckebach vs. Mobitz

vagal maneuver

2:1 AV block   if Wenckebach, more cycles/series   **3:2 Wenckebach**

if Mobitz, it becomes 1:1 conduction   **1:1 AV conduction**

Differentiation of 2:1 Wenckebach (AV Node block) and Mobitz (AV conduction system block) is important clinically. In order to determine which type of 2:1 (2° AV) block a patient has, we can carefully employ vagal maneuvers (see page 61).

Note: Occasionally an EKG of 2:1 block (like the one on the cover of this book) has criteria (i.e., for PR length and QRS width) that fit both Wenckebach and Mobitz. This may require the judicious use of a vagal maneuver to differentiate between the two.

The AV Node is richly supplied with parasympathetic innervation, so vagal _____ inhibit the AV Node, making it more refractory.

maneuvers

Therefore, vagal maneuvers increase parasympathetic inhibition of the AV _____, increasing the number of cycles/series to produce 3:2 or 4:3 Wenckebach.

Node

But if the 2:1 block is Mobitz (i.e., the block is in the His _____), vagal maneuvers either eliminate the block, producing 1:1 AV conduction, or they have no effect.

bundle

On every EKG check:

1. PR Interval

- **increased consistently in 1° AV block**
- **progressively increases in each series of cycles with Wenckebach**
- **totally variable in 3° AV block**
- **decreased in WPW and LGL syndromes**

2. P without QRS response

- **Wenckebach and Mobitz 2° AV blocks**
- **3° AV block - independent atrial and ventricular rates**

Let's take a moment to see why routine EKG examination requires both checking the *PR interval* and looking for *P waves missing their QRS response*. Routinely checking these two parameters can reveal the entire spectrum AV conduction problems.

A prolonged *PR interval* can alert you to the existence
of 1° AV block, 2° AV block, and 3° AV _____.   block

An EKG with *P waves lacking a QRS response*
can expose 2° AV blocks and 3° ___ block.   AV

Note: Let's pause to contemplate how these two diagnostic parameters relate to each type of AV block. Really, take a moment and try this. It's not just a meaningless exercise. You have consumed a great deal of practical knowledge about AV blocks. Now you can easily detect these blocks by checking both parameters on every EKG you see. In each instance, you should consider not only the anatomical origin of the problem, but its prognostic significance to the patient as a person. Congratulations on your progress; you should take pride in your knowledge.

Practice Tracing

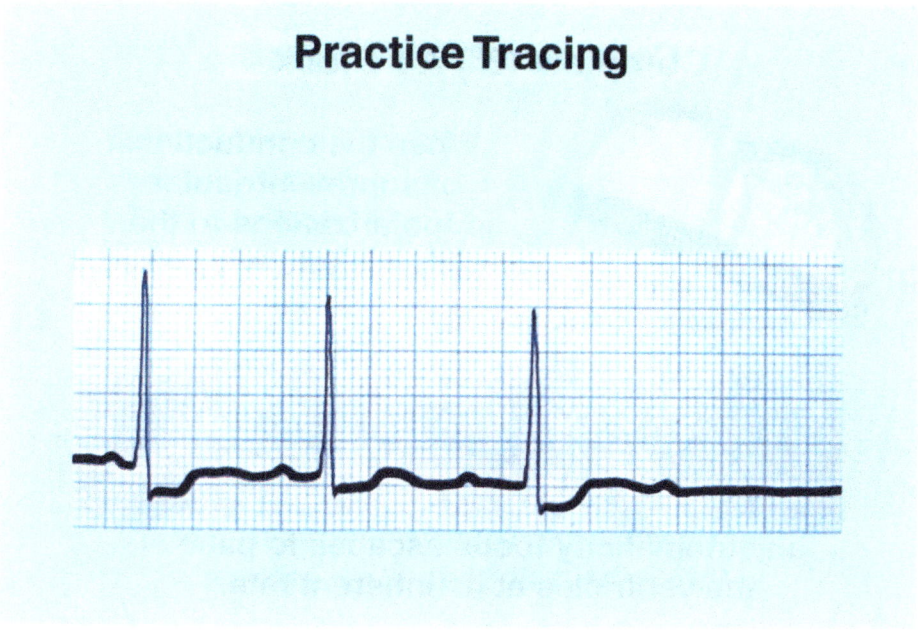

An examining physician noticed that a patient had an irregular pulse. The doctor was surprised to feel a group of three pulse beats followed by a pause, and this group of beats seemed to repeat over and over. Let's share the patient's EKG.

First we scan the *PR intervals* and discover that the third cycle has a PR interval that exceeds .2 sec., so we suspect some kind of ___ Block.   AV

While looking for *P waves that lack a QRS response,* we notice a lone P wave with no ____ response following   QRS the last complete cycle.

Upon close examination, we see that the PR interval is normal at first, but becomes progressively longer with each successive cycle. We now recognize a _____ block.   Wenckebach

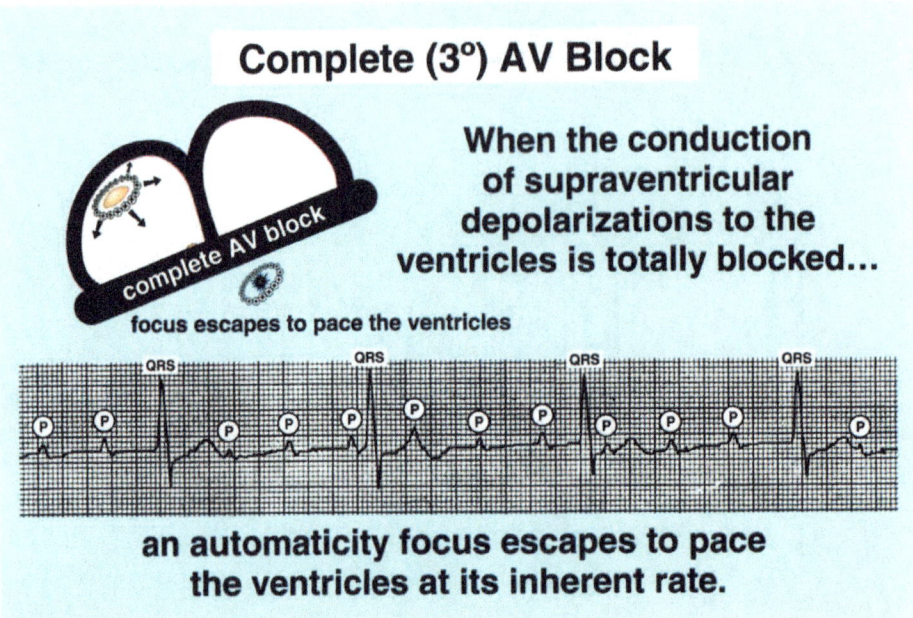

Complete (3°) AV Block

When the conduction of supraventricular depolarizations to the ventricles is totally blocked...

focus escapes to pace the ventricles

an automaticity focus escapes to pace the ventricles at its inherent rate.

Complete (3°) AV block is a total block of conduction to the ventricles, so atrial depolarizations are *not* conducted to the ventricles. Therefore, an automaticity focus below the complete block escapes to pace the ventricles at its inherent rate.

3° block is a complete block that prevents sinus-paced atrial depolarizations from reaching the _____.

ventricles

A single block of the AV Node or the His Bundle can be "complete," but more distally in the ventricular conduction system, there must be complete blocks of all subdivisions (branches) to eliminate _____ to the ventricles.

conduction

Absent paced depolarizations from above, an automaticity focus below the complete block escapes to pace the ventricles at its inherent _____.

rate

Note: The location of the escaping focus depends on the location of the complete (3°) block. Next, let's look at the possibilities.

Forms of Complete (3°) AV Block

Junctional foci spared

Complete block in the upper AV Node leaves Junctional foci to escape and pace the ventricles.	Complete block of the entire AV Node or in the His Bundle leaves only a ventricular focus to pace.	Below the His Bundle, all paths are completely blocked, so a ventricular focus escapes.

Complete (3°) AV block occurs either in the upper AV Node, allowing a Junctional focus (below the block in the AV Node) to escape and pace the ventricles, or... the complete block may be below the AV Node, leaving only a ventricular focus to escape and pace the ventricles. To be a "complete block," all avenues of AV conduction must be blocked.

If a complete block is high in the AV Node, a Junctional focus (the fastest-pacing focus below the block), escapes to pace the _____ at its inherent rate.   ventricles

If a complete block destroys the entire AV Node or is below the AV Node (for instance in the His Bundle), that leaves only ventricular foci to assume pacing responsibility...

...so a ventricular focus escapes to pace at its (slow) _____ rate.   inherent

Note: Regardless of the location of the focus that escapes to pace the ventricles, the atria remain *independently* paced by the SA Node. So on EKG, we see a Sinus-paced atrial (P wave) rate and a totally *independent*, focus-paced, slow ventricular (QRS) rate. Complete AV block produces this *"AV dissociation"* that records on EKG as a (usually normal) P wave rate superimposed over an independent, slower QRS rate. The AV dissociation (on EKG or cardiac monitor) tips us off that there is probably a complete AV block.

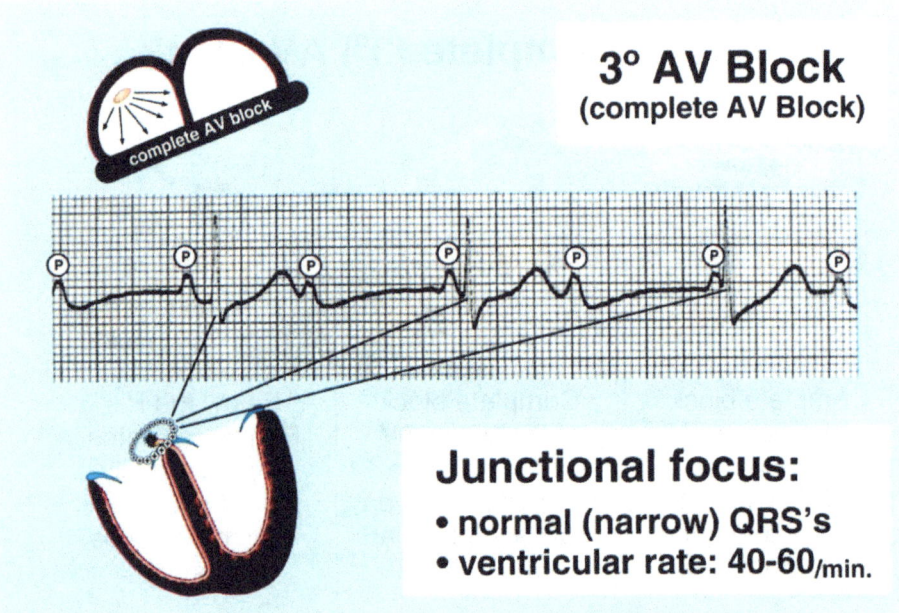

3° AV Block
(complete AV Block)

complete AV block

Junctional focus:
• **normal (narrow) QRS's**
• **ventricular rate: 40-60/min.**

If a complete AV block occurs above the AV Junction (i.e., in the upper AV Node), then a Junctional focus, no longer overdrive-suppressed, escapes to pace the ventricles. On EKG, we see Sinus-paced P waves and a slower, independent QRS rate, usually with normal QRS complexes.

Note: If the complete AV block is in the AV Node, above the AV Junction, then a Junctional focus, no longer overdrive-suppressed, escapes to pace the ventricles. This is an "idiojunctional rhythm."*

With a complete AV block, if the QRS's appear normal (because each pacing stimulus passes down the ventricular conduction system), we know that a Junctional focus must be pacing the _____.   ventricles

Note: Sometimes paced depolarizations from a Junctional focus may have to pass through diseased regions in the ventricular conduction system, delaying depolarization in some areas of the ventricles, producing wide QRS complexes.

If the ventricular rate ranges between 40 and 60, then a focus in the ___ _____ is probably pacing the ventricles.   AV Junction

* Pacing by a Junctional focus may accelerate to become an *accelerated idiojunctional rhythm.*

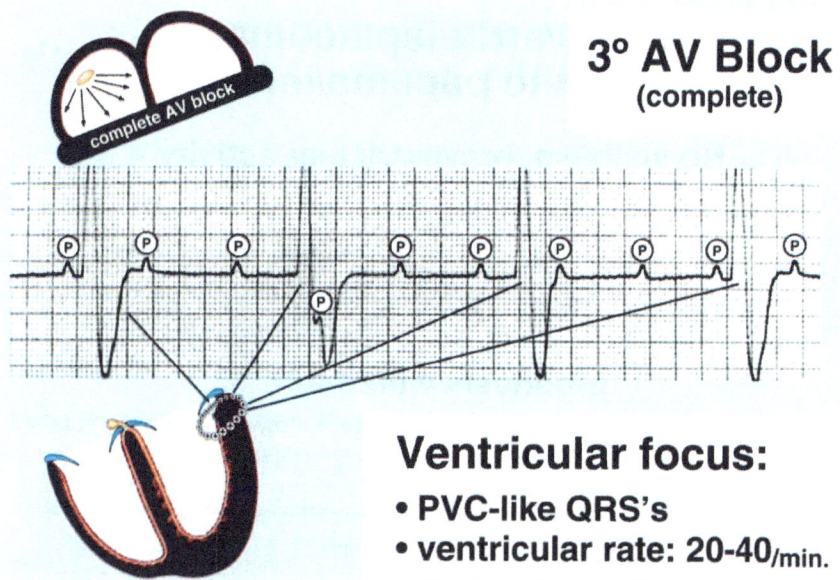

3° AV Block
(complete)

Ventricular focus:
- **PVC-like QRS's**
- **ventricular rate: 20-40/min.**

When a complete AV block occurs *below* the AV Junction, a ventricular focus escapes overdrive suppression to pace the ventricles at its slow inherent rate of only 20 to 40 per min.; so slow, in fact, that cerebral blood flow is compromised and syncope may ensue.

Noticing AV Dissociation (separate atrial P wave) and ventricular (QRS) rates, you should check the morphology of the QRS's. When we see large, wide, PVC-like complexes, we know that the ventricles are probably being paced by a _____ focus.   ventricular

We also see that the ventricular rate is within the inherent rate range (20 to 40 / min.) of a ventricular _____.   focus

Note: We understand that a ventricular focus could only escape to pace if there were no Junctional focus available above it. So the complete AV block either obliterated the entire AV Node or it occurred below the AV Junction (i.e., below the AV Node).

Note: In 3° (complete) AV block the ventricular rate may be so slow that blood flow to the brain is inadequate, and the patient may lose consciousness (syncope). This is *Stokes-Adams Syndrome*. Patients with complete AV block need continuous surveillance and maintenance of airway… many die needlessly without. Respond! Patients with 3° AV block eventually need an artificial pacemaker.

Downward displacement
of the pacemaker

No visible supraventricular activity

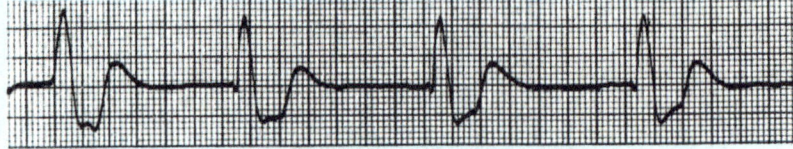

prognosis worse for:

• wider complexes • diminished amplitude • slower ventricular rate

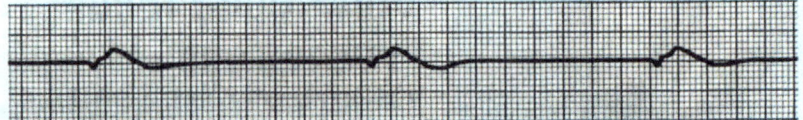

The above tracing is not caused by a 3° AV block. Don't be trapped by assuming that wide complex bradycardia is always due to a 3° block. Can you see signs of independent atrial activity? In practice, you should check all leads.

Bradycardia with wide ventricular complexes is not always pathognomonic for complete AV block, so identify AV dissociation (independent atrial and ventricular activity) before calling any wide complex bradycardia a 3° AV _____.   block

Note: The absence of atrial activity with wide complex bradycardia indicates that neither the SA Node nor supraventricular foci are viable enough to pace the atria. This failure of all automaticity centers above the ventricles, called *"downward displacement of the pacemaker"* usually carries an unfavorable prognosis. Before pronouncing this "downward displacement," make certain that the flat baseline is not due to atrial fibrillation.

Note: Extremely high serum K⁺ concentrations "hyperkalemia" can severely depress the SA Node and supraventricular foci, producing the same EKG findings. Hyperkalemia can cause cardiac asystole, a form of cardiac arrest.

Why don't we all take a break. Then, a little refreshed, we can look at Bundle Branch Block... next page.

Bundle Branch Block

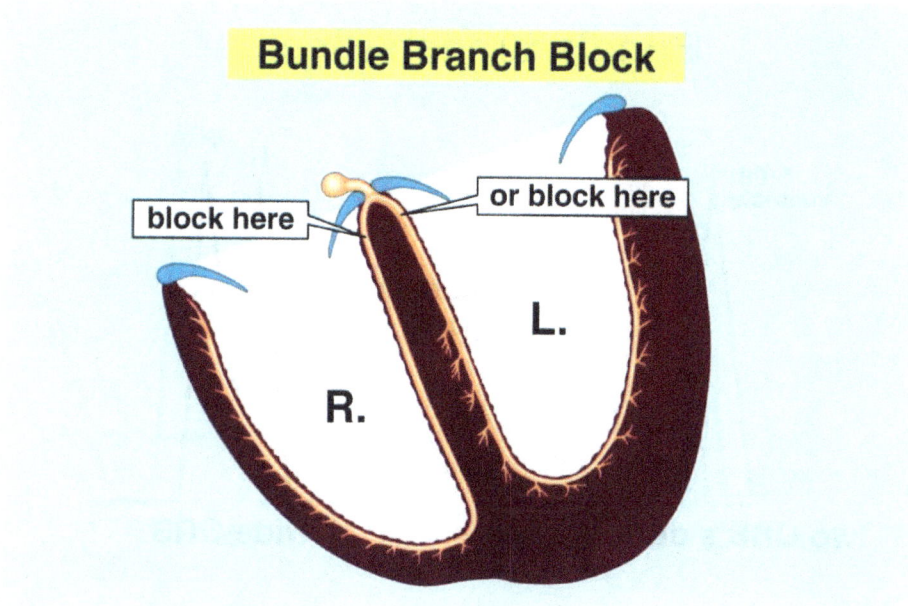

block here

or block here

L.

R.

Bundle Branch Block (BBB) is caused by a block (of conduction) in the Right or in the Left Bundle Branch. The blocked Bundle Branch delays depolarization to the ventricle that it supplies.

Normally, the Right Bundle Branch quickly conducts the stimulus of depolarization to the right ventricle, and the Left Bundle Branch does the same to the _____ ventricle. The depolarization stimulus is conducted to both ventricles at the same time (i.e., simultaneously).

left

A block of one of the Bundle Branches produces a _____ of depolarization of the ventricle that it supplies.

delay

Note: Ordinarily both ventricles are depolarized simultaneously. But with Bundle Branch Block, the unblocked Bundle Branch conducts normally, while depolarization in the blocked Bundle Branch has to creep slowly through the surrounding muscle (which conducts more slowly than the specialized Bundle Branch) to stimulate the Bundle Branch below the block. After the delay, depolarization proceeds rapidly again below the block. However, the delay in the blocked Bundle Branch allows the unblocked ventricle to begin depolarizing before the blocked ventricle (see next page).

Bundle Branch Block

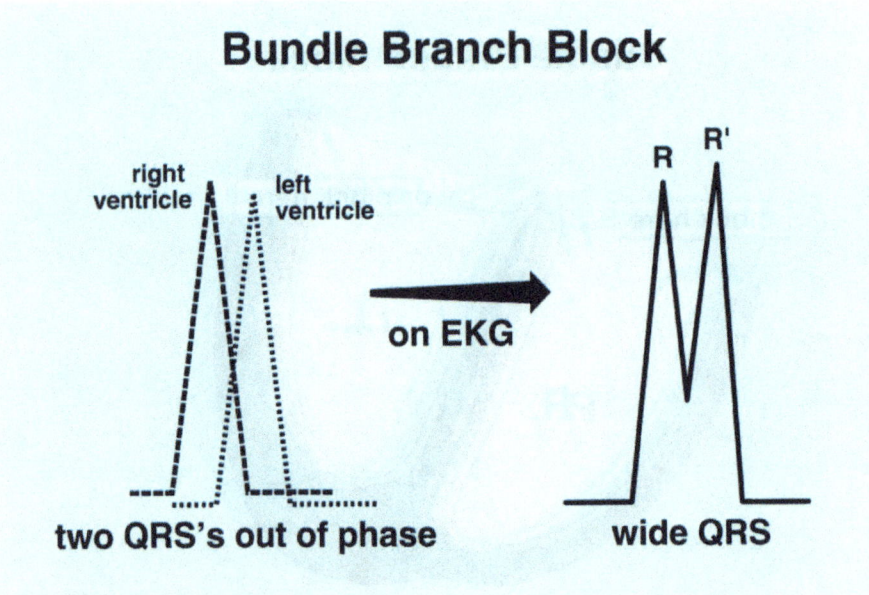

Therefore in Bundle Branch Block, one ventricle depolarizes slightly later than the other, causing two "joined QRS's" to appear on EKG.

When a Bundle Branch Block is present, either the left or the right ventricle may depolarize late, depending on which Bundle _____ is blocked.   Branch

Note: Individual depolarization of the right ventricle and depolarization of the left ventricle are still of normal duration. Because the ventricles do not depolarize simultaneously, this produces the "widened QRS" appearance that we see on the EKG. The two "out-of-sync" QRS's are superimposed on one-another, and the machine records this combined electrical activity as a widened QRS with two peaks.

Note: Because the "widened QRS" represents the non-simultaneous depolarization of both ventricles (one punctually depolarized, the other slightly delayed), we usually see two R waves named in sequential order: R and R'. The R' (pronounced "R-prime") represents delayed depolarization of the blocked ventricle.

Bundle Branch Block

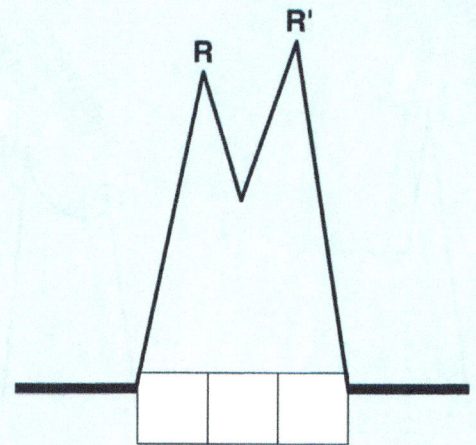

In Bundle Branch Block the "widened QRS" increases in duration to three small squares (.12 sec.) or greater, and two R waves (R and R') appear. The R' designates the delayed depolarization of the blocked ventricle.

Note: Simultaneous depolarization of the ventricles normally occurs in less than twelve hundredths second, producing a QRS that is less than three small squares in duration.

The diagnosis of Bundle Branch Block is mainly based on the widened _____ (.12 sec. or more duration).   QRS

In order to make the diagnosis of Bundle Branch Block, the QRS complex should be at least _____ small squares wide   three (3) (.12 second). Check the QRS width of every EKG that you read!

Note: The needle that records the EKG tracing moves rapidly enough to record most of the heart's electrical activity accurately. However, with great deflections the needle lags a bit mechanically, sometimes giving us an exaggerated duration on the tracing. Therefore, it is best to check the limb leads for QRS duration (where QRS amplitude is minimal), rather than the chest leads where the QRS deflections are often great.

Note: If a patient with BBB develops a supraventricular tachycardia, the rapid succession of widened QRS's may imitate Ventricular Tachycardia. Careful!

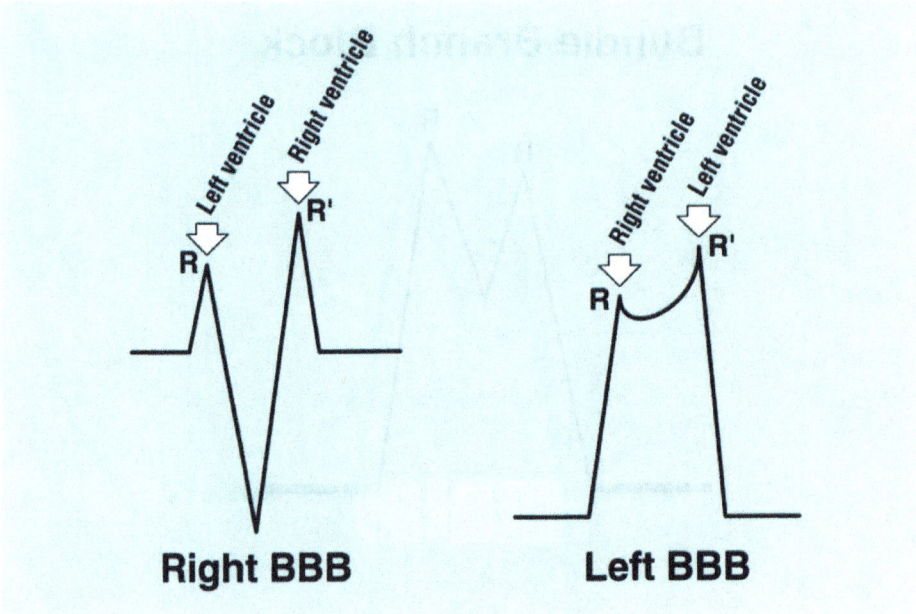

In *Left Bundle Branch Block* (LBBB), left ventricular depolarization is delayed.
In *Right Bundle Branch Block* (RBBB), right ventricular depolarization is delayed.

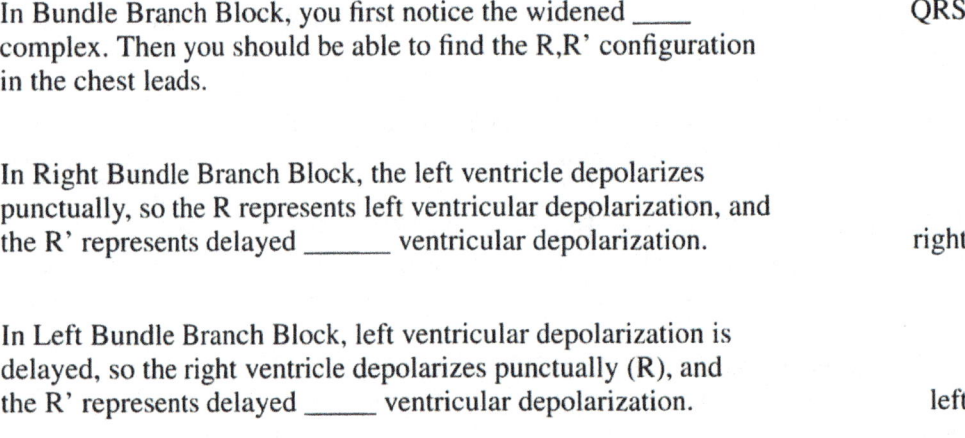

In Bundle Branch Block, you first notice the widened ____   QRS
complex. Then you should be able to find the R,R' configuration
in the chest leads.

In Right Bundle Branch Block, the left ventricle depolarizes
punctually, so the R represents left ventricular depolarization, and
the R' represents delayed _____ ventricular depolarization.   right

In Left Bundle Branch Block, left ventricular depolarization is
delayed, so the right ventricle depolarizes punctually (R), and
the R' represents delayed _____ ventricular depolarization.   left

Kind of easy to understand, isn't it?

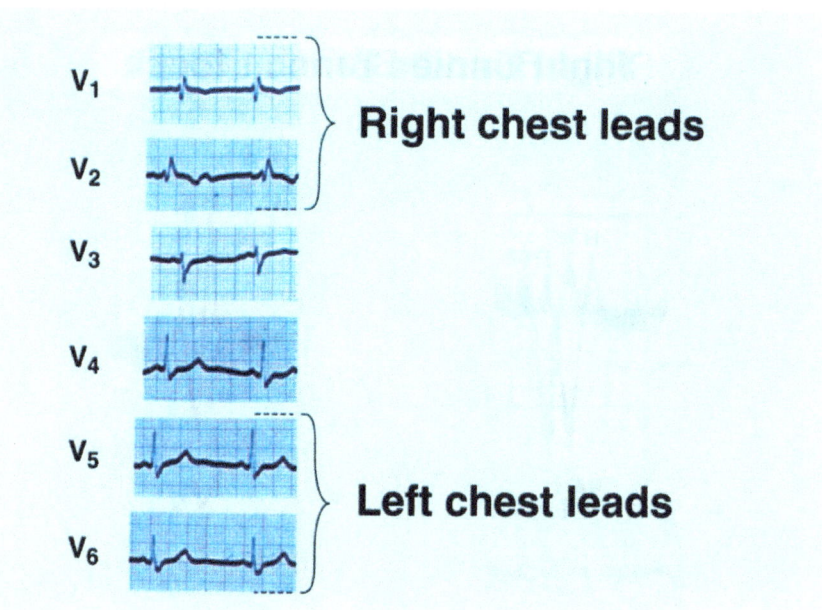

If there is a Bundle Branch Block, look at leads V_1 and V_2 (right chest leads) and leads V_5 and V_6 (left chest leads) for the R,R'.

When the QRS complex is wide enough (.12 sec. or more) to make the diagnosis of **BBB**, we immediately look at the right and left chest leads for the ____.   R,R'

Note: During ventricular depolarization and just afterward (up to the peak of the T wave), any additional stimulus cannot depolarize the ventricles, that is, they are *refractory* to a premature stimulus. The Bundle Branches have a refractory period, but the Left and Right Bundle Branch refractory periods are not identical, so with a supraventricular tachycardia one Bundle Branch is receptive to stimulation before the other. At a certain *critical* rapid rate, one Bundle Branch conducts before the other, producing non-simultaneous depolarization of the ventricles. So this *rate-dependent* Bundle Branch Block produces a tachycardia with wide QRS's that imitates Ventricular Tachycardia.

The right chest leads are V_1 and ____. V_2

Right Bundle Branch Block

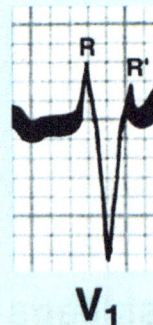

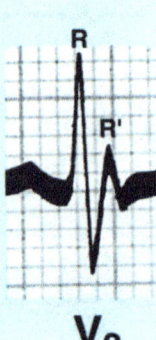

Right Bundle Branch Block produces an R,R' in the right chest leads, V_1 or V_2.

With a wide ____ (and a diagnosis of BBB), check   QRS
the right and left chest leads for R,R'.

Then, if there is an R,R' in the right chest leads V_1 or V_2
there is probably a _____ Bundle Branch Block.   Right

In Right Bundle Branch Block, the right ventricle is
depolarizing slightly later than the left ventricle, so the R'
in the above illustration represents the delayed depolarization
to the (blocked) _____ ventricle.   right

Left Bundle Branch Block

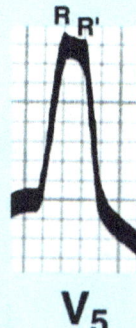

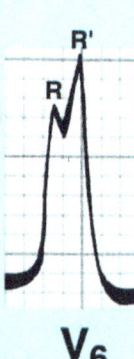

With a BBB, an R,R' in the left chest leads V₅ or V₆ means that Left Bundle Branch Block is present. The R' represents delayed depolarization of the *left* ventricle.

The chest electrode is located over the left ventricle in left chest leads ___ and V₆.

V₅

Occasionally, the R,R' in V₅ or V₆ will appear only as a flattened peak with two tiny points in _____ Bundle Branch Block. (Examine the QRS in V₅ in the illustration).

Left

In LBBB the right ventricle depolarizes before the left ventricle, so the first portion of the wide QRS represents _____ ventricular depolarization.

right

Note: Make a mental note of the typical QRS pattern (i.e., shape) of Right and Left BBB. A diagnosis is often made by appearance alone. These patterns are important because sometimes a PVC or the ventricular complexes in VT are said to have a "RBBB" or "LBBB" pattern; you should understand what that means. The same is true of the ventricular complexes (on EKG) produced by artificial pacemaker electrodes.

Note: The Left Bundle Branch has two subdivisions ("fascicles"); blocks of these fascicles are called *Hemiblocks* (pages 295 - 305).

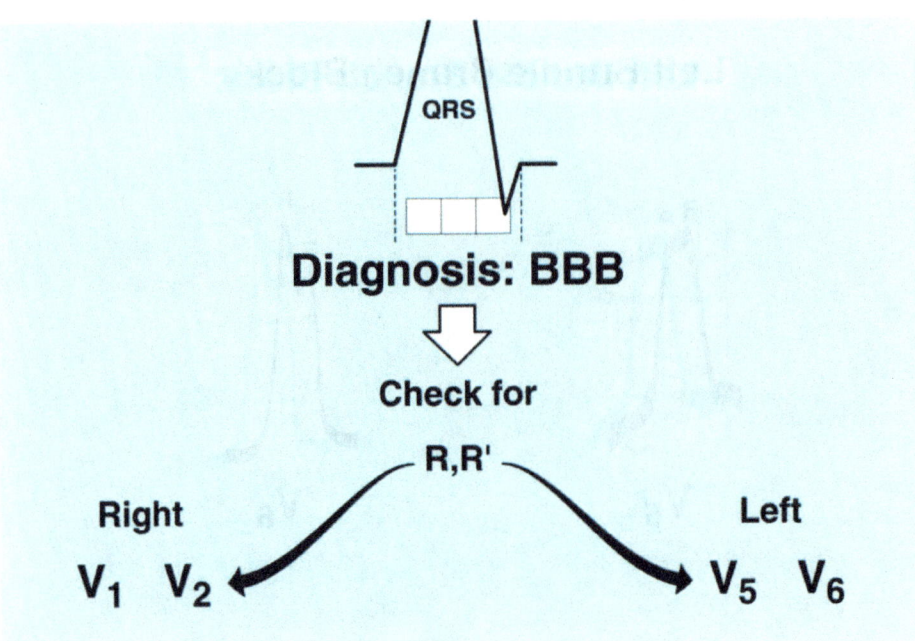

Remember, a wide QRS (three small squares) indicates BBB, and you should identify which Bundle Branch is blocked by checking the left and right chest leads.

To diagnose BBB, the QRS complex must be at least ___ of a   .12
second in duration. Now, just for smiles, let's identify the type
of BBB in the illustration on page 193.

Note: In some individuals recovery from refractoriness (during the
last stage of repolarization) differs slightly in duration between bundle
branches. So only at a particular critical rate of tachycardia, one
ventricle depolarizes after the other to produce a *rate-dependent* Bundle
Branch Block (see Note, page 195).

The R,R' pattern may occur in only one chest _____. It is   lead
often difficult to see the R', but usually it can be found in the
right chest leads V_1 or V_2 or in the left chest leads V_5 or V_6.

Note: Occasionally you will see an R,R' in a QRS of normal duration.
This is called *"incomplete"* BBB.

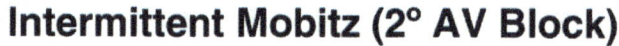

Intermittent Mobitz (2° AV Block)

Intermittent
dropped
QRS

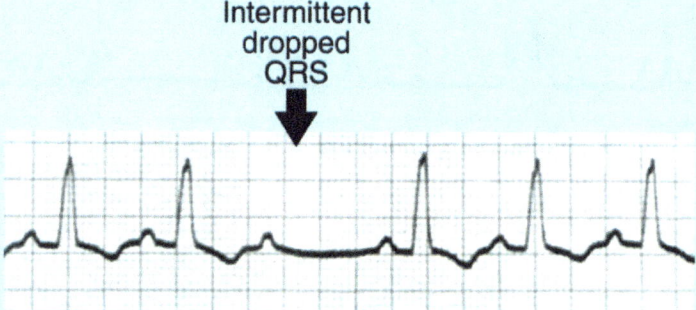

Occasional dropped QRS due to permanent BBB (one side) with intermittent BBB of the other side.

Simultaneous RBBB and LBBB prevents depolarization from reaching the ventricles; this is a complete (3°) AV block. So, block of one Bundle Branch with intermittent block of the other produces intermittent complete AV block, **intermittent Mobitz**.

Right BBB plus intermittent Left BBB will record on EKG
as continuous Right BBB pattern QRS's with intermittent
episodes of complete AV block (P waves without ____ response).   QRS

Left BBB plus intermittent Right BBB will record on EKG as
continuous Left BBB pattern QRS's with intermittent episodes
of complete AV block (P waves without ____ response).   QRS

Note: An EKG tracing or cardiac monitor display with a continuous BBB pattern QRS with an occasional missing QRS indicates *intermittent* complete AV block. The intermittent block may worsen, eventuating in a constant complete AV block. This *intermittent Mobitz* (exactly what it is) flashes an important warning sign. *Intermittent Mobitz* is the heart's warning that eventually it will need an artificial pacemaker to drive the ventricles at a normal rate. Don't let it slip by you unnoticed... for the patient's sake!

Innocuous Imitators of Intermittent Mobitz

dropped QRS at the end of a long Wenckebach series

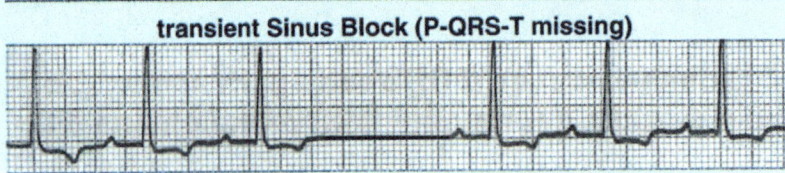

non-conducted Premature Atrial Beat (P')

transient Sinus Block (P-QRS-T missing)

Since intermittent Mobitz may herald a complete AV block requiring a pacemaker, it is important that we recognize its characteristic span of clear baseline after a normal P wave. But, *innocuous* conditions can also produce a span of empty baseline.

A Wenckebach series (innocuous) produces a barren span of baseline after the terminal, punctual P _____, which is not conducted (review page 180).

wave

A non-conducted Premature Atrial Beat (innocuous) strikes the AV Node while it is still refractory, so no stimulus is conducted to the _____ (page 128); notice the peculiar, premature P' before the barren baseline.

ventricles

A transient Sinus Block (usually innocuous, but the patient should be followed) can produce a pause before pacing resumes, or an automaticity focus may respond to the pause with an escape _____; in either case there is never an isolated P wave preceding the pause (review page 174).

beat

Note: Simply stated:

- punctual P wave (no QRS response)... 2° AV block; Mobitz vs. Wenckebach

- premature P' wave (no QRS response)... non-conducted PAB

- missed P-QRS-T cycle... SA Node transiently blocked (Sinus Block)

Rhythm: always observe

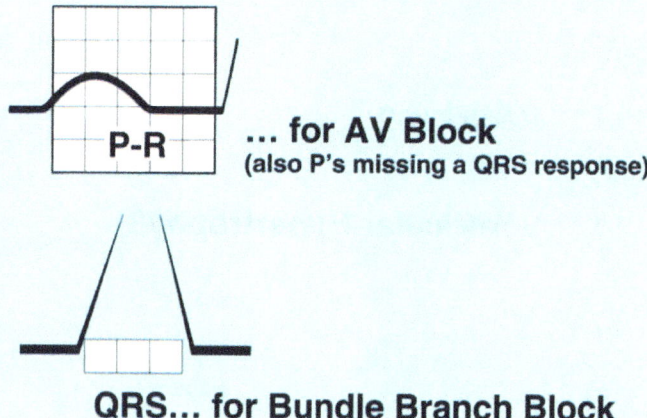

P-R

... for AV Block
(also P's missing a QRS response)

QRS... for Bundle Branch Block

Remember that you must always *visually* measure* the duration of the PR intervals and the duration of the QRS complex when examining the rhythm on an EKG. Observation will suffice.

On all EKG's, you must always measure* the PR intervals because if <u>any</u> is prolonged more than one large square, then there is some kind of ___ Block present (and, of course, look for missing QRS's, which indicate that a 2° or 3° AV Block is present).

AV

On all EKG's, the QRS duration must be measured* for if it is prolonged to .12 second or _____ there is a Bundle Branch Block.

more

Note: Always check the PR intervals and the QRS duration when scrutinizing the rhythm on any EKG. This must be part of any EKG interpretation. The spontaneous appearance of Mobitz AV block or Bundle Branch Block may be an early warning of impending infarction.

Note: *Hemiblocks* commonly occur with infarction, so they are described in the Infarction chapter. A hemiblock is a block of one of the two subdivisions ("fascicles") of the Left Bundle Branch.

* Once you <u>visually</u> check these criteria on EKG, you should record the precise PR and QRS duration.

Bundle Branch Block

Vector = ?

Ventricular Hypertrophy?

The Mean QRS Vector, "Axis", (we'll get to this in the next chapter) and ventricular hypertrophy cannot be determined accurately in the presence of Bundle Branch Block.

Note: Because the Mean QRS Vector represents the general direction of the simultaneous depolarization of the ventricles, with BBB it is very difficult to represent such a vector. This is because with BBB the ventricles do not depolarize simultaneously, so there are really two separate (right and left) ventricular vectors.

Note: The criteria for ventricular hypertrophy (enlargement) are based on a normal QRS. Bundle Branch Block produces large QRS deflections because each ventricle lacks the (usual) simultaneous electrical opposition from depolarization of the other ventricle. Therefore the EKG diagnosis of ventricular hypertrophy should be very guarded with BBB. However, atrial hypertrophy can be diagnosed in the presence of BBB.

Note: Let's review all the illustrations in this chapter. Then see "Blocks" in the **P**ersonal **Q**uick **R**eference **S**heets on page 339, and relate this to the simplified methodology that is summarized on page 334.

Chapter 7: Axis

Before you begin, look at this chapter's summary on pages 334 and 340.

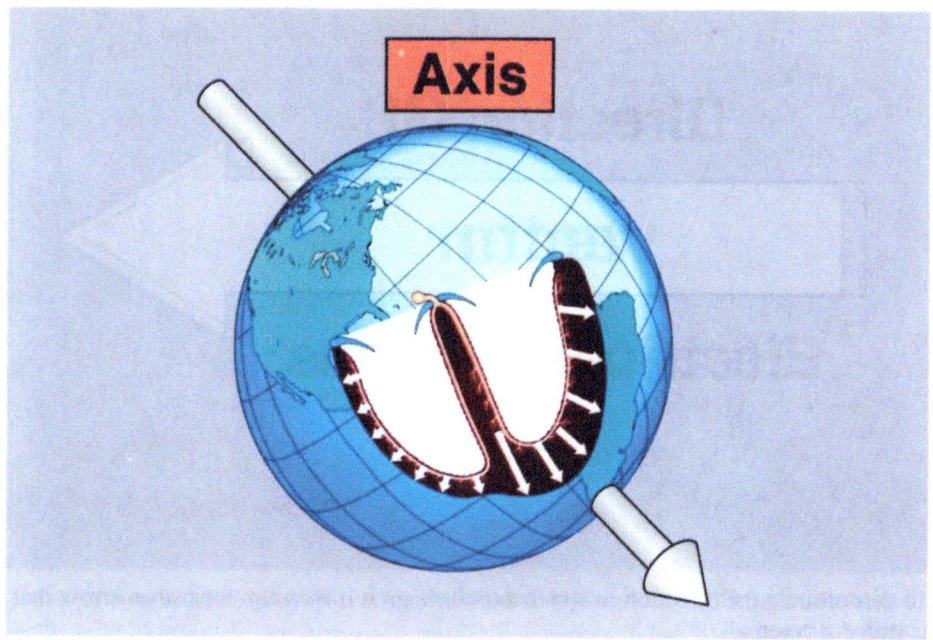

*Axis** refers to the direction of the movement of depolarization, which spreads throughout the heart to stimulate the myocardium to contract.

Note: The axis around which the earth rotates has nothing to do with electrocardiography, but we can borrow the large arrow ("Axis") in the illustration.

The progressive depolarization of the _____   myocardium
moves in a certain direction.

Axis refers to the _____ of   direction
depolarization as it passes through the heart.

   * Sometimes called "electrical axis."

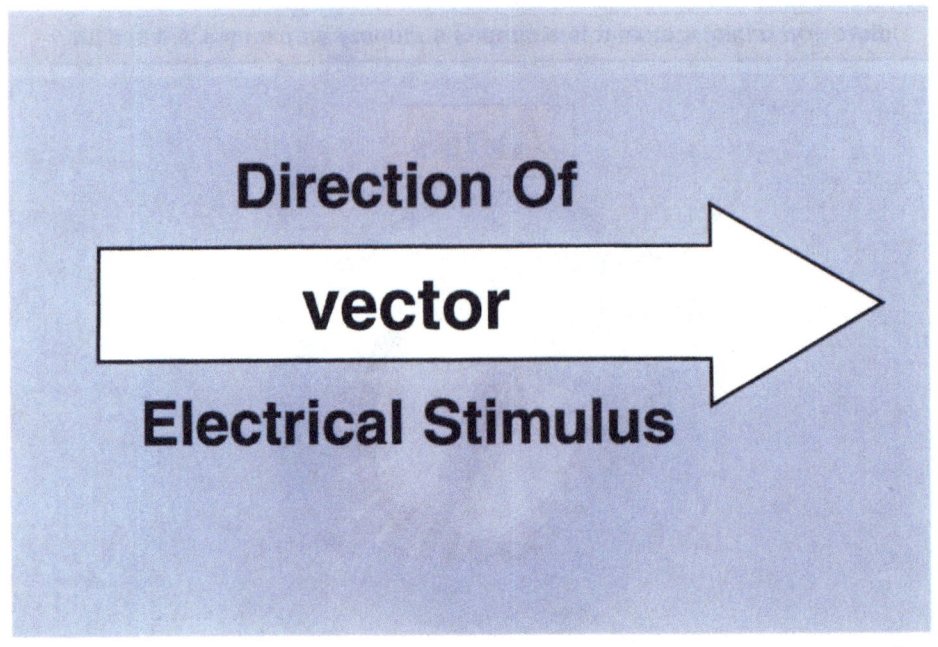

To demonstrate the direction in which depolarization is moving, we use an arrow that is called a "vector."

We can demonstrate the general direction of the
movement of depolarization by using a _____.   vector

The vector shows the direction in which
_____ is moving.   depolarization

When interpreting EKG's, a vector shows the
general _____ of depolarization in the heart.   direction

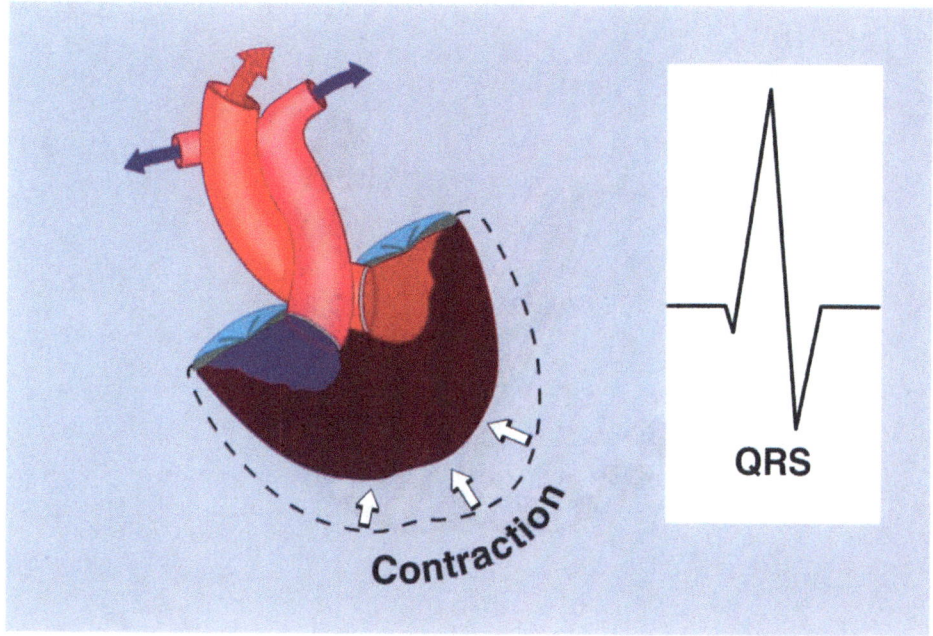

The QRS complex represents the depolarization of the ventricular myocardium.

The QRS complex represents the simultaneous depolarization of both _____.

ventricles

Ventricular depolarization and contraction can be said to occur at the same time, (but we know that _____ lasts a little longer).

contraction

Depolarization of the ventricles and their contraction is represented by the _____ complex.

QRS

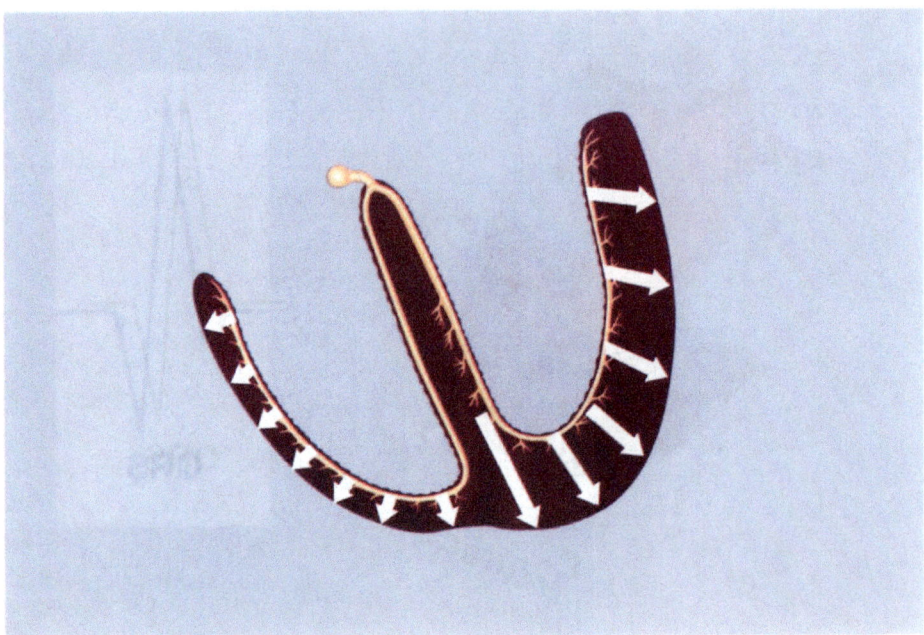

We can use small vectors to demonstrate ventricular depolarization, which begins at the endocardium that lines both ventricles and proceeds toward the outside surface (epicardium) in all areas at once.

Note: Once depolarization is beyond the AV Node, the ventricular conduction system conducts this stimulus to the ventricles with great speed. In this way, ventricular depolarization begins at the endocardial lining of the ventricles and proceeds through the thickness of the ventricular wall in all areas at about the same time. (We will not yet address depolarization of the ventricular septum).

The Purkinje fibers transmit depolarization to the myocardial cells just beneath the endocardium that lines both ventricles; this occurs so fast, that depolarization begins at the general level of the _____ in all areas at about the same time.   endocardium

Depolarization of the ventricles generally proceeds from the endocardial lining to the outside (epicardial) surface through the full thickness of the_____ wall in all areas at once.   ventricular
(See small vectors in the illustration).

Note: Notice that the thicker left ventricular wall has larger vectors.

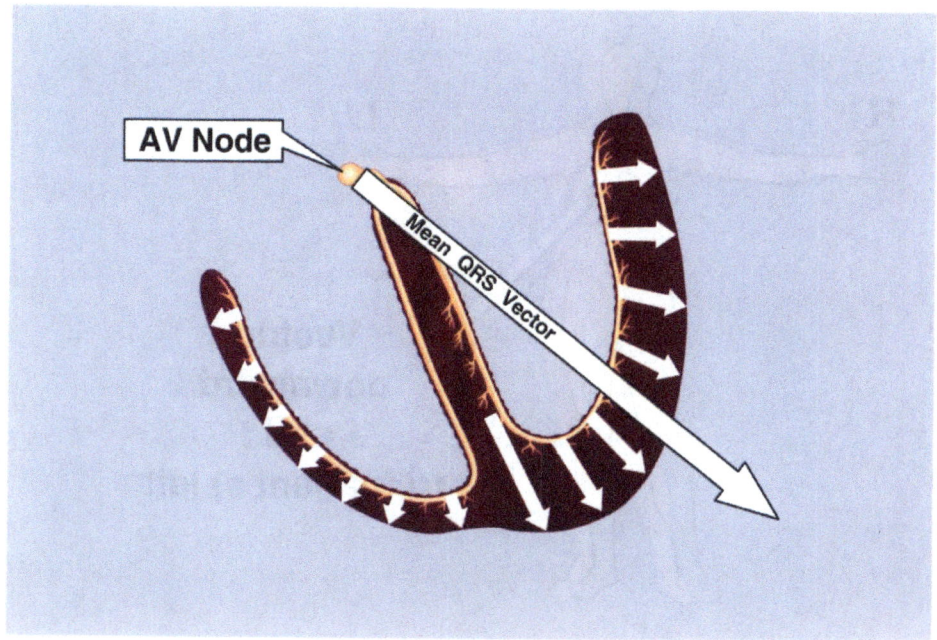

If we add up all the small vectors of ventricular depolarization (*considering both direction and magnitude*), we have one large "Mean QRS Vector" that represents the general direction of ventricular depolarization.

The Mean QRS Vector is the sum of all the
smaller vectors of _____ depolarization.   ventricular

By convention we consider the origin of the Mean
QRS Vector to be the AV Node, so the "tail" of
the Vector is always the ___ _____.   AV Node

Because the small depolarization vectors of the
thicker left ventricle are larger (previous page), the
Mean QRS Vector points more toward the _____.   left

Note: Remember that a vector represents both direction and magnitude
of depolarization… bigger vectors represent greater magnitude.

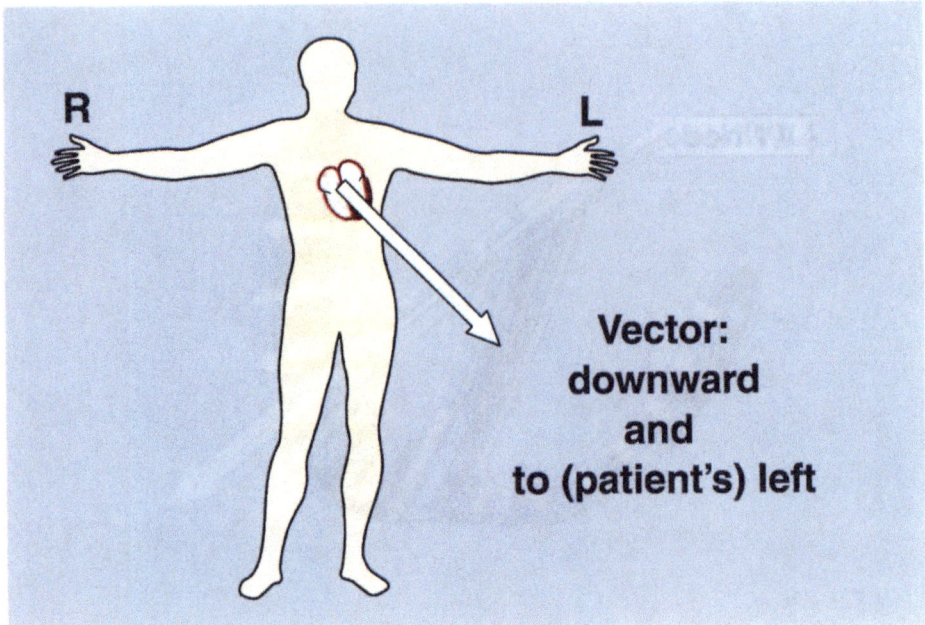

The Mean QRS Vector normally points downward and to the patient's left, because this is the general direction of ventricular depolarization.

The ventricles are in the left side of the chest and
angle downward and to the _____.   left

The _____ ____ Vector points downward and   Mean QRS
toward the patient's left side.

Note: From now on, we occasionally will use the word "Vector"
(with a capital "V") to represent the Mean QRS Vector, which depicts
the general direction and magnitude of ventricular depolarization.
Visualize the Vector over the patient's chest, and remember that it
begins in the AV Node.

Note: Depolarization is an advancing wave of Na^+ ions.

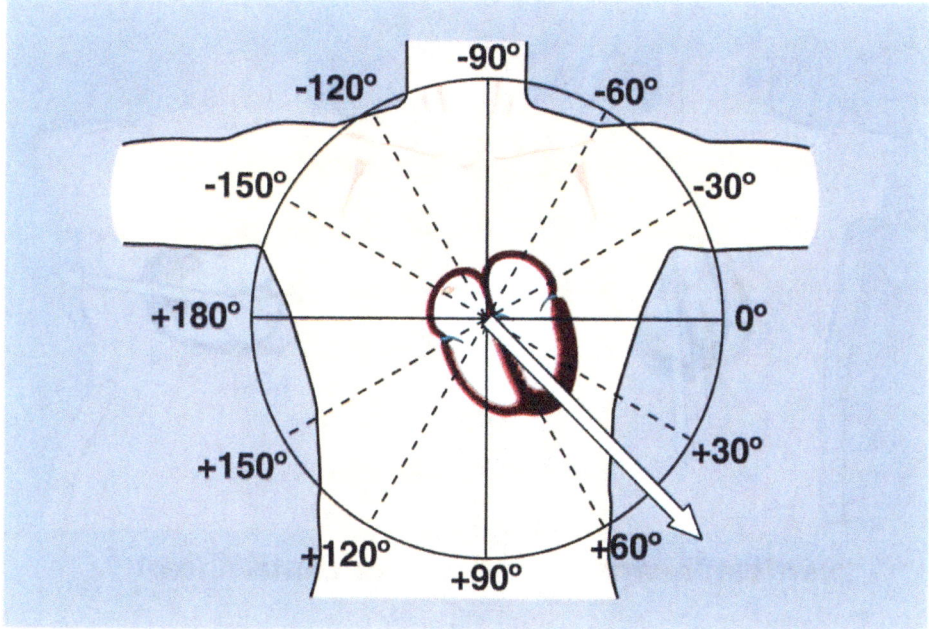

The position of the Mean QRS Vector is described in degrees within a circle drawn over the patient's chest. This circle is in the *frontal* plane. The limb leads are used to determine the position ("Axis") of the Mean QRS Vector in the frontal plane.

We can locate the position of the Mean QRS Vector within a large _____ around the heart.

circle

The center of the circle is the ____ _____.

AV Node

The Vector normally points downward and to the patient's left, that is, between 0 and ____ degrees.

+90
(don't forget the +)

Note: The "axis" of the heart is simply the Mean QRS Vector when located by degrees in the frontal plane. For example, the axis of the heart in the above illustration is about +45 degrees. Review the illustration and note that 0° is on the patient's left, and that the lower half of the circle is "positive" degrees. The top half of the circle is "negative" degrees. Axis is often denoted in medical literature by an "A" as in "A +30°" or "A = +30°", and it may be called "electrical axis."

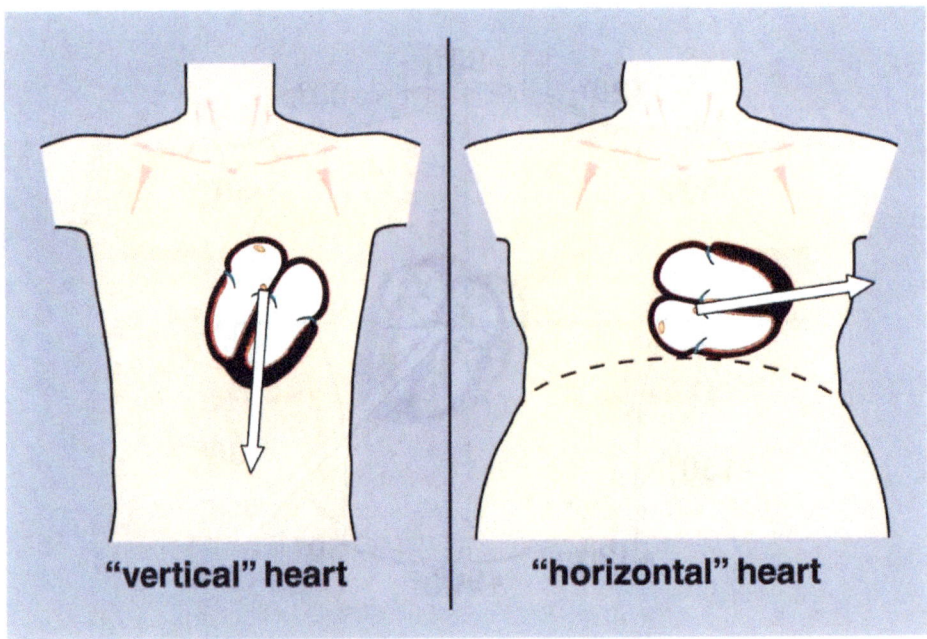

"vertical" heart   "horizontal" heart

If the heart is displaced, the Mean QRS Vector is also displaced in the same direction.
The AV Node is always the tail of the Vector.

If the heart is rotated toward the patient's right side,
then the Mean QRS Vector moves toward the _____ as well.   right
This is common in tall, slender individuals (see illustration).

In very obese people the diaphragm is pushed up
(and also the heart), so the Mean QRS Vector
may point directly to the patient's _____.   left
(See illustration).

The tail of the Vector is the ____ _____.   AV Node

Note: In obese individuals the increased abdominal pressure
often pushes the diaphragm upward so the position of the displaced
heart may be called a "horizontal heart". By the same token, a tall,
slender individual may have a so called "vertical heart".

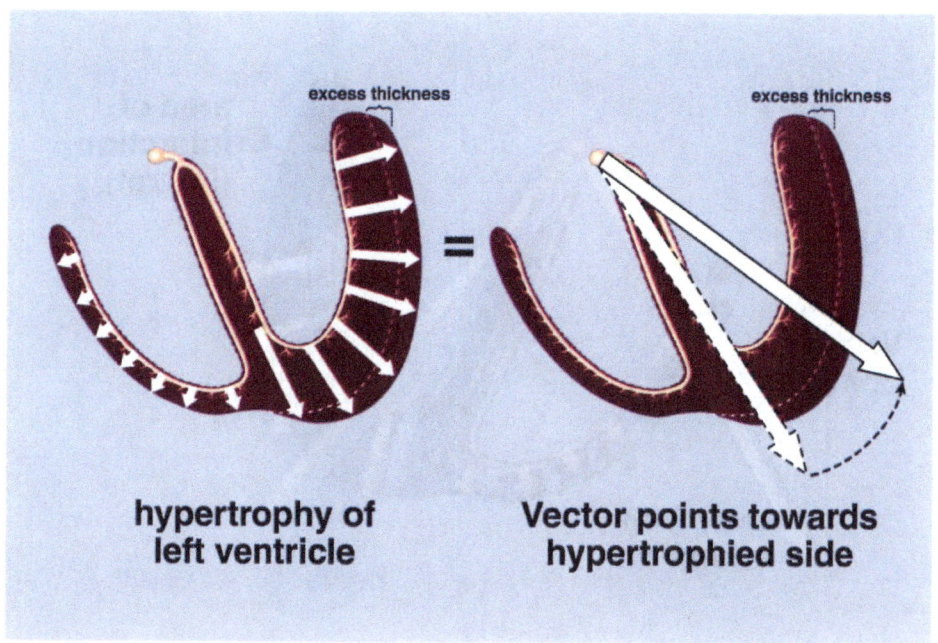

hypertrophy of
left ventricle   **Vector points towards**
hypertrophied side

With hypertrophy (enlargement) of one ventricle, the greater depolarization activity of the hypertrophied side displaces the Mean QRS Vector toward the hypertrophied side.

There is increased depolarization in a _____   hypertrophied
ventricle.

So, the Mean QRS Vector deviates toward the _____   ventricle
that is hypertrophied.

Note: A hypertrophied ventricle has more (and larger) vectors,
which draw the Mean QRS Vector in that direction.

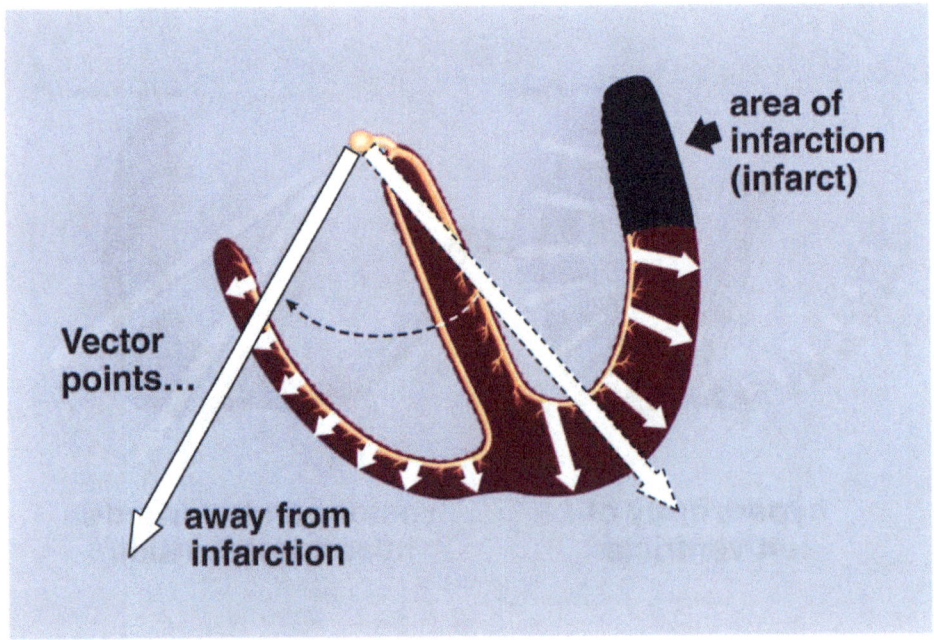

In myocardial infarction there is a necrotic (dead) area of the heart that has lost its blood supply and does not depolarize. The unopposed vectors from the other side draw the Mean QRS Vector away from the infarct.

Note: Myocardial infarction occurs when a branch of one of the coronary arteries (the heart's own source of blood supply) becomes occluded. The area of myocardium supplied by this blocked coronary artery has no blood supply and becomes electrically dead (can't depolarize).

In myocardial infarction (coronary occlusion) there is an area in the ventricles that has no _____ supply. This infarcted area cannot depolarize, and therefore it has no vectors.

blood

Since there is no depolarization (and no vectors) in the infarcted area, the vectors from the opposite side are unopposed, so the Mean QRS Vector tends to point away from the _____.

infarct

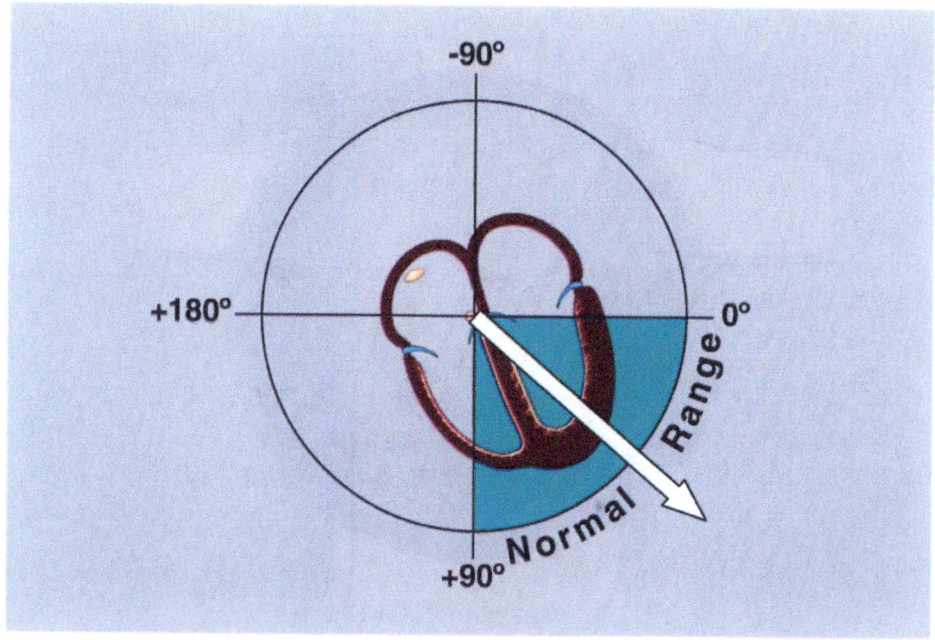

Now you understand why the Mean QRS Vector is diagnostically so valuable. "Axis" is the Mean QRS Vector when given in degrees, and the normal axis range is 0° to +90° in the frontal plane.

The Mean QRS Vector should point downward and to the patient's _____, that is, in the 0° to +90° range. This is the range of normal axis.

left

The Mean QRS Vector gives us valuable information about the position of the _____, and...

heart

... insight into ventricular _____, and it also provides us with valuable information concerning myocardial _____.

hypertrophy

infarction

Note: The Mean QRS Vector tends to point <u>toward ventricular hypertrophy</u>, and <u>away from myocardial infarction</u>. These basic principles of axis are so logical and easy to understand that you should employ this diagnostic* tool whenever a twelve lead EKG is available.

* The diagnosis of Hemiblocks (pages 295-305) is based on changes in QRS Axis.

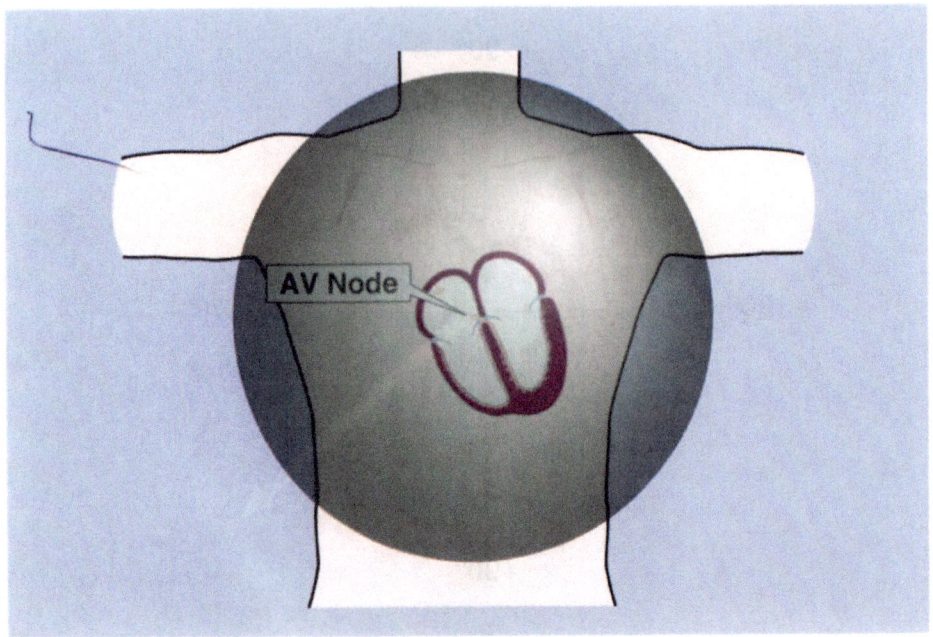

To determine the direction of the Vector, visualize a sphere surrounding the heart, with the AV Node at the center of the sphere.

Visualize a large _____ surrounding the heart.   sphere

The AV Node is the _____ of the sphere.   center

Note: The Mean QRS Vector has the AV Node as its tail, and the tip of the arrow touches somewhere on the surface of this hypothetical sphere.

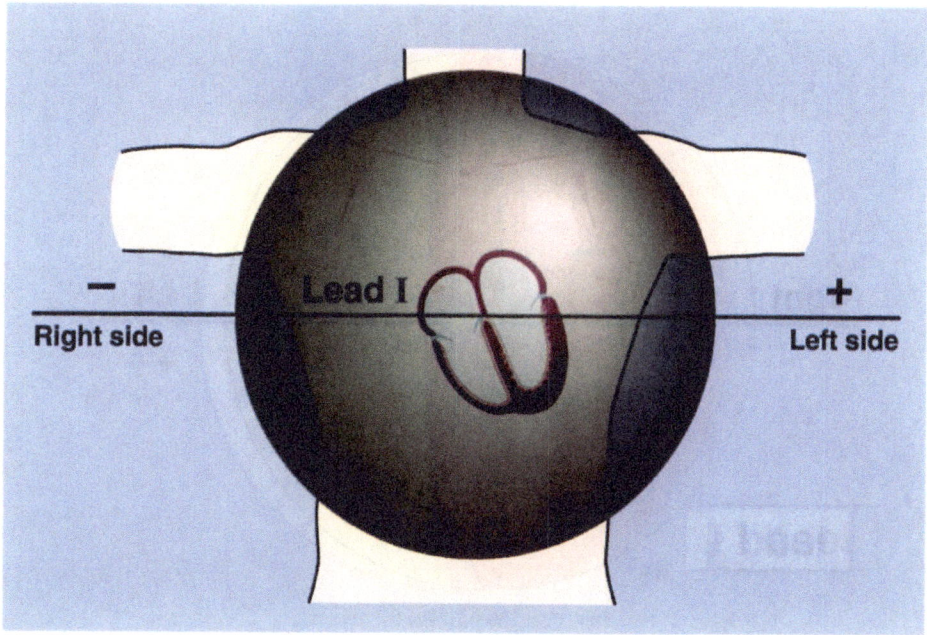

With the sphere in mind, consider lead I (left arm with the positive electrode, right arm with the negative electrode).

Lead I uses the right and left _____ for recording.   arms

If lead I is introduced into the sphere, the patient's left side
(left arm) is _____.   positive

In lead I the right arm is _____.   negative

Note: Lead I passes through the center of the sphere,
which is the AV Node.

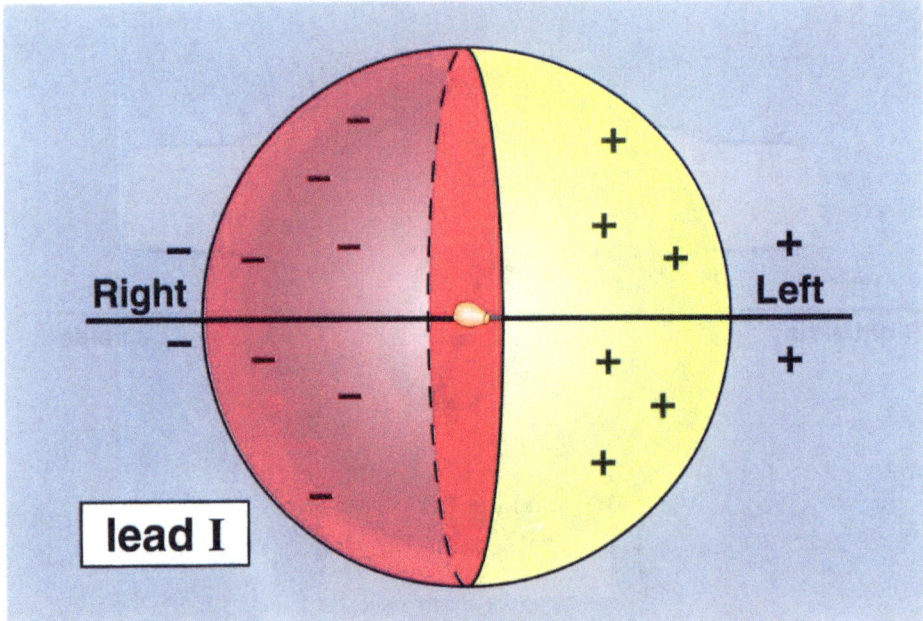

Still considering lead I, the patient's left-hand side of the sphere is positive, and the right half is negative. The center of the sphere is the AV Node.

We are considering only lead ___ at this time.   I

We will now consider the lead I sphere in two _____.   halves

The patient's right half of the sphere is _____.   negative

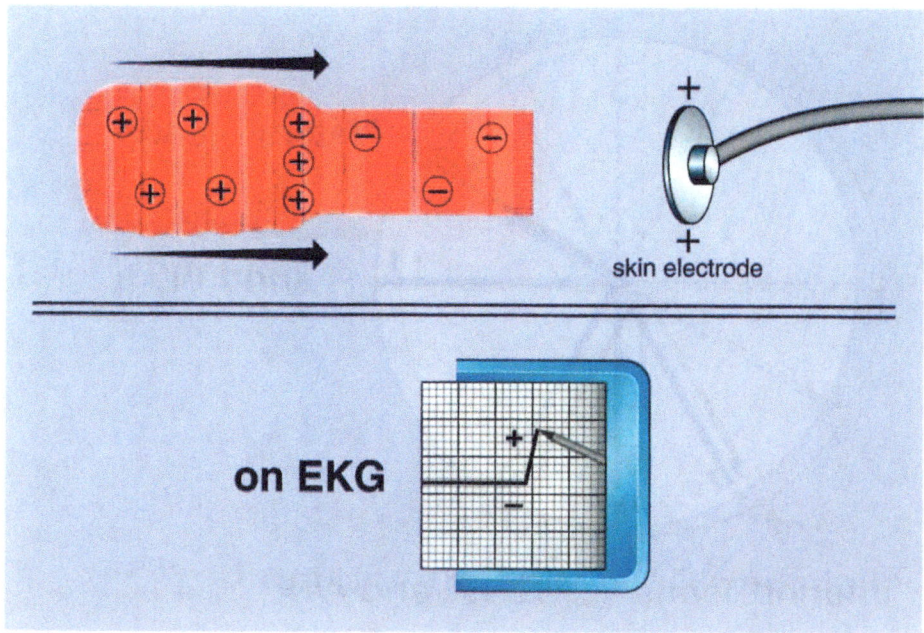

As the positive wave of depolarization within the myocardial cells moves toward a positive (skin) electrode, there is a simultaneous upward (positive) deflection recorded on EKG.

An advancing wave of depolarization may be considered a moving wave of _____ charges.

positive

When this wave of positive charges is moving toward a _____ skin electrode, there is a simultaneous upward (positive) deflection recorded on the EKG.

positive

If you see a _____ (upward) wave on EKG, it means at that instant a depolarization stimulus is moving toward a positive skin electrode that is being used to record the EKG.

positive

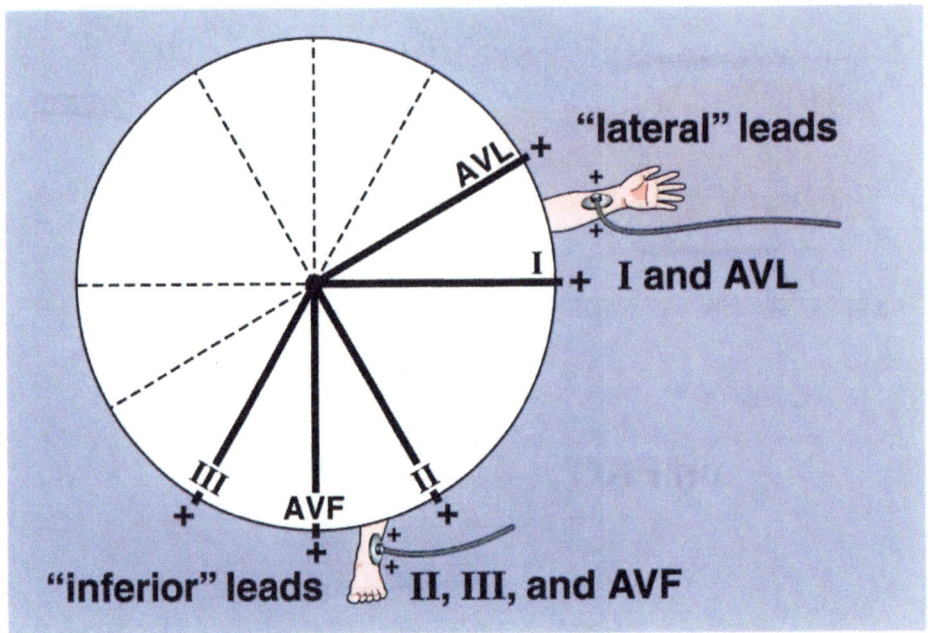

The positive electrode used to record the *inferior* limb leads, II, III, and AVF, is on the left "foot." The positive electrode that is used to record the *lateral* limb leads, I and AVL, is on the left arm.

Let's focus our attention on the only horizontal lead, that is,
lead I, which uses a positive electrode on the _____ arm.   left

Next, we will look at the only vertical lead, AVF,
which uses a _____ electrode on the left leg ("Foot").   positive

That was fast... let's move on.

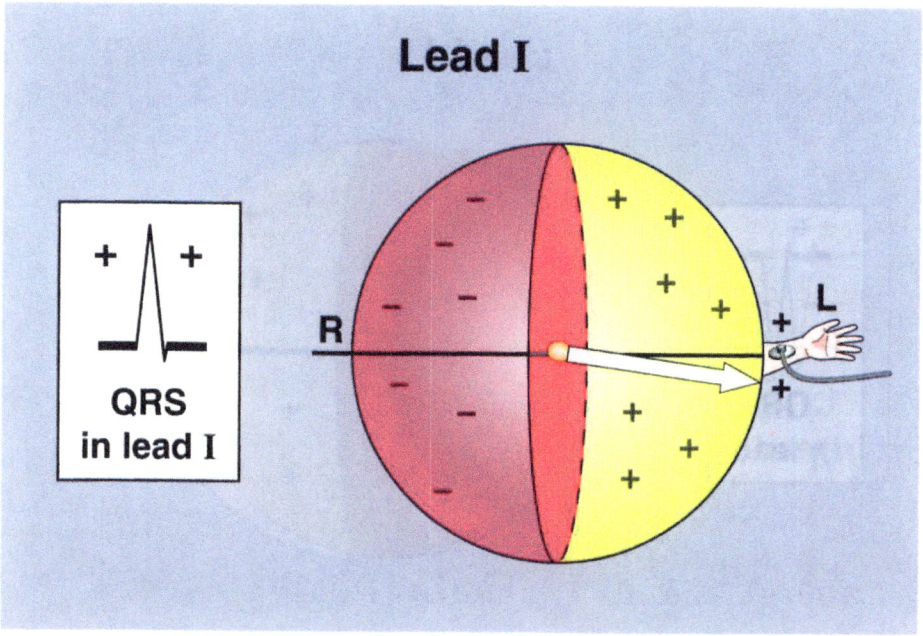

If the QRS complex is *positive* (mainly upright) in lead I, the Mean QRS Vector is pointing somewhere into the patient's *left* half (i.e., the positive half) of the sphere.

Obtain an EKG tracing and check the _____ complex in lead I.   QRS

> Note: We check the QRS complex because it represents ventricular depolarization on the EKG tracing.

If the QRS in lead I is mainly upright,
it is _____ (positive or negative)...   positive

... and if the QRS is positive in lead I, then the Mean QRS Vector points positively, that is, into the _____ half of the sphere   left
(toward the positive skin electrode on the patient's left arm).

> Note: This point becomes clearer if you go back and reread the previous page and continue directly with this page. It comes into focus better on the second go 'round.

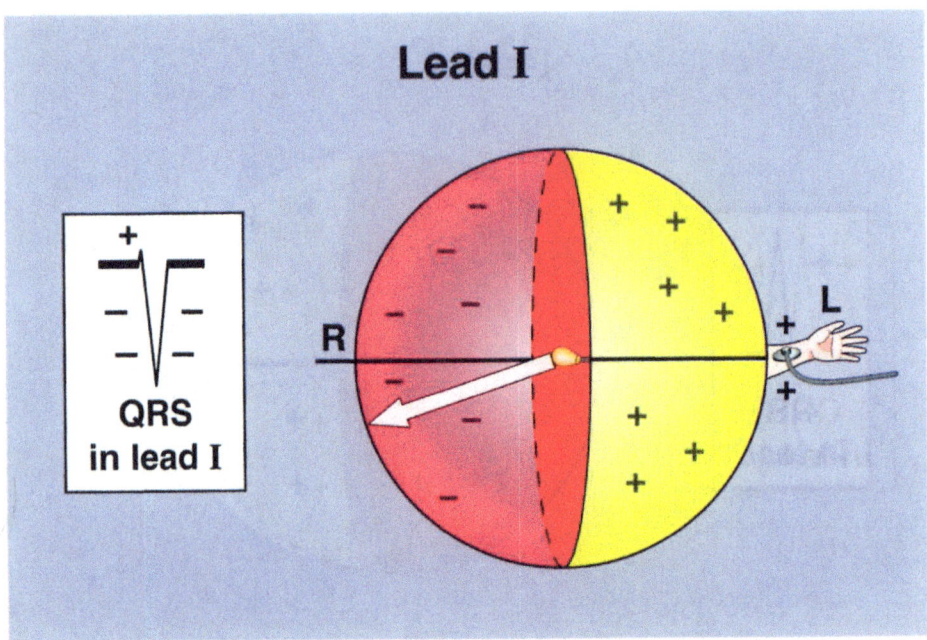

Still considering lead I on the tracing, if the QRS complex is mainly *negative*
(downward), the Vector points to the patient's *right* side.

In lead I, if the QRS complex is mainly below the baseline,
it is _____ (positive or negative).   negative

Now checking the lead I sphere surrounding the patient,
a Vector pointing into the negative half of the sphere
points to the patient's _____ side.   right

So if the QRS in lead I is mainly negative, then the Mean
_____ Vector points to the patient's right side (away from   QRS
the positive electrode on the patient's left arm).

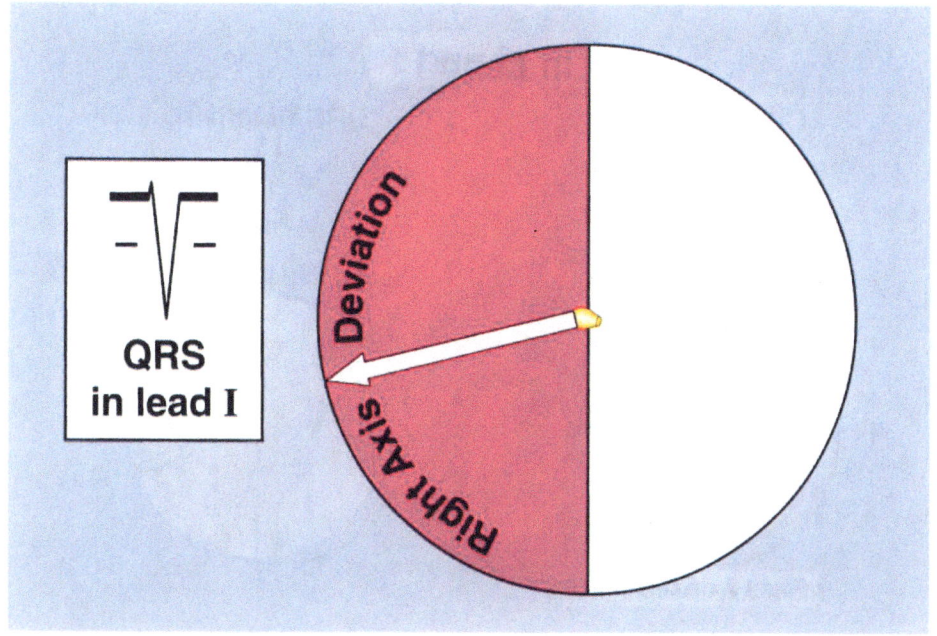

If the QRS is negative in lead I (Vector toward the right), this is *Right Axis Deviation*.

If the Mean QRS Vector points toward the right, we expect
the QRS complex in lead I to be _____.   negative

If the Mean QRS Vector points to the patient's right side
(to the right of a vertical line drawn through the AV Node),
this indicates Right _____ Deviation.   Axis

So if the QRS complex is negative in lead ___, this indicates   I
that there is Right Axis Deviation (R.A.D.).

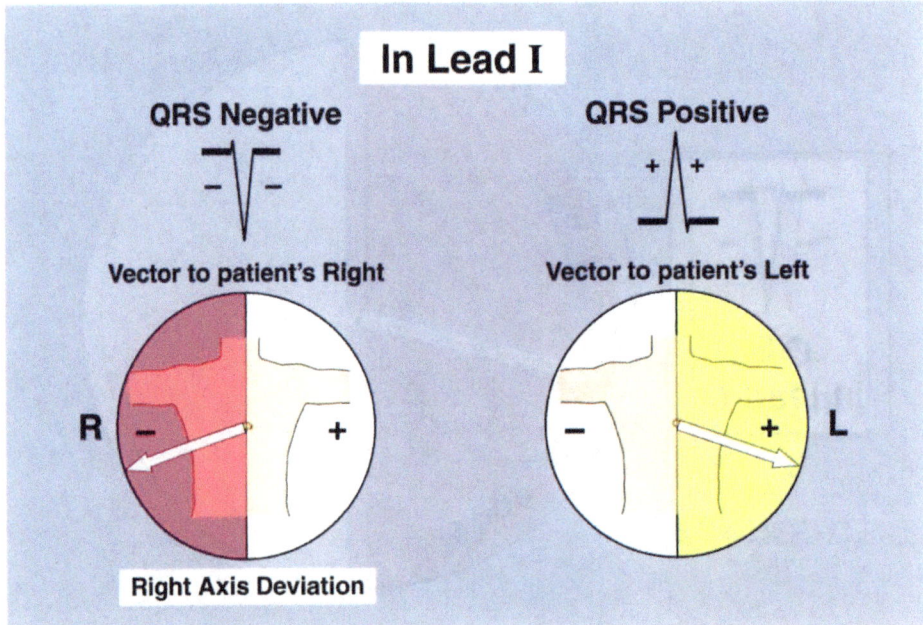

By simple observation, we can tell whether the Mean QRS Vector points to the patient's left or right side.

Lead I is the best lead for detecting Right _____   Axis
Deviation.

If the QRS complex is positive in lead I (which it usually
is), this indicates that there is no R.A.D., because the Vector
is pointing to the _____ side of the patient.   left

When we record lead I on an EKG, the patient's left arm
has the _____ electrode.   positive

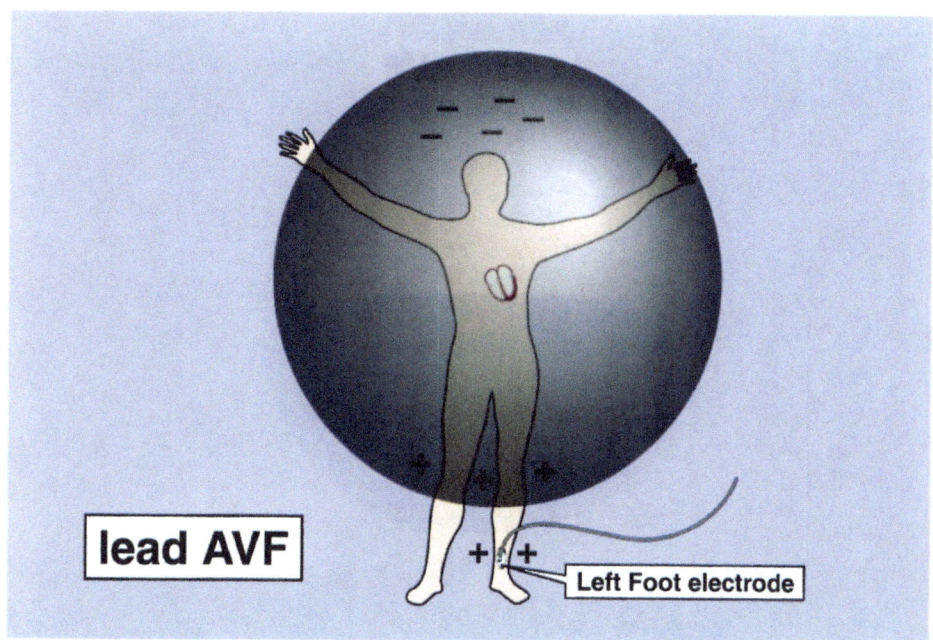

The left foot has a positive electrode in lead AVF. Imagine a sphere around the patient for lead AVF.

Ignore the lead discussed on the previous page. We are considering only lead _____ at this time.   AVF

Note: We are now considering a completely different sphere – the one that surrounds the body when we record lead AVF on the EKG machine. We need to re-orient ourselves as to the positive and negative halves of the sphere in AVF.

When we switch the EKG machine to monitor lead AVF, the machine makes the electrode on the left _____ positive.   foot

The lower half of this sphere is _____.   positive

The center of this sphere is the ___ _____.   AV Node

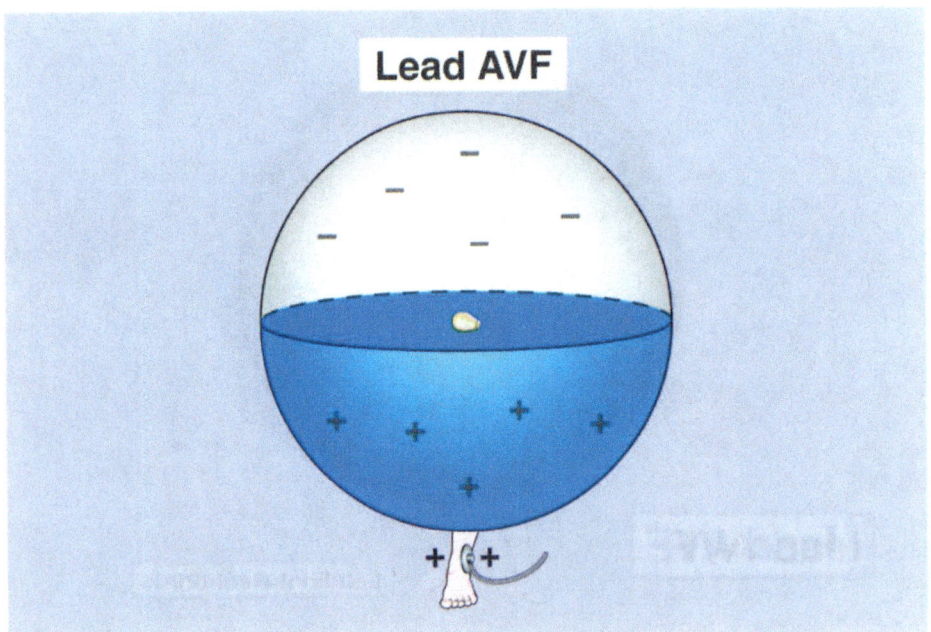

Lead AVF

For AVF the lower half of the sphere is positive, and the upper half is negative.

The lower half of the AVF sphere is the location of the
positive left foot electrode, so we know that the lower
half of this sphere is _____.   positive

The upper portion of the sphere (above the AV Node)
is _____ (positive or negative).   negative

The sphere in AVF has two halves, the upper half
is _____…   negative

… and the lower half of the AVF sphere is _____.   positive

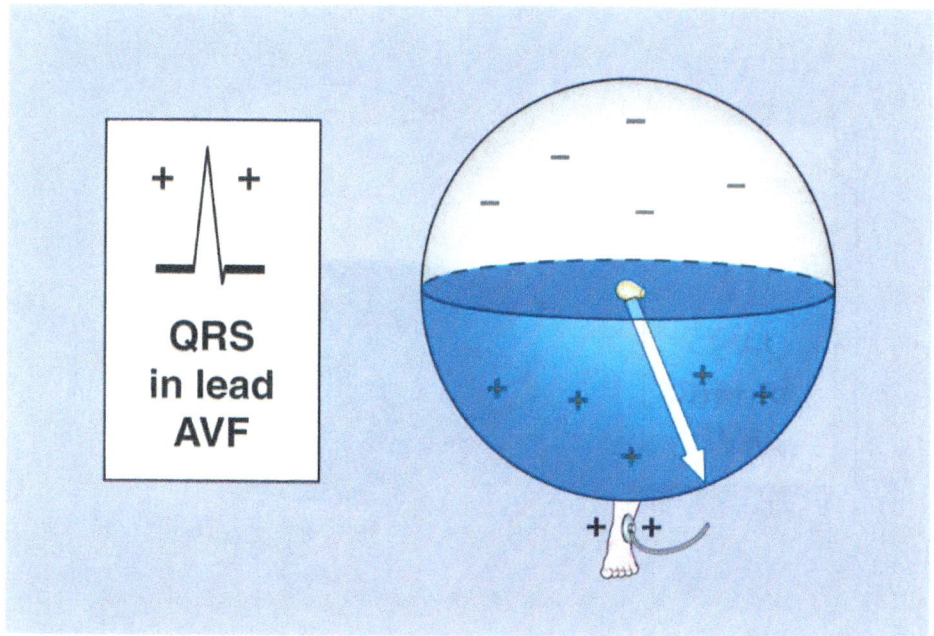

Considering lead AVF of the EKG, if the QRS is mainly positive on the tracing, then the Mean QRS Vector points downward into the positive half of the sphere, toward the positive (lead AVF) electrode.

If the Mean QRS Vector points downward, then
the QRS complex in lead AVF is _____.   upright (or positive)

Note: Don't get confused just because the positive QRS is upright, yet the Vector points downward. You must remember that the Vector points into the positive half of the sphere (toward the positive left foot electrode) when the QRS is positive. The lower half of the sphere just happens to be the positive half in lead AVF.

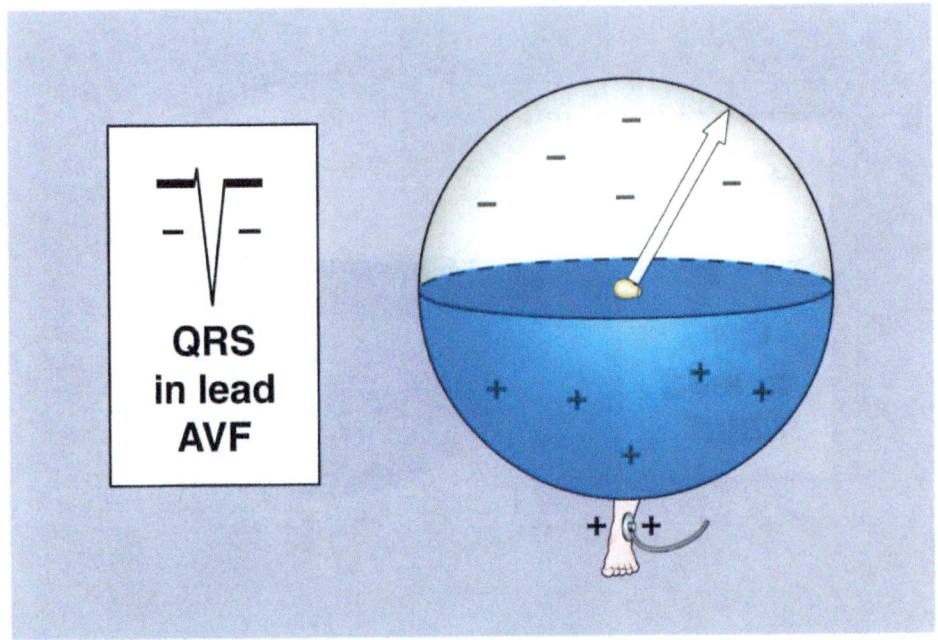

In AVF, if the QRS is negative, the Vector points into the negative half of the sphere.

The center of the sphere is the ___ _____.   AV Node

The upper half of the (lead AVF) sphere is _____.   negative

A negative QRS complex in lead AVF tells us that the
Mean QRS Vector points _____ into the negative   upward
half of the sphere (i.e., it is pointing away from the positive
electrode on the left foot).

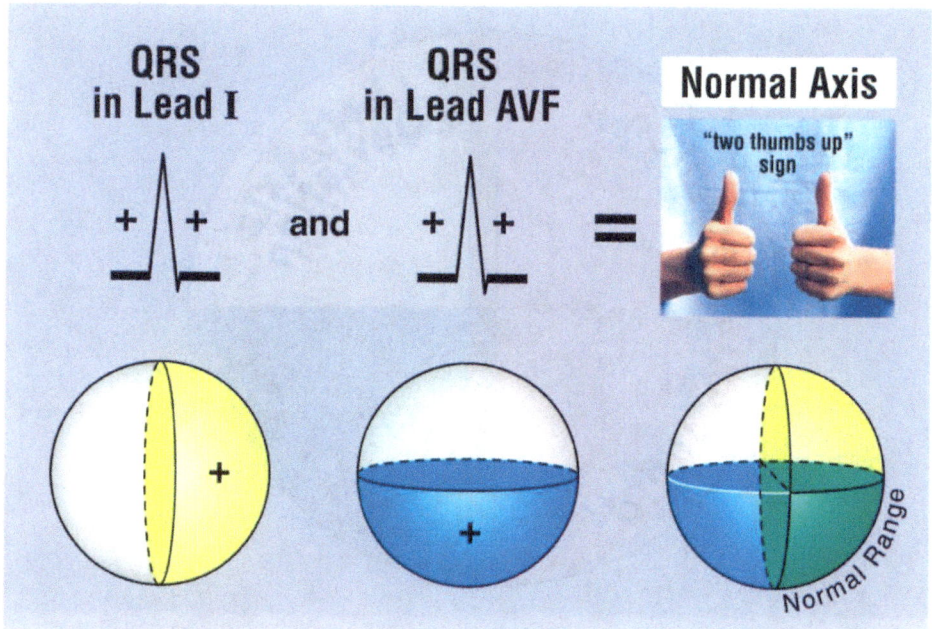

Follow the illustration closely. If the QRS is positive in lead I and also positive in AVF, the Vector points downward and to the patient's left. This is the normal axis range; the area that is both yellow and blue (yellow plus blue equals green).

A mainly positive QRS in lead I indicates that the Mean
QRS Vector points to the _____ side of the patient, and...   left

... a mainly positive QRS complex in lead AVF means
that the Vector points _____.   downward

In the same patient, if the Vector points leftward and also
points downward, the Vector must be in the only quadrant
of the _____ that satisfies both criteria (and it happens   sphere
to be the normal range).

Note: Since the ventricles angle downward to the left, and ventricular
depolarization moves downward and leftward, it should not surprise
you that this is the normal range of the Vector. Remember, Vector
position is stated in terms of the patient's left or right. If the QRS is
upright in both lead I and AVF (the "two thumbs up" sign), the Vector
("Axis") is within the normal range.

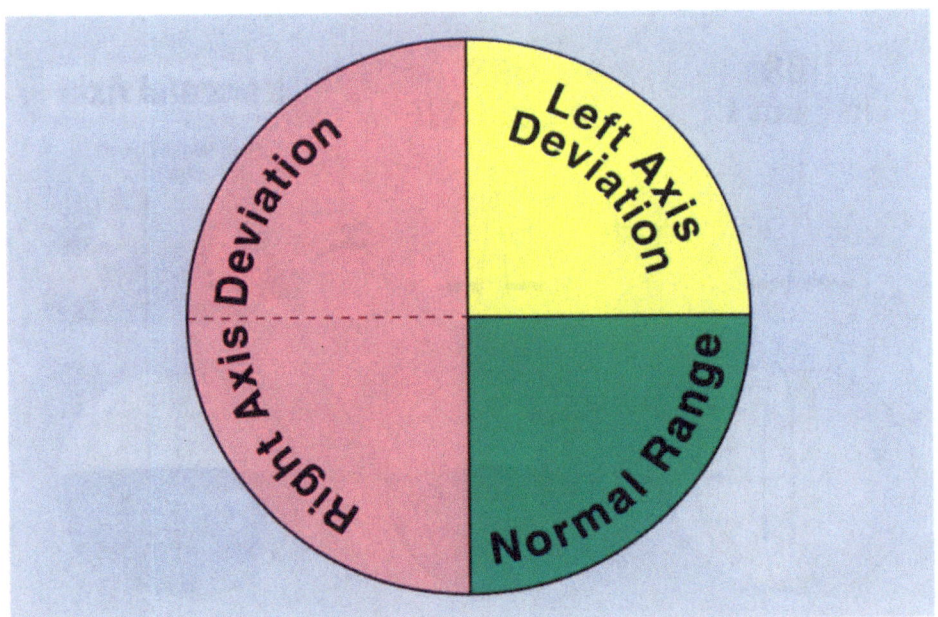

In the frontal plane, there are four possible axis quadrants where the Mean QRS Vector may point. Visualize this large circle on the patient's chest in the frontal plane.

Note: In the *frontal* plane, we determine if there is any *Deviation* of Axis out of the normal range.

If the Vector points upward (from the AV Node) and to the patient's left, this is Left _____ Deviation (L.A.D.).

Axis

If the Vector points to the patient's right side, this is _____ Axis Deviation (R.A.D.).

Right

If the Vector points downward to the patient's left, it is in the _____ range (i.e., Normal Axis).

normal

Note: Remember, Axis is merely the position (that is, the direction) of the Mean QRS Vector, which indicates the general direction of ventricular depolarization.

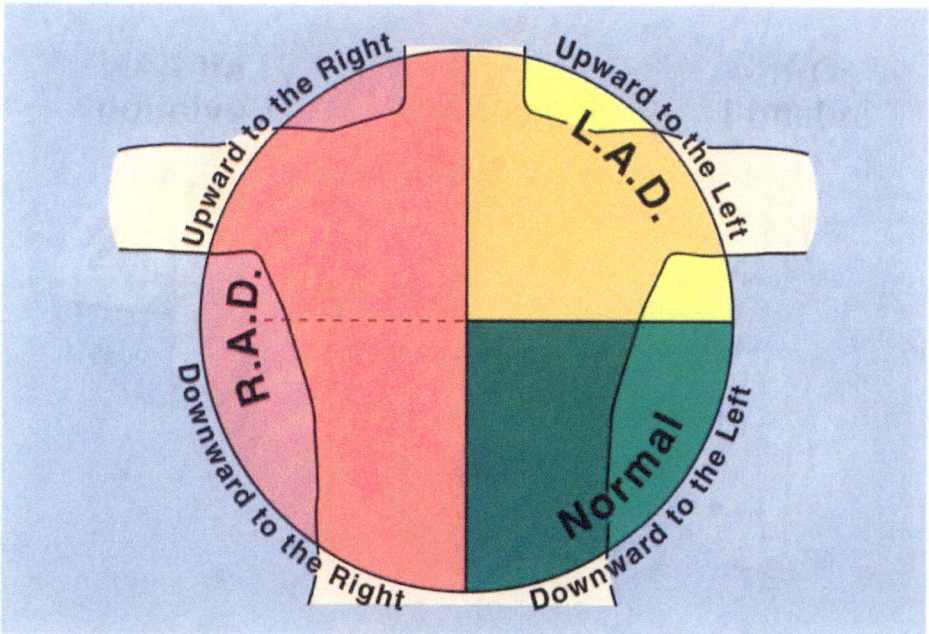

For any patient, when we find into which quadrant (of the frontal plane) the Vector points, we know in which direction the ventricular depolarization is going. The small type in the illustration relates to the patient's right or left.

Note: This is how you should visualize the four axis quadrants in a large circle (AV Node is the center) drawn on the patient's chest in the frontal plane. On some EKG charts the Mean QRS Vector is depicted in a similar circle (which represents the frontal plane).

The upper left quadrant represents _____ Axis Deviation   Left
(L.A.D.).

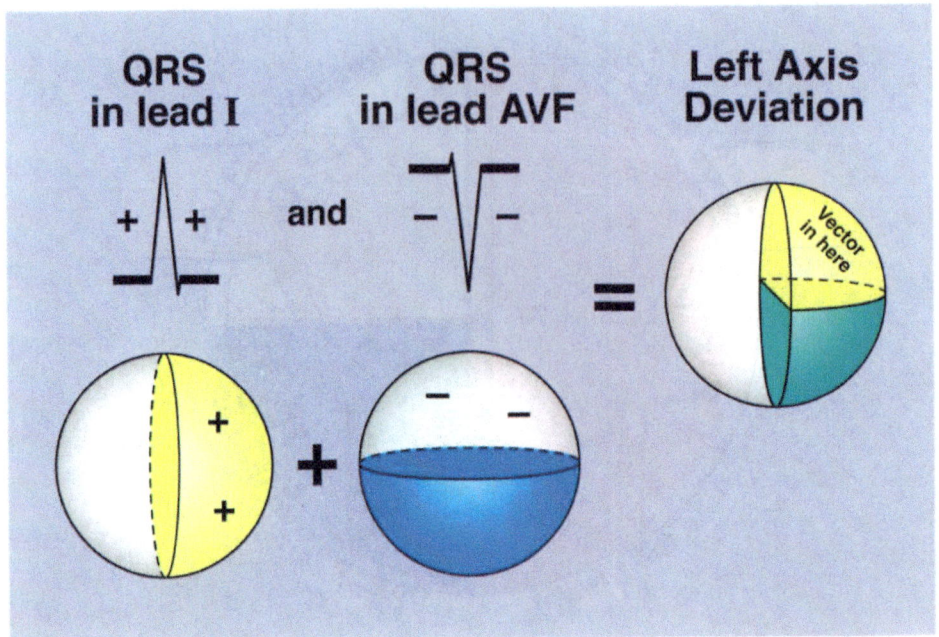

If the QRS is *positive* in lead I, and *negative* in AVF, that places the Vector in the upper left quadrant. This is *Left Axis Deviation.*

If the QRS in lead I is upright, the Vector points
to the patient's _____.   left

If the Vector is pointing upward, then the QRS in
lead AVF is mainly _____ the baseline.   below

And when the Vector points upward and to the patient's left,
this is Left _____ Deviation (L.A.D.).   Axis

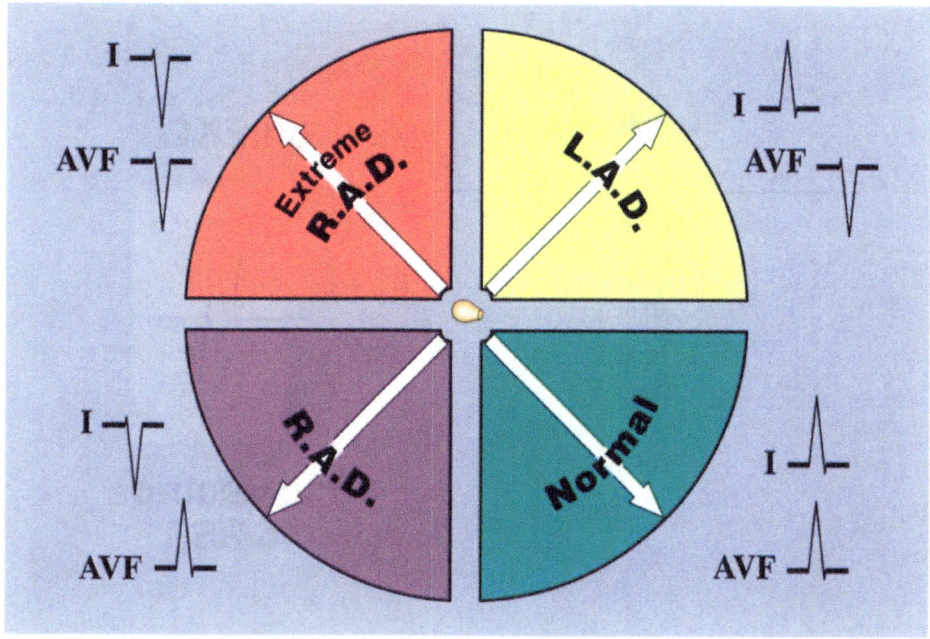

Now, by looking at the QRS complex in I and AVF, you can locate the Mean QRS Vector in an Axis quadrant (in the frontal plane as it relates to the patient).

Any time the QRS complex is negative in lead I, there is
_____ Axis Deviation (R.A.D.); and when the Vector   Right
also points upward (and to the patient's right), this is commonly
called "Extreme" R.A.D.

But if the QRS is positive in lead I and negative in lead AVF,
there is Left Axis _____.   Deviation

So if the Mean QRS Vector points downward and to the patient's left,
we expect the QRS complexes in leads I and AVF to be
mainly _____ (upright). And of course, they usually are,   positive
since this is normal.

Note: You also can calculate the vector for a portion of a QRS complex
(for instance, the initial or terminal .04 sec.) in exactly the same
manner as for the Mean QRS Vector.

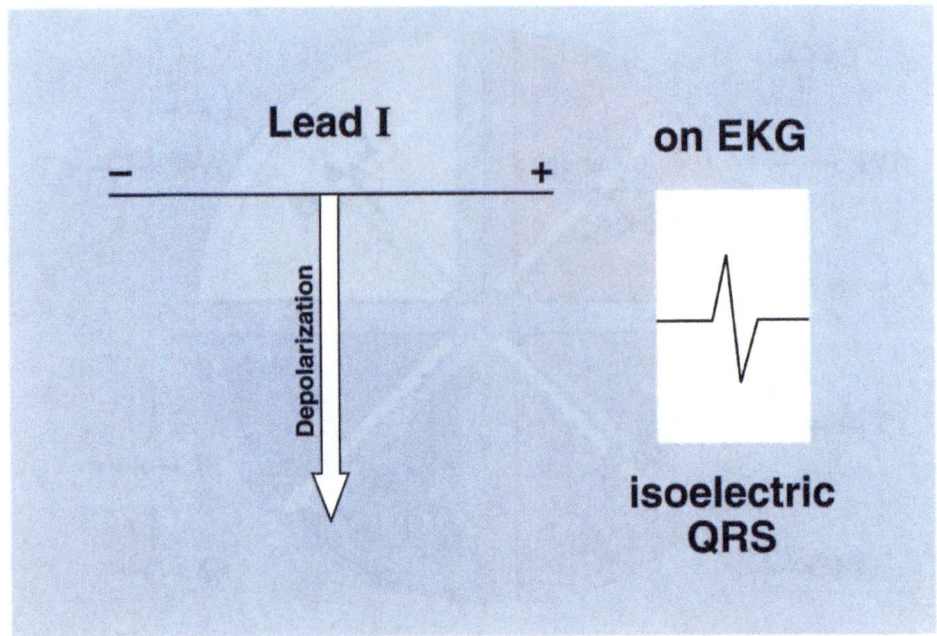

When depolarization moves in a direction perpendicular to the orientation of a lead, the deflection is minimal and/or "isoelectric." An isoelectric QRS records equal magnitudes of upward (positive) and negative (downward) deflection.

Depolarization that moves perpendicular to the orientation of a lead, is directed negligibly toward either electrode, so the recorded deflection is as much negative as positive and is called _____.   isoelectric

The word "isoelectric" literally means "same voltage," so it is used when the positive and the negative portions of the QRS complex are about _____.   equal

Although the positive and negative deflections of an isoelectric QRS are equal in amplitude, they are generally small in the limb _____.   leads

Note: First, locate the Mean QRS Vector in an axis quadrant (i.e., Normal, L.A.D., R.A.D., or Extreme R.A.D.). Then, find the limb lead in which the QRS is the most isoelectric, so you can more precisely locate the Vector in degrees (Axis). The Axis is about 90° from the orientation of the most isoelectric lead. It is really very easy... next page.

Left Axis Deviation

most isoelectric	Axis
I	-90°
AVR	-60°
II	-30°
AVF	0°

Normal Range

most isoelectric	Axis
AVF	0°
III	+30°
AVL	+60°
I	+90°

To locate the position of the Vector (Axis) more precisely (i.e., in degrees) in the frontal plane: first locate the axis quadrant, and then note the limb lead in which the QRS is most isoelectric.

Note: Please refer to the illustration on this page (and the page that follows) to determine the exact position of the Mean QRS Vector (Axis) in degrees. For exams and in "real life" situations you need a reference. Accuracy is far more important than memory. You may copy page 340; it's yours for real life use.

Note: Let's review. First, locate the appropriate axis quadrant. Then, to determine the exact position of the Vector (Axis), find the lead where the QRS is most isoelectric. Refer to the illustration as you contemplate the hypothetical examples below.

A patient with Left Axis Deviation has a Mean QRS Vector of between 0 and ____ degrees (QRS positive in I and negative in AVF). Check the illustration.

-90
(don't forget the negative)

A young lady has a Mean QRS Vector in the normal range. If the QRS in lead III is isoelectric, then she has an electrical axis of ____. Please don't proceed to the next page until you feel comfortable with this exercise.

+30°

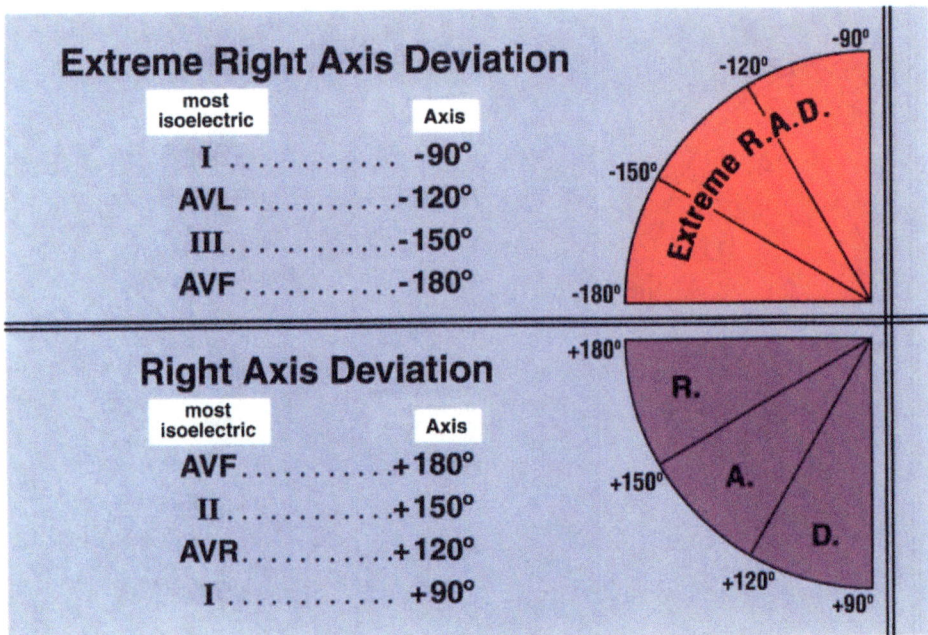

The exact position of the Vector (Axis) can be located in a similar way for Right Axis Deviation and Extreme Right Axis Deviation. Refer back to the illustration for each sentence below.

Note: After the axis quadrant is determined, the limb lead with the most isoelectric QRS is noted.*

Consider a patient with R.A.D. You find that the QRS is isoelectric in lead II, so the Axis is ____.   +150°

You have a patient with numerous widened, premature QRS's, and you need to know whether it is a PVC or an aberrant Junctional beat. The wide QRS is negative in I and AVF, which places its Vector in the Extreme ____ quadrant (how could that be?)...   R.A.D.

... the wide QRS is also isoelectric in AVL, so its Axis is ____. For ventricular depolarization to progress in that direction,   -120°
it must have originated in a focus (or pacemaker electrode) at the apex of the left ventricle, rather than from a Junctional focus. Let's think about that.

Note: An Axis of 180° is either + or - depending on whether the Vector is in the R.A.D. or Extreme R.A.D. quadrant respectively.

* This is summarized for you (page 340) of your Personal Quick Reference Sheet.

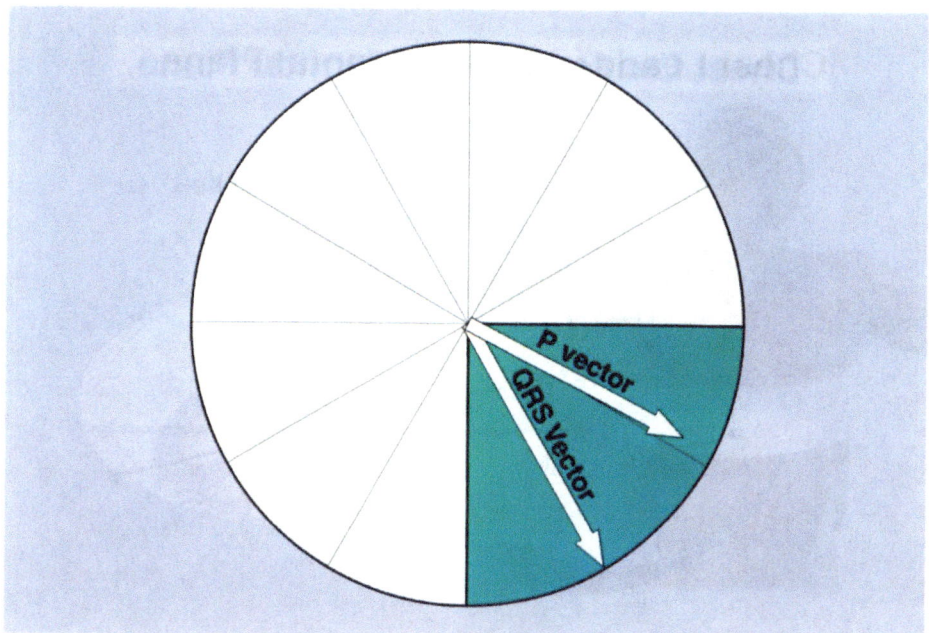

The Mean QRS Vector, which represents normal biventricular depolarization, points downward and to the patient's left. The P wave vector, which represents normal biatrial depolarization, points downward to the left side of the patient.

A vector is used to represent the general direction of depolarization. When depolarization (a wave of positive charges) moves toward a positive electrode, it records _____-ly (upward) on the EKG.   positive

Note: The P wave vector points generally downward, toward the positive electrode on the patient's left foot (for *inferior* leads II, III, and AVF), so the P waves are usually upright in those leads. The P wave vector also points leftward, toward the positive electrode on the patient's left arm (for leads I, and AVL), producing generally upright P waves in those leads. So, if we see an inverted "P wave" in any of those leads, it is probably a P' depolarizing upwards from a low atrial focus, or retrograde atrial depolarization moving upward from the AV Node.

Note: Most PVC's emanate from a peripheral focus in a ventricular wall, depolarizing the ventricles in a general bottom upward direction, so they are usually mostly negative in the *inferior* and *lateral* limb leads where the QRS is usually upward. Exception: PVC's that are mainly upward like the QRS's in those leads, probably originate in a septal ventricular focus and follow a near-normal path.

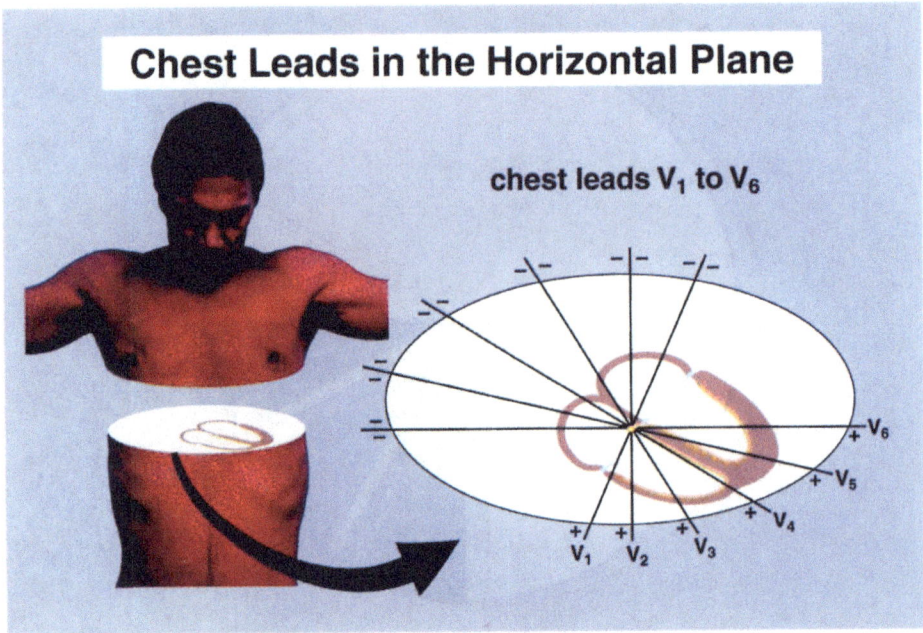

The sphere has three dimensions, so it is important to note the general position of the Mean QRS Vector in the *horizontal* plane as well.

The horizontal _____ divides the body into top   plane
and bottom halves.

The chest leads form the _____ plane.   horizontal

Note: To determine changes ("rotation") of the Mean QRS Vector in the horizontal plane, we examine the chest leads.

Note: Although the Axis may "deviate" in the frontal plane, the Vector is said to "rotate" in the horizontal plane. This is conventional (universally accepted) terminology used in communication and in medical literature.

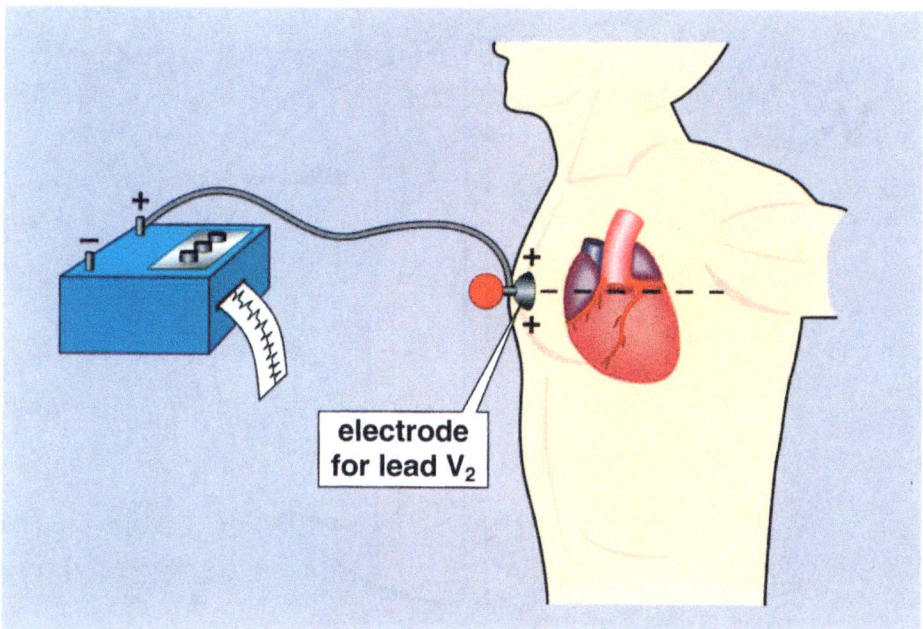

electrode
for lead V$_2$

Chest lead V$_2$ is obtained by placing a positive electrode on the chest along the left side of the sternum (at the fourth interspace).

The chest electrode used for recording lead V$_2$ is always _____ (positive or negative).   positive

Note: The electrode for the chest leads is a suction cup that is moved to a different position on the chest for each of the six chest leads (which form the horizontal plane). In each case, the suction cup electrode is positive.

The position of the (suction cup) electrode for recording lead V$_2$ places it in front of the heart, at the fourth interspace to the left of the sternum, so it is just _____ to the AV Node.   anterior

Note: We already know that metal electrodes affixed with conductive gel are often used for recording the chest leads, so let's refocus on the conceptual material.

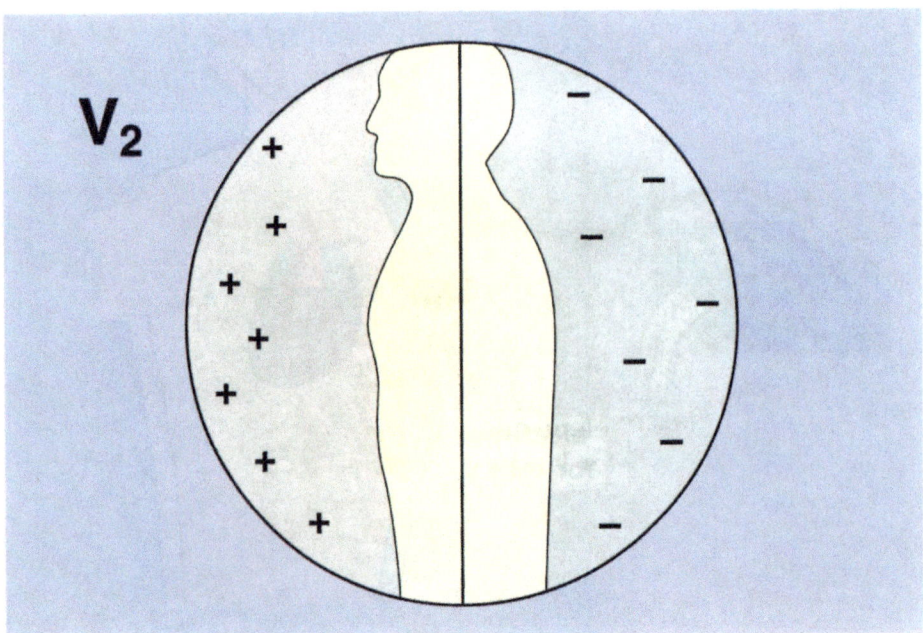

Considering the sphere for lead V_2 we can see that the front half is positive and the back half is negative.

Considering a lead V_2 sphere, we view the patient from the side. The center of the _____ is still the AV Node.

sphere

The patient's back is _____ (negative or positive), when considering lead V_2.

negative

The front half of the sphere is _____ in lead V_2.

positive

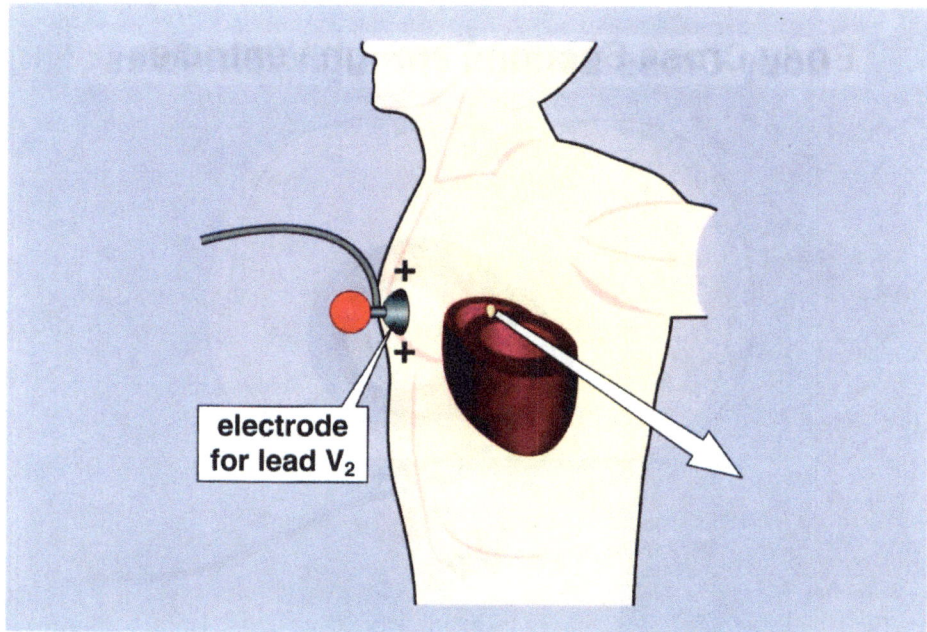

Normally the QRS in lead V_2 is negative. Therefore, the Mean QRS Vector points backward, because of the (generally) posterior position of the thick left ventricle.

Considering lead V_2 on the standard EKG, the QRS complex is usually _____ (below the baseline).

negative

Therefore, the Mean QRS Vector usually points _____ into the negative half of the sphere.

backward
(posteriorly)

Normally, most of the ventricular depolarization moves away from the positive V_2 electrode, toward the thicker and more posteriorly positioned _____ ventricle.

left

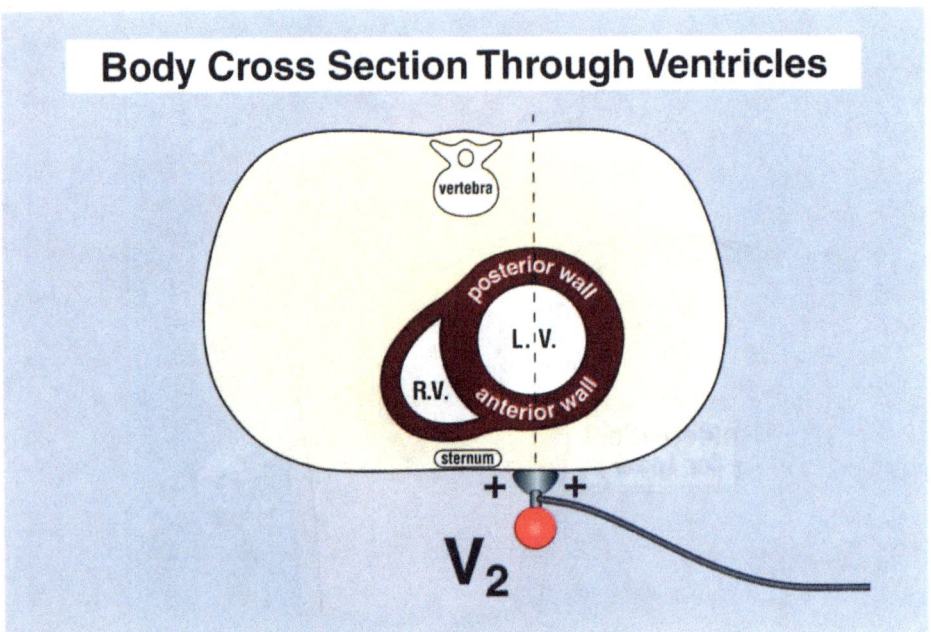

The orientation of chest lead V_2 makes it the most informative lead for the
determination of both Anterior and Posterior Infarction.

The orientation of lead V_2 projects through the anterior wall
and the posterior wall of the _____ventricle.   left

So V_2 reflects the most reliable information concerning Anterior
Infarction and _____ Infarction of the left ventricle.   Posterior

Note: As you will soon see, both ventricular depolarization and
repolarization should be scrutinized in the right chest leads, because
they reveal subtle vector changes caused by both anterior and posterior
infarctions (of the left ventricle).

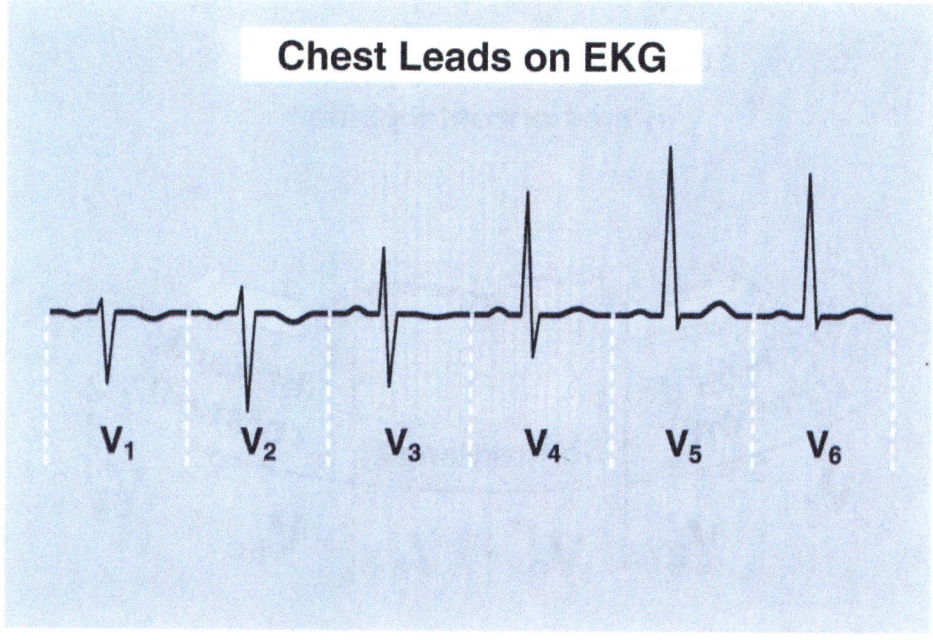

Chest Leads on EKG

V_1 V_2 V_3 V_4 V_5 V_6

In the chest leads, there is a gradual transition from the generally negative QRS in V_1 to the generally positive (upright) QRS in V_6.

The QRS is mainly negative in lead V_1 and mostly _____ in lead V_6.

positive

Examining chest leads V_1 through V_6 to observe the gradual transition of QRS complexes, we notice that the QRS usually becomes as much positive as negative or "_____" in lead V_3 or V_4. This is the *transitional zone*.

isoelectric

Note: You will recall that an isoelectric QRS is 90° away from the Mean QRS Vector. So a shift ("rotation") of the Vector in the horizontal plane is reflected as a similar change in position of the "transitional" (isoelectric) QRS in the chest leads. You will better understand and appreciate this, when you see the next page.

As the Vector changes its position (rotates) in the horizontal plane, the Vector's tail remains anchored to the ___ _____.

AV Node

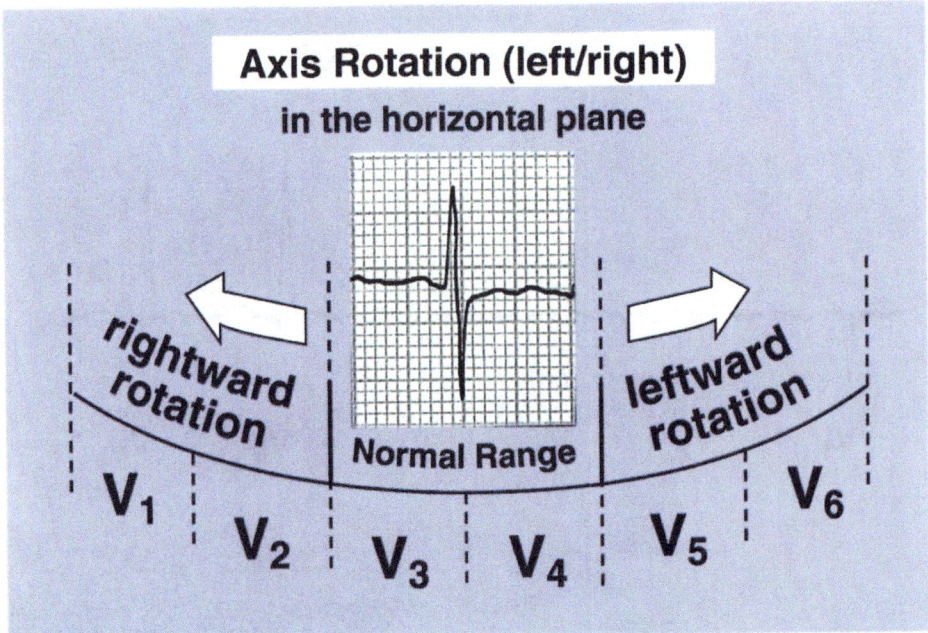

Rotation of the Vector in the horizontal plane is described from the patient's point of view as "rightward" or "leftward." Check the chest leads for the isoelectric QRS.

Note: The Vector can *rotate* in the horizontal plane with its tail anchored to the AV Node. When the isoelectric ("transitional") QRS has rotated to the patient's right (into leads V_1 or V_2) this is *rightward* rotation. But if the transitional QRS is found in the patient's left chest leads, V_5 or V_6 this is *leftward* rotation. Anatomically speaking the heart is not capable of much rotation in the horizontal plane. But, we know that the Vector shifts toward Ventricular Hypertrophy and away from Infarction.

Note: In older literature you may still see the terms "clockwise" (meaning leftward) rotation or "counterclockwise" (meaning rightward) rotation of the Vector in the horizontal plane. These terms have become obsolete since they do not relate well to clocks, and much confusion resulted.

Reminder: Axis deviation is in the frontal plane.
              Axis rotation is in the horizontal plane.

Note: Please observe the simplified technique for determining *Axis* by turning to page 340. A quick review of the methodology may be found in the **Personal Quick Reference Sheets** on page 334.

Chapter 8: Hypertrophy

Before you begin, look at this chapter's summary on pages 334 and 341.

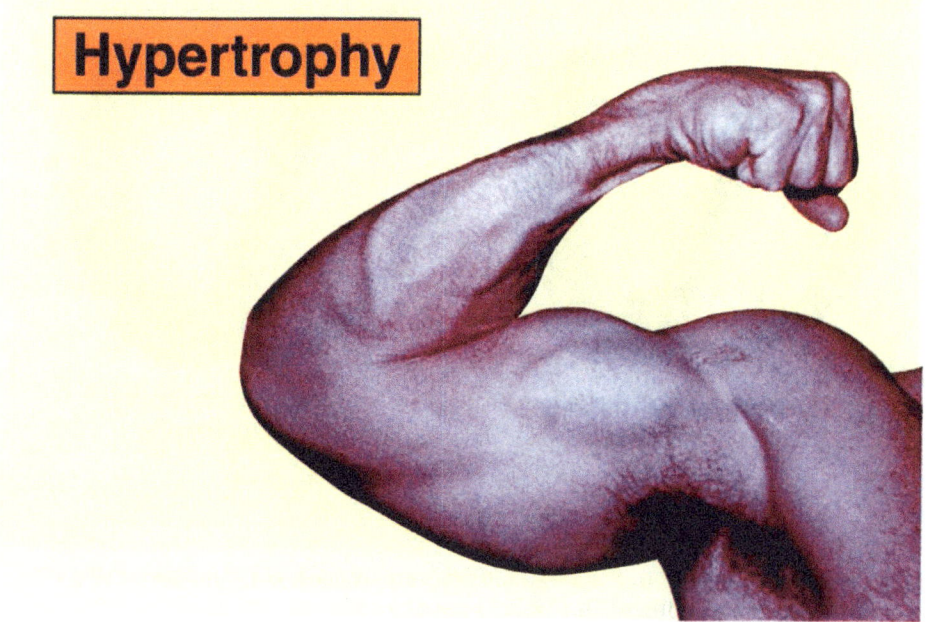

Hypertrophy

Hypertrophy usually pertains to an increase in size, but when relating to muscle as in myocardium, this term refers to increase in muscle mass.

Note: The photo above is the arm of a weight-lifter. I had contemplated using a photo of my own arm, but I soon abandoned the idea because then I would have to title this section "hypotrophy" (if there is such a word).

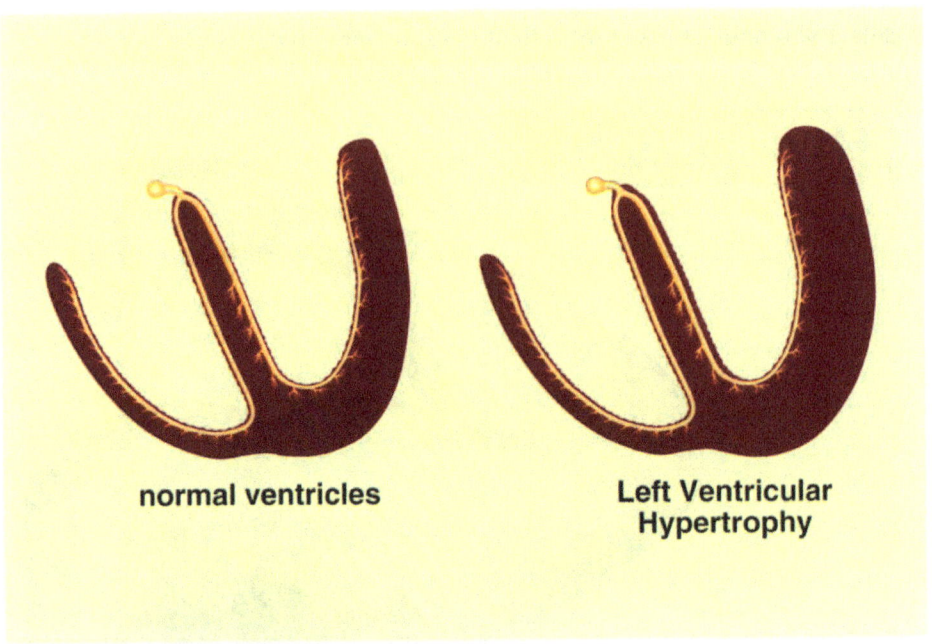

normal ventricles   **Left Ventricular
                                          Hypertrophy**

Hypertrophy of a chamber of the heart implies an increase in the thickness of the
chamber wall, but some dilation is always present also.

Hypertrophy of a chamber of the heart means that the
muscular wall of that chamber has dilated and thickened
beyond _____ thickness.   normal

Hypertrophy may increase the volume that the
_____ contains, and the wall of that chamber   chamber
is thicker than normal.

The increase in the muscular thickness of the wall of
a hypertrophic chamber, as well as dilation of a chamber
of the heart may be diagnosed on _____.   EKG

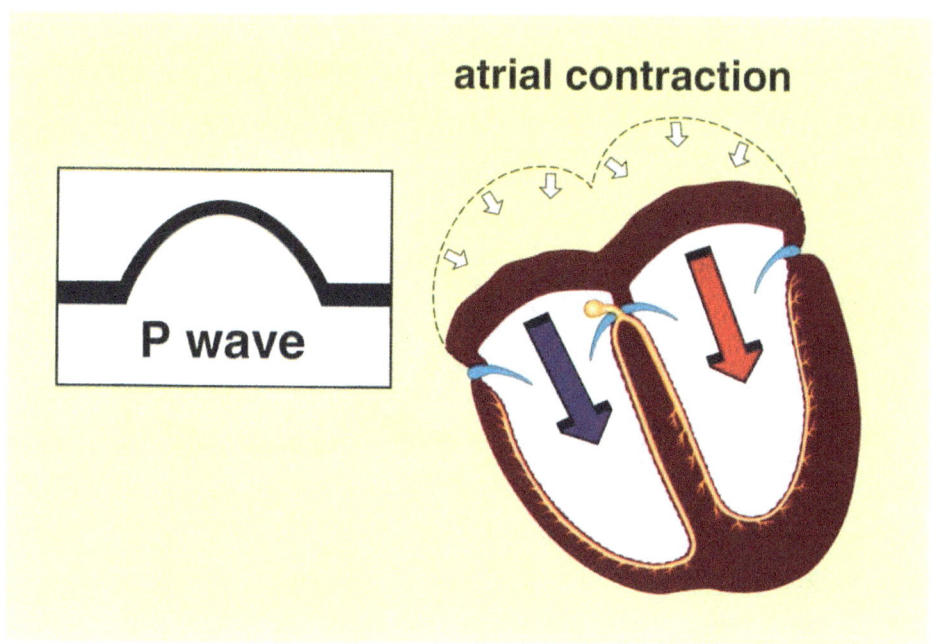

Since the P wave represents the depolarization and contraction of both atria, we examine the P wave for evidence of atrial enlargement. (See Note.)

The depolarization of both atria causes their
simultaneous _____.   contraction

The depolarization of both atria is recorded on
EKG as a ___ wave.   P

Signs of atrial enlargement can be detected by examining
the P wave on the twelve lead _____.   EKG

Note: Although the designation "atrial hypertrophy" is commonly used, enlargement of an atrium is usually due to dilation of the atrium. Therefore, the general term *atrial enlargement* is preferred, since it includes both dilation and hypertrophy. Whereas when referring to the ventricles, "ventricular hypertrophy" predominates.

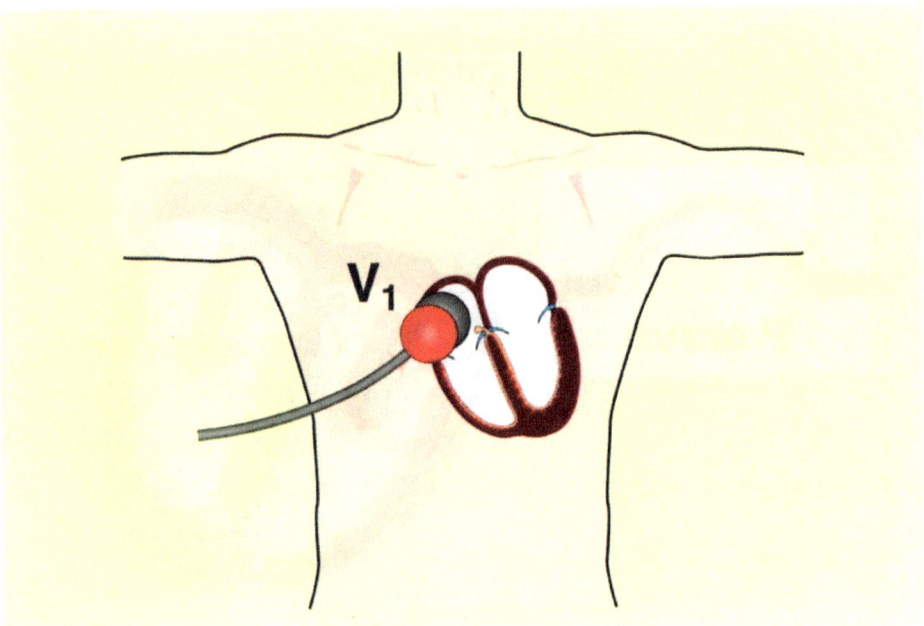

Lead V_1 is directly over the atria, so the P wave in V_1 is our best source of information about atrial enlargement.

The chest electrode that records lead V_1 is considered
_____ (positive or negative).   positive

When lead V_1 is recording, the electrode is positioned just
to the right of the sternum in the 4th interspace; this places
the electrode directly over the _____.   atria

Because the V_1 electrode is close to the atria, the
P wave in lead V_1 gives us the most accurate information
about atrial _____.   enlargement

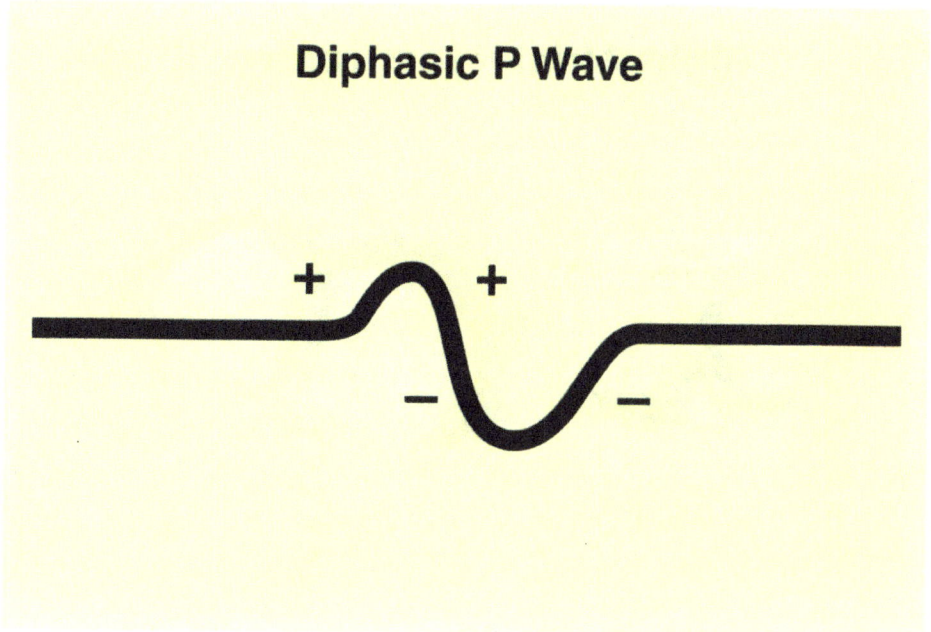

Diphasic P Wave

With atrial enlargement, the P wave is usually *diphasic* (both positive and negative).

A wave that has both positive and negative portions is
called a _____ wave (two phased wave).   diphasic

A diphasic P wave has deflections above and
below the _____.   baseline

The diphasic P wave is characteristic of atrial enlargement,
but we want to know which of the two _____ is enlarged.   atria

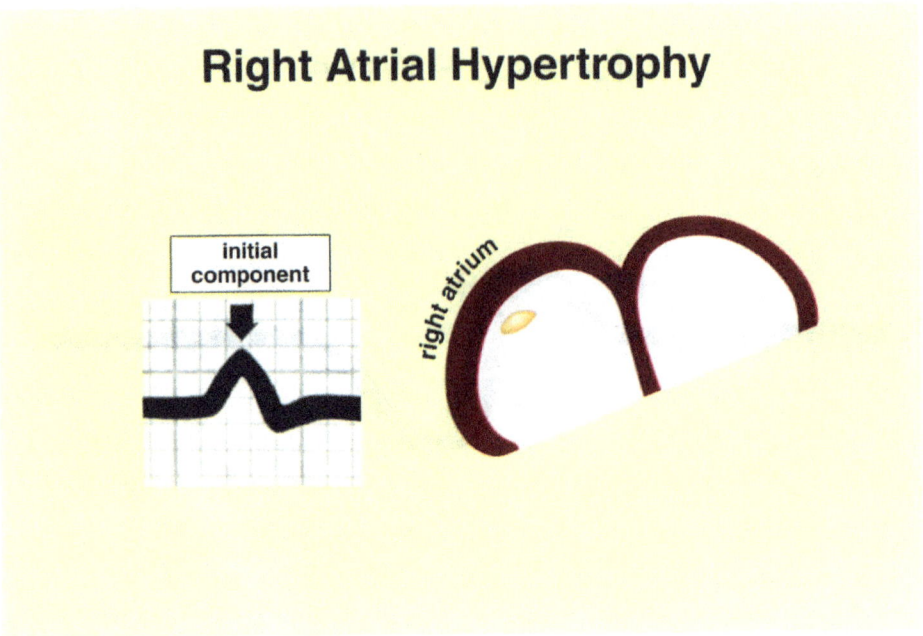

If the initial component of a diphasic P wave (in lead V_1) is the larger, then this is *Right Atrial Enlargement.*

If the P wave in lead V_1 is _____, then we know that one of the atria is enlarged.   diphasic

If the initial portion of the diphasic P wave is the _____ of the two phases, then there is Right Atrial Enlargement.   larger

A diphasic P wave in V_1 with a large, often peaked, initial component tells us that this patient's _____ atrium is probably thicker and more dilated than the left.   right

Note: If the height of the P wave in any of the limb leads exceeds 2.5 mm (even if it's not diphasic), suspect Right Atrial Enlargement.

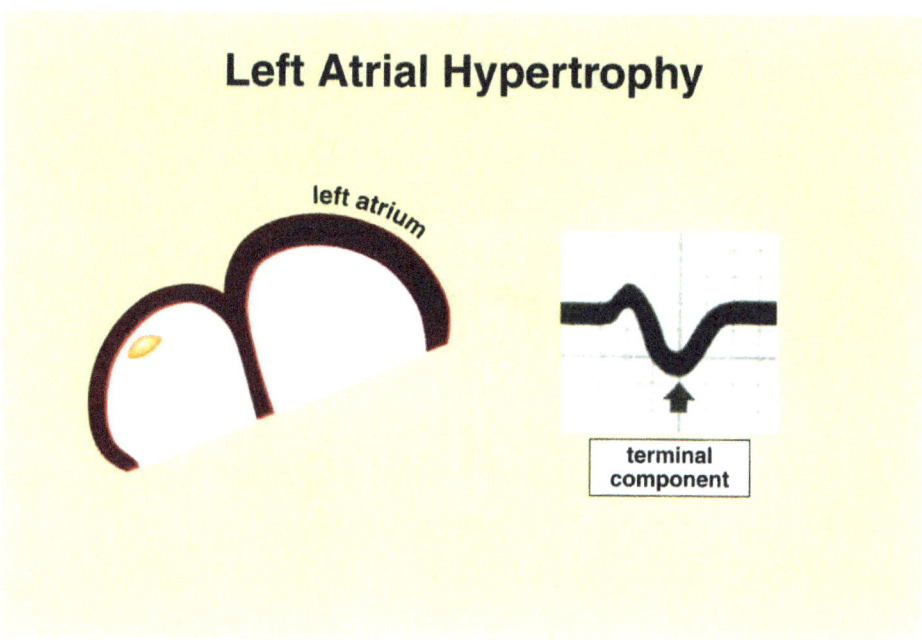

Left Atrial Hypertrophy

left atrium

terminal
component

If the terminal portion of a diphasic P wave in V_1 is large and wide, there is
Left Atrial Enlargement.

A patient who has enlargement of the left atrium,
because the mitral valve is stenosed*, will have
a diphasic P wave in lead ___. V_1

This patient's diphasic P wave in lead V_1 has a small initial
component and a larger _____ component.   terminal

The terminal component of a diphasic P wave in lead V_1
is usually _____ (positive or negative).   negative

* *Mitral stenosis* (narrowed mitral valve opening) can cause left atrial enlargement,
  but systemic hypertension is the most common cause.

Normal QRS in Lead V₁

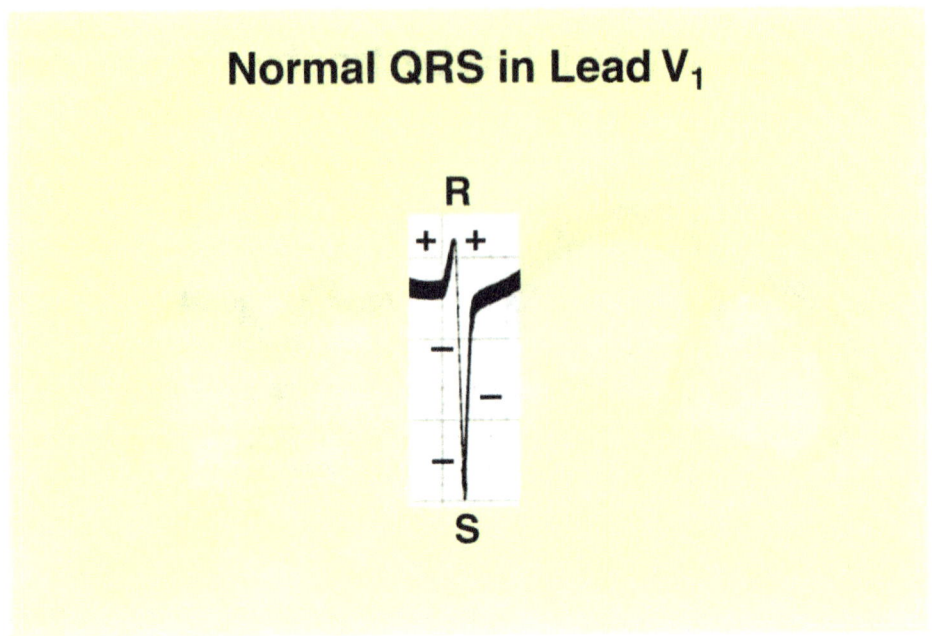

Now let's consider the QRS complex in V_1. Normally the S wave is much larger than the R wave in this lead.

The QRS complex represents ventricular depolarization, so we would expect the QRS to reflect the presence of ventricular _____.

hypertrophy

In lead V_1 the QRS complex is mainly _____, and therefore the R wave is usually very short.

negative

Note: The V_1 electrode is positive. Ventricular depolarization moves downward to the patient's left side and also posteriorly (the thicker left ventricle is more posteriorly located). Because ventricular depolarization is moving away from the (positive) V_1 electrode, the QRS in V_1 is usually mainly negative. Remember that the positive wave of depolarization moving toward a positive electrode records a positive deflection on EKG. By the same token, depolarization moving away from a positive electrode records negatively.

Right Ventricular Hypertrophy

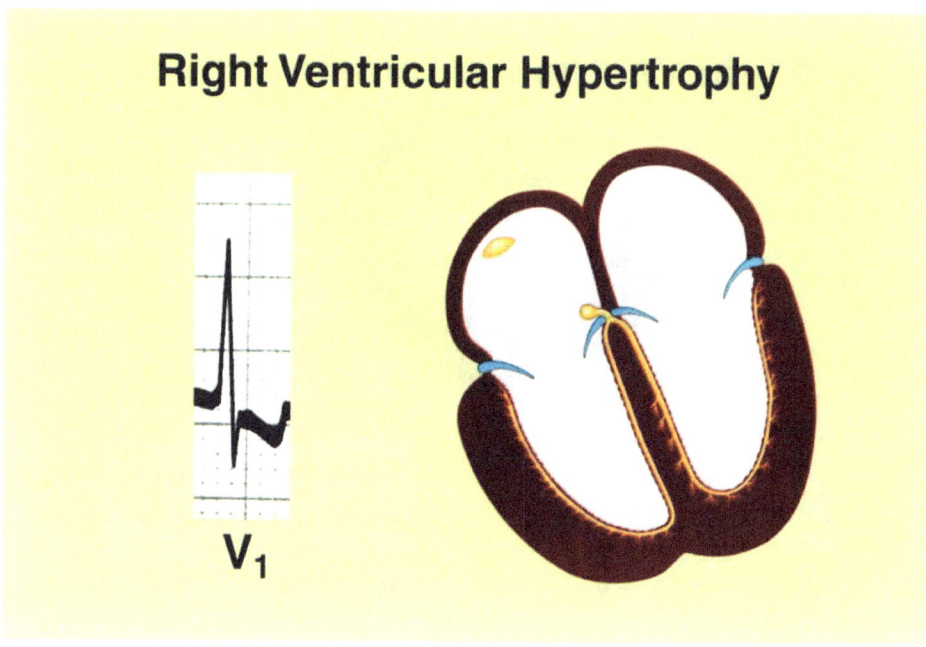

V_1

However, with *Right Ventricular Hypertrophy* (RVH) there is a large R wave in V_1.

In Right Ventricular Hypertrophy there is a large ___   R
wave in lead V_1.

Note: With Right Ventricular Hypertrophy, the wall of the right
ventricle is very thick, so there is much more (positive) depolarization
(and more vectors) toward the positive V_1 electrode. We would
therefore expect the QRS in lead V_1 to be more positive (taller)
than usual.

The S wave in lead V_1 is smaller than the ___ wave   R
in Right Ventricular Hypertrophy. (See illustration).

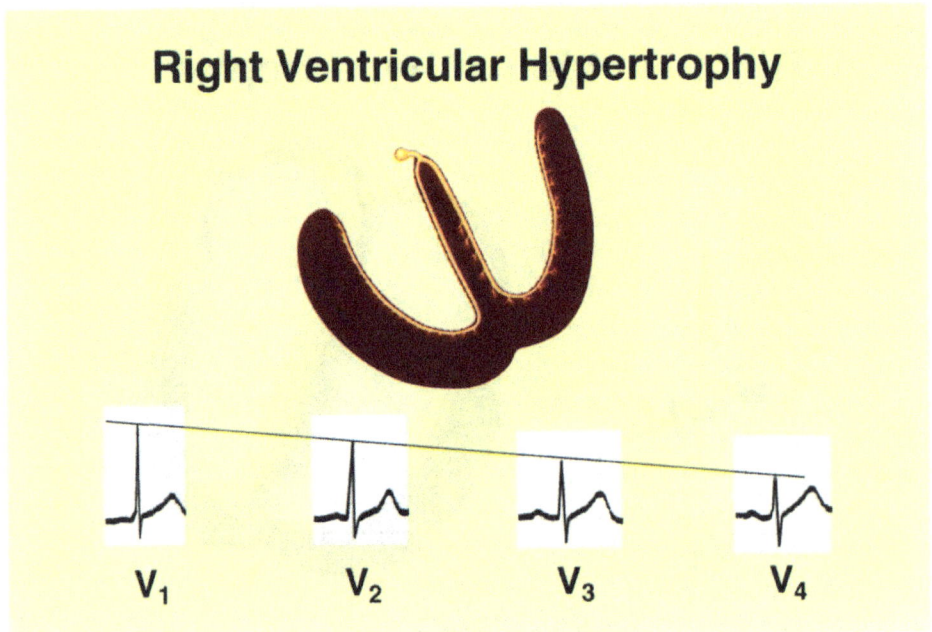

Right Ventricular Hypertrophy

V₁   V₂   V₃   V₄

With Right Ventricular Hypertrophy, the large R wave of V_1 gets progressively smaller from V_2 to V_3 to V_4 etc.

When Right Ventricular Hypertrophy is present, there is a large R wave in lead ___ that becomes progressively smaller in chest leads V_2, V_3, and V_4.

V_1

The progressive decrease in the height of the ___ wave is gradual, proceeding from the right chest leads to the left chest leads.

R

Note: The enlarged right ventricle adds more vectors toward the right side, so there is Right Axis Deviation (in the frontal plane), and in the horizontal plane there is rightward rotation of the (Mean QRS) Vector. Visualize the reasons for these (Mean QRS) Vector shifts and the criteria will become very logical.

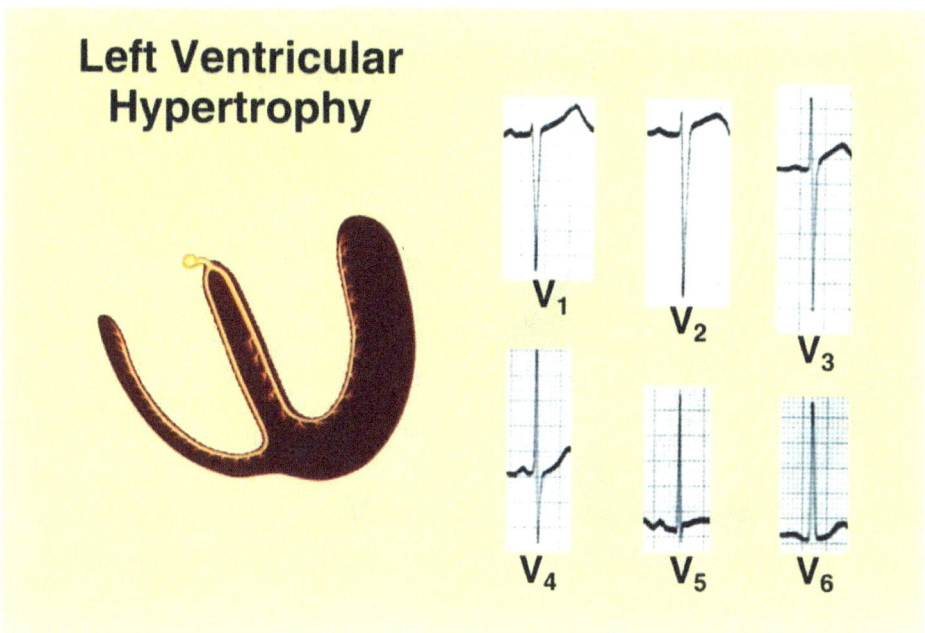

Left Ventricular Hypertrophy

With *Left Ventricular Hypertrophy* (LVH), the left ventricular wall is very thick, causing great QRS deflections in the chest leads.

The heart chamber with the thickest muscular walls is the _____ ventricle.

left

Hypertrophy of the left ventricle produces QRS complexes that are exaggerated amplitude, both in height and in depth, especially in the _____ leads.

chest

Note: Normally the S wave in V_1 is deep. But with Left Ventricular Hypertrophy, even more depolarization is going downward to the patient's left – away from the positive V_1 electrode. Therefore, the S wave is even deeper in V_1. There is Left Axis Deviation, and often the Vector is displaced in a leftward direction in the horizontal plane. Visualize and understand the reason for these shifts of the Vector. Lasting knowledge results from understanding.

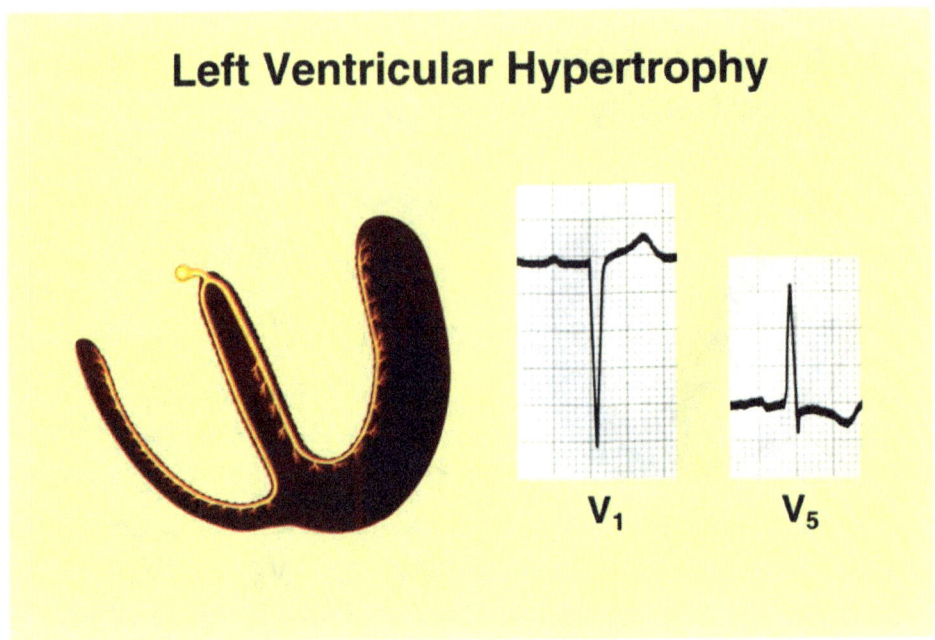

Left Ventricular Hypertrophy

V₁   V₅

With Left Ventricular Hypertrophy there is a large S in V$_1$ and a large R in V$_5$.

With Left Ventricular Hypertrophy there is a very tall ____
wave in lead V$_5$.

R

Note: Lead V$_5$ is over the left ventricle, so the increased depolarization is going toward the electrode of V$_5$ when there is L.V.H. This results in more (positive) depolarization going toward the (positive) electrode of V$_5$ which produces a very tall R wave in that lead.

In Left Ventricular Hypertrophy, there is a very tall R wave
in lead ____, and this excessive depolarization moving away
from the V$_1$ electrode produces a deep S wave in lead V$_1$.

V$_5$

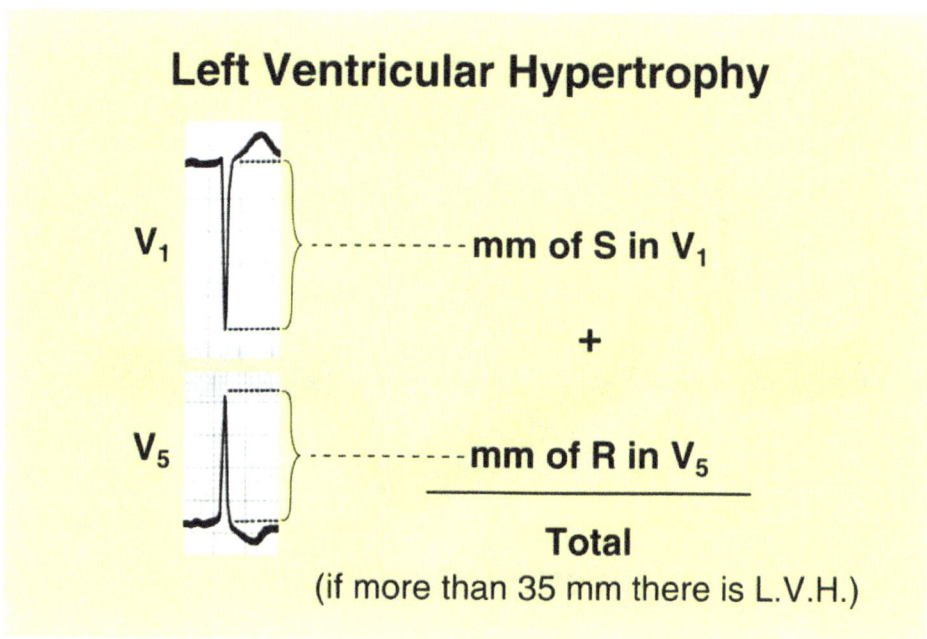

Left Ventricular Hypertrophy

V₁ ·············· **mm of S in V₁**

+

V₅ ·············· **mm of R in V₅**

Total

(if more than 35 mm there is L.V.H.)

Depth (in mm) of S in V_1 plus the height of R in V_5... if greater than 35 mm, there is Left Ventricular Hypertrophy.

To check an EKG for Left Ventricular Hypertrophy, just add the depth of the S wave in V_1 to the height of the____ wave in V_5.   R

If the depth (in mm) of the S wave in V_1 added to the height (in mm) of the R wave in V_5 is greater than 35 (mm), then _____ Ventricular Hypertrophy is present.   Left

Note: The sum of the S in V_1 plus the R in V_5 should be routinely checked (mere observation will usually suffice) with every twelve lead EKG. When providing a written EKG interpretation, however, one should measure and document the amplitude of these waves in millimeters.

Left Chest Leads in LVH

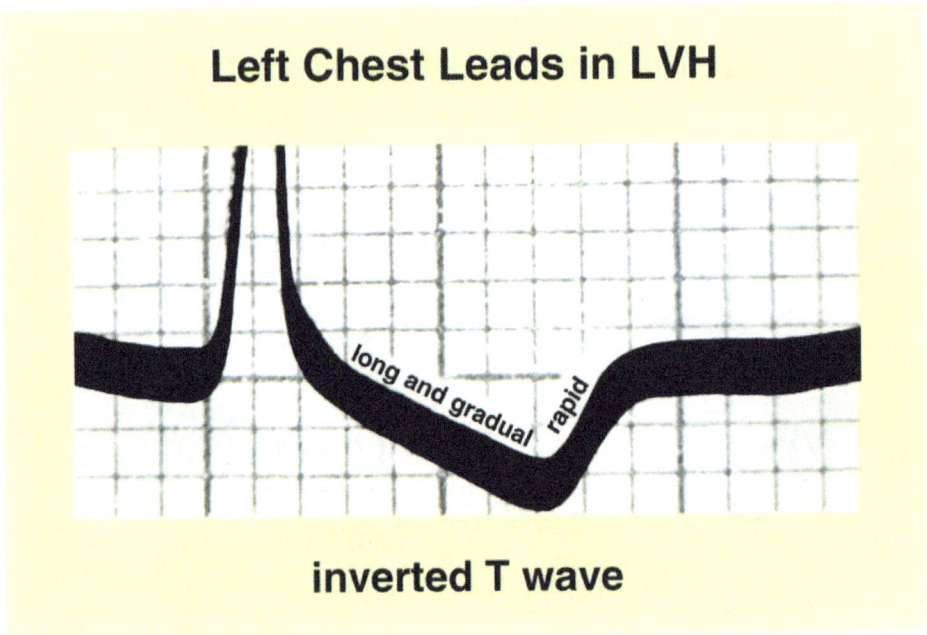

long and gradual rapid

inverted T wave

The T wave may show "Left Ventricular Hypertrophy" characteristics. Often there is T wave *inversion* with T wave *asymmetry*.

There is a characteristic T wave that is commonly associated with _____ Ventricular Hypertrophy.

Left

Since the left chest leads (V_5 or V_6) are over the left _____, these are ideal leads to check for this characteristic T wave that we find with LVH.

ventricle

With LVH, the *inverted* T wave has a gradual downslope (often including the ST segment) and a very steep return to the _____, making it *asymmetrical*.

baseline

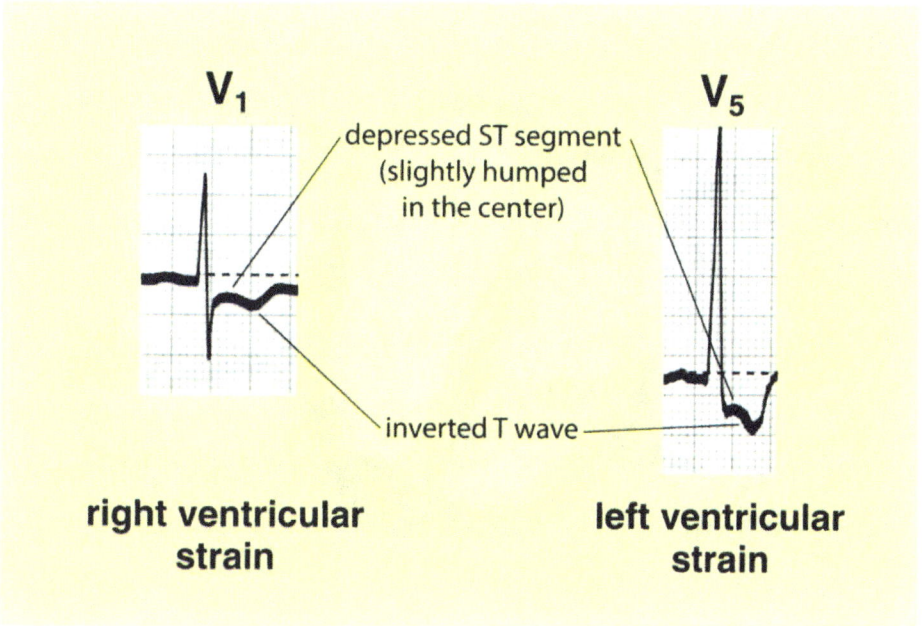

Ventricular hypertrophy may be associated with a *strain* pattern. With *ventricular strain*, the ST segment becomes depressed and the mid-portion of ST segment is slightly humped upward. Also, the T wave is usually inverted.

Ventricular strain is characterized by T wave inversion
with depression of the ST _____.   segment

Note: Strain is usually associated with ventricular hypertrophy, which is logical, since a ventricle that is straining against some kind of resistance (e.g., increased resistance from a narrowed valve or from hypertension) will become hypertrophied in its attempt to compensate.

Ventricular strain depresses the ST segment, which generally
humps upward in the middle of the _____.   segment

Note: As you will soon see, T wave inversion is characteristic of ischemia (page 264).

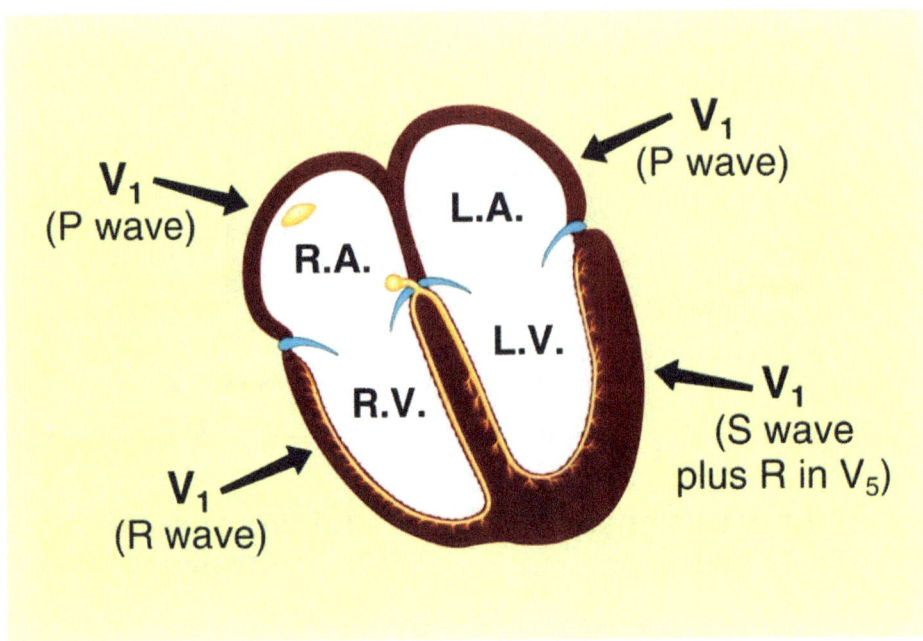

Note that lead V_1 provides most of the information concerning hypertrophy of the heart's chambers.

When routinely reading a 12 lead EKG, you should check
to see if there is _____ of any of the chambers.   hypertrophy

First, check lead V_1 to see if the P waves are _____.   diphasic

Second, check the R wave in V_1... and then check
the S wave in V_1 and the ___ wave in V_5.   R

Note: You may now review *Hypertrophy* by turning to the **Personal
Quick Reference Sheets** on page 341 and relate this to the simplified
methodology that is summarized on page 334.

Chapter 9: Infarction (includes Hemiblock)

Before you begin, look at this chapter's summary on pages 334, 342, and 343.

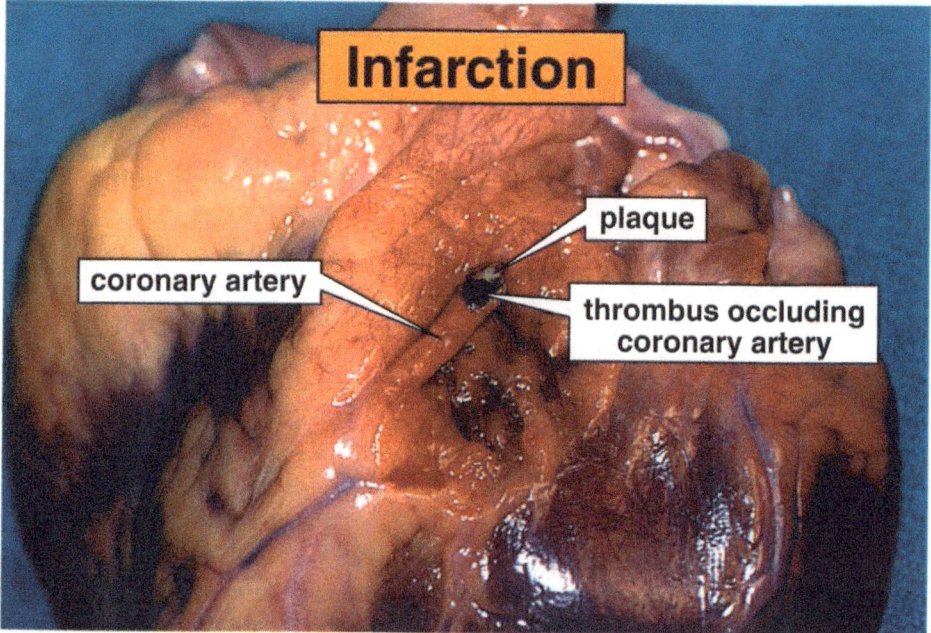

Infarction

plaque

coronary artery

thrombus occluding coronary artery

Myocardial Infarction (M.I.) results from the complete occlusion of a coronary artery. The infarcted area of myocardium becomes *necrotic* (dead), so it can't depolarize or contract.

Note: Although the heart's chambers are filled with blood, the myocardium's own blood supply is provided exclusively by the coronary arteries. A coronary artery can be gradually narrowed by lipid deposits that become *atheromatous plaque* beneath the *intima* lining of the vessel. The intima may eventually rupture, exposing the plaque to the blood within the artery. This initiates the immediate formation of a clot (*thrombus*). The vessel, already narrowed by the plaque, becomes totally occluded by the thrombus. Instantly the infarcted area of the ventricle (without a blood supply) becomes necrotic. Ventricular foci in the hypoxic area around the infarct become very irritable; this can produce deadly ventricular arrhythmias.

Note: Myocardial Infarction implies the complete occlusion of a coronary artery, which we can diagnose with the EKG. The electrocardiogram will also tell us which coronary artery (or coronary branch) is occluded, and it can even reveal any blocks in the ventricular conduction caused by the infarction. By careful interpretation of the EKG, we can also determine if a coronary vessel is narrowed, rendering a decreased blood supply to the heart. Practical lifesaving knowledge. Let me show you…

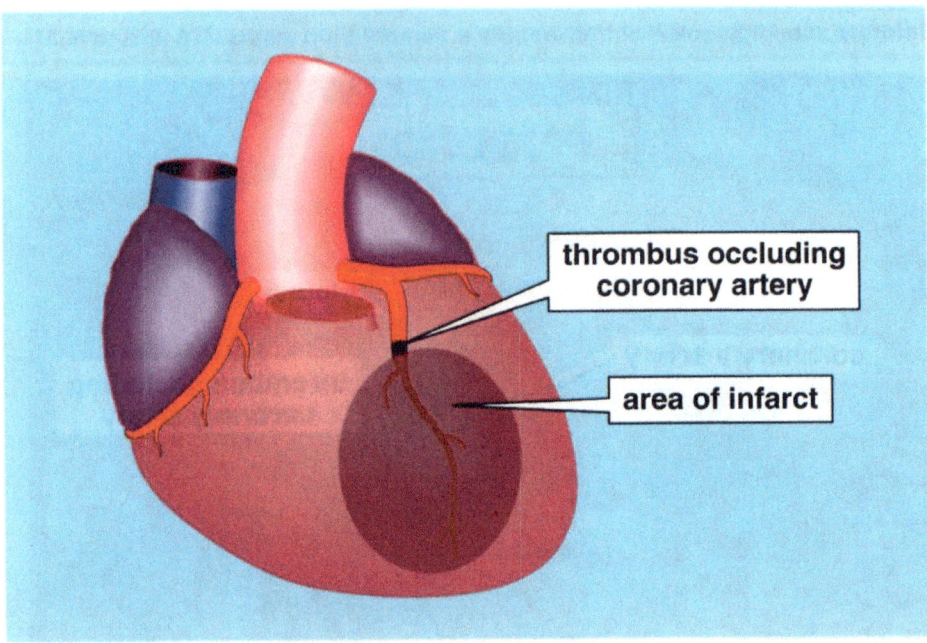

Myocardial infarction is due to the occlusion of a coronary artery supplying the left ventricle, so an area of the heart* is without a blood supply and suffers necrosis.

The terms "myocardial _____," "coronary occlusion,"   infarction
and "heart attack" refer to the same serious problem.

The heart derives its own blood supply from the _____   coronary
arteries, so when a coronary artery or one of its major branches
is occluded, an area of the myocardium is without blood supply.

The infarcted (necrotic) area is primarily in the _____ ventricle;   left
deadly arrhythmias may result.

Note: We understand that the coronary arteries also supply the right
ventricle, so there is often some involvement of the right ventricle. But
since most of the critical problems originate in left ventricular infarcts,
myocardial infarction is usually conceptualized in terms of the left
ventricle.

* In this illustration, the pulmonary artery has been "surgically" removed to show the origin of
  the coronary arteries at the base of the aorta.

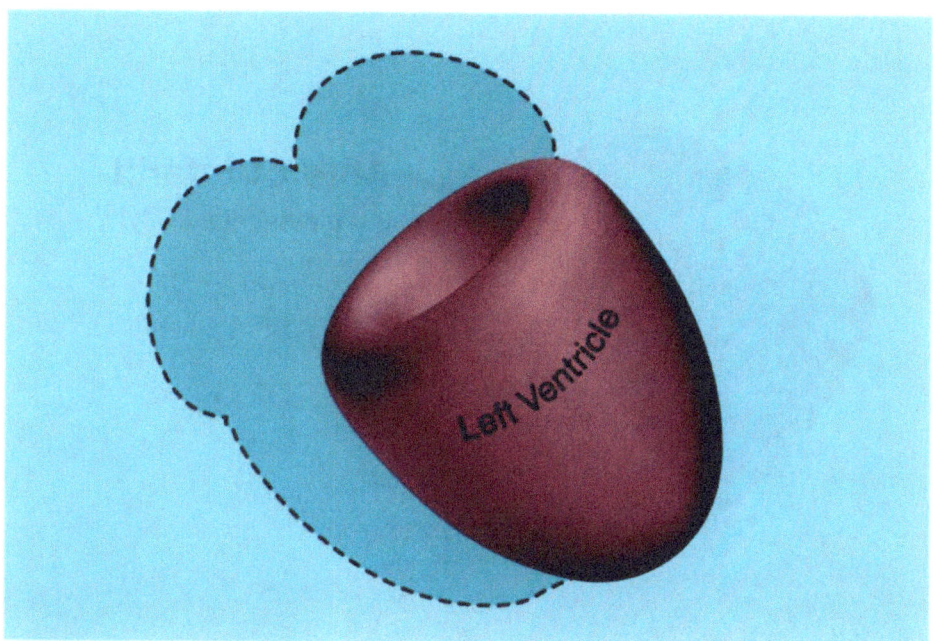

Commonly, it is the thick left ventricle that suffers myocardial infarction.

The left ventricle is the thickest chamber of the heart; so if
the coronary arteries are narrowed, the left ventricle (which
uses the greatest blood supply) is the first to suffer from
an obstructed coronary _____.   artery

Blood is pumped to all parts of the body by the powerful,
thick, _____ ventricle.   left

Note: When we describe infarcts by location, we are speaking of an
area within the left ventricle. Coronary arteries to the left ventricle
usually send smaller branches to other regions of the heart, so an
infarction of the left ventricle can include a small portion of another
chamber.

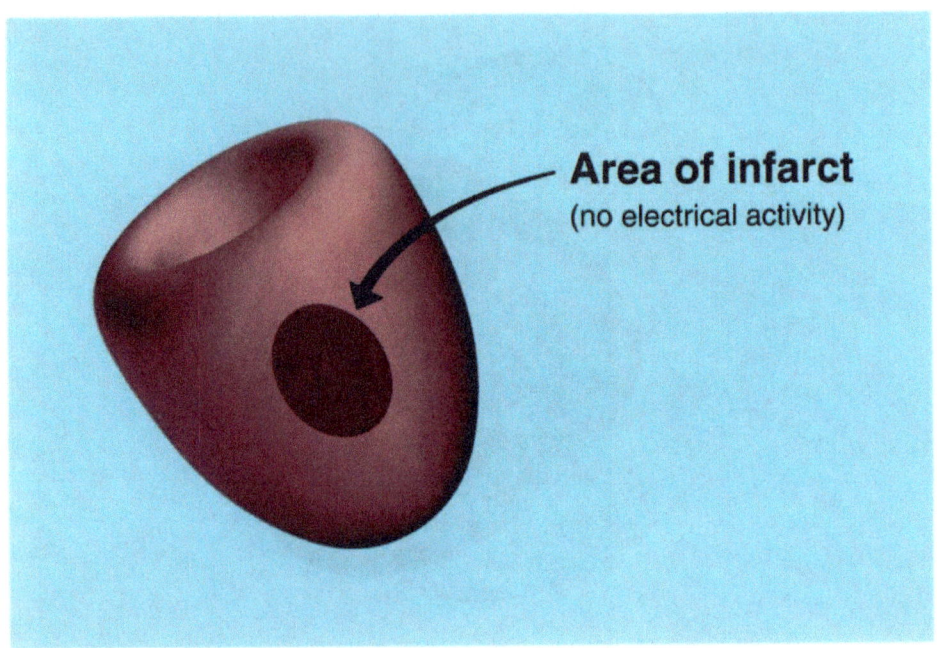

Area of infarct
(no electrical activity)

The necrotic infarcted area of the left ventricle (that has no blood supply) is
electrically dead and cannot depolarize.

Infarctions usually involve an area of the wall of the
left _____.   ventricle

An area of infarction cannot be depolarized because
the cells there are without a _____ supply, so they   blood
are necrotic (functionally dead).

Note: This necrotic infarcted area produces an electrical void, while
the rest of the heart (with an adequate blood supply) functions
as usual. The infarcted region does not depolarize, so it does not
contract, thereby impairing the muscular function of the left ventricle.
Also, hypoxic ventricular foci nearby are often the source of serious
ventricular arrhythmias.

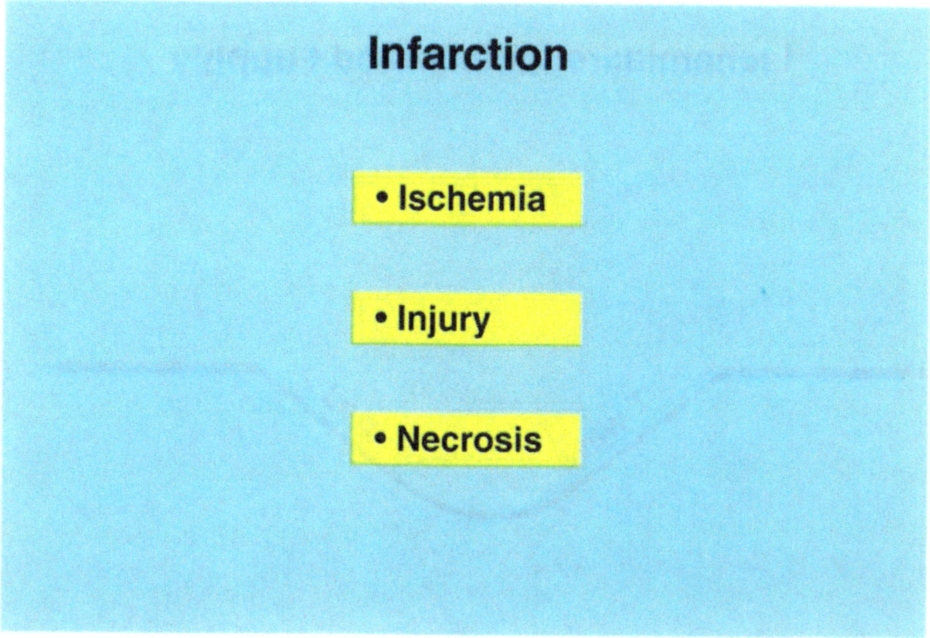

Infarction

• Ischemia

• Injury

• Necrosis

The myocardial infarction triad is "**ischemia**," "**injury**," and "**necrosis**," but any of the three may occur alone.

Note: Necrosis (death) of a ventricular region produces dead myocardial cells that cannot depolarize.

The myocardial infarction triad is the basis for recognizing and diagnosing a _____ infarction.   myocardial

The word *hypoxia* means decreased oxygen; in the heart it is usually caused by *ischemia,* which literally means reduced _____ supply (diminished blood flow).   blood

Note: *Ischemia, injury,* and *necrosis* need not all be present at once in order to establish the diagnosis of myocardial infarction. Routine EKG interpretation requires checking these infarction criteria.

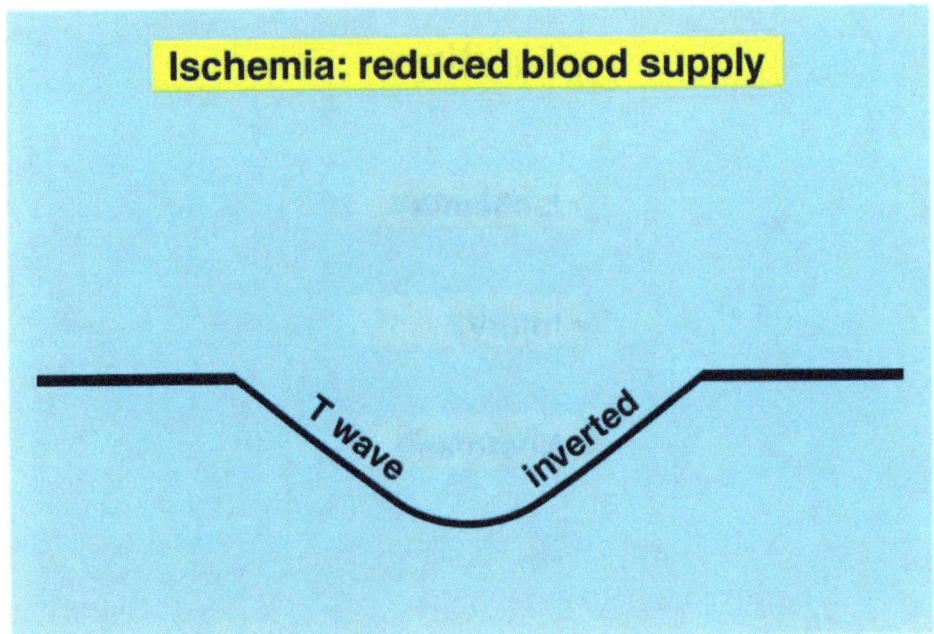

Ischemia (decreased blood supply) is characterized by inverted T waves.

Ischemia means reduced _____ supply (from the
coronary arteries); the ischemic area is at the periphery
of the infarct.   *blood*

The characteristic sign of ischemia is the _____
T wave. It may vary from a slightly inverted
to a deeply inverted T wave.   *inverted*

Inverted ___ waves may indicate ischemia in the absence
of myocardial infarction. Coronary blood flow can decrease
without producing an infarction.   *T*

Note: Cardiac ischemia alone can cause chest pain known as *angina*,
which is usually associated with transient T wave inversion.

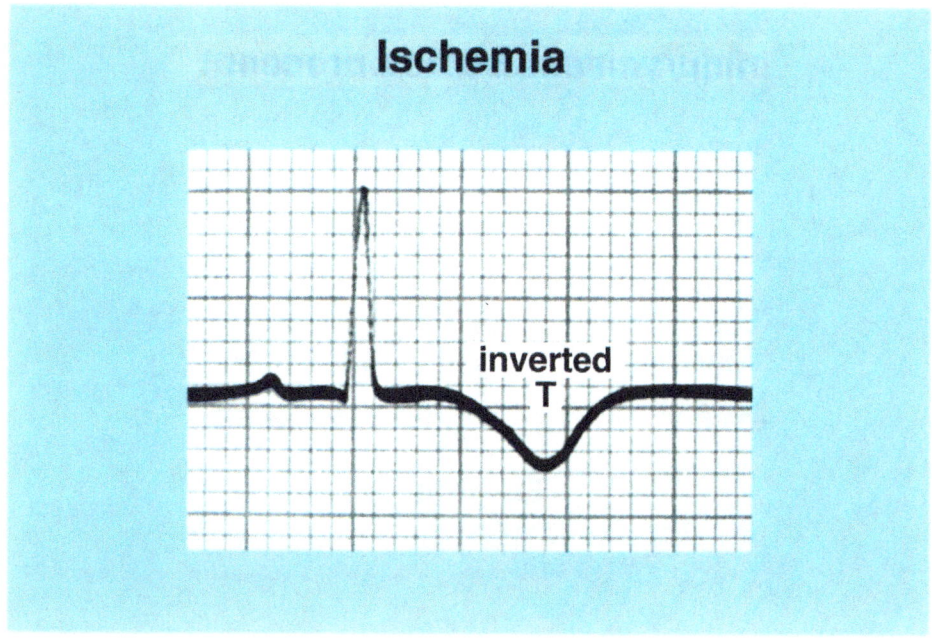

The typical ischemia T wave is symmetrically inverted.

Note: You should check every EKG that you read for T wave inversion. Since the chest leads are nearest the ventricles, T wave changes are most pronounced in these leads. Always run down V_1 to V_6 (as well as the limb leads) and check for T wave inversion to see if there is diminished coronary flow.

The T wave of ischemia is both inverted and _____; that is, the right and left sides   symmetrical of the inverted T wave are mirror images.

Note: In adults flat (nonexistent) T waves or minimal T wave inversion may be a normal variant in any of the limb leads (frontal plane). However, any T wave inversion in leads V_2 through V_6 is considered pathological. Marked T wave inversion in leads V_2 and V_3 the hallmark of **Wellens syndrome**, alerts us to *stenosis* of the anterior descending coronary.

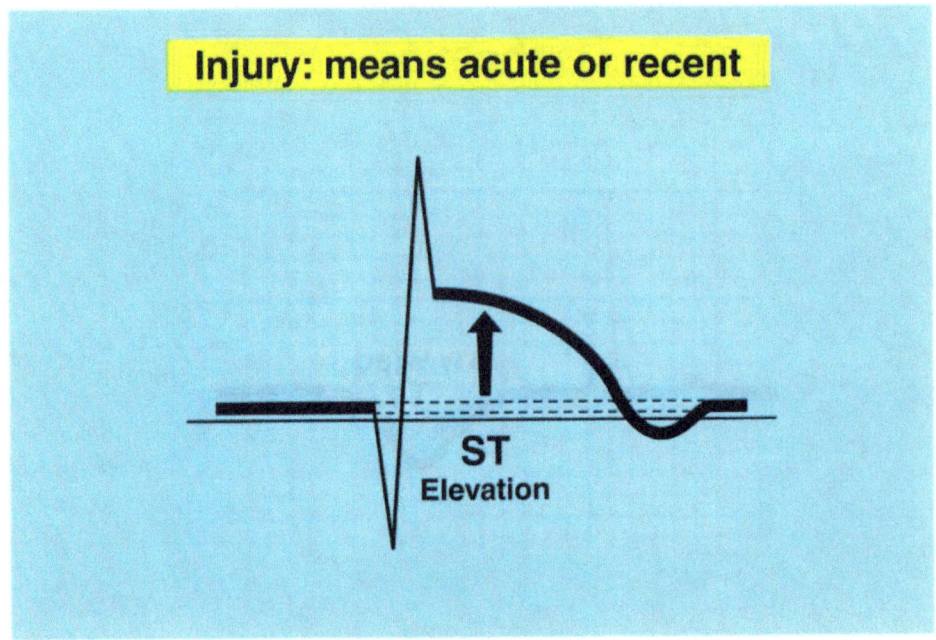

Injury indicates the acuteness of an infarct. Elevation of the ST segment denotes "injury" sometimes called the "current of injury."

"Acute" means recent or new.

The ST segment is that section of baseline between the QRS complex and the ___ wave. The ST segment contains no waves.

T

Elevation of the ST segment signifies "injury." The ST segment may be elevated only slightly, or as much as ten or more millimeters above the _____.

baseline

ST segment elevation tells us that a myocardial infarction is _____. It is the earliest consistent sign of infarction to record on EKG.

acute

Angina without exertion, "*Prinzmetal's*" angina, can cause transient ST elevation in the absence of an infarction.

ST Elevation

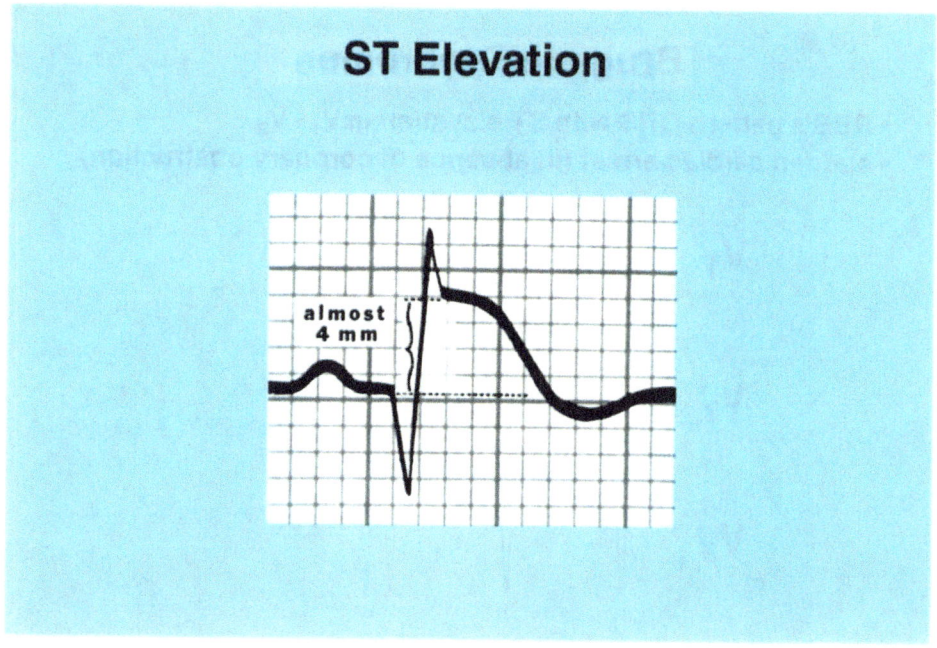

almost
4 mm

If there is ST elevation, this indicates that the infarction is acute. ST elevation, alone, can indicate an infarction.

Note: Once you have made a diagnosis of infarction, it is important to know whether the infarction just occurred and needs immediate treatment, or if the infarction is old — maybe years old.

The ST _____ rises above the baseline with an acute   segment
infarction, in fact it is usually the earliest EKG sign of an
infarction. With time, the ST segment returns to the baseline.

Note: If the ST segment is elevated without associated Q waves, this may represent *non-Q wave infarction*, which is usually a small infarction that may herald an impending larger infarct. Significant ST changes require enzyme studies and close scrutiny.

Note: A *ventricular aneurysm* (the outward ballooning of the wall of a ventricle) can cause persistent ST elevation in most of the chest leads; but in this case, the ST segment does *not* return to the baseline with time. *Pericarditis* (next page) produces a unique type of ST segment elevation that may also elevate the T wave off the baseline.

Brugada Syndrome

- **RBBB pattern QRS with ST elevation in V₁ - V₃**
- **sudden cardiac arrest (in absence of coronary obstruction)**

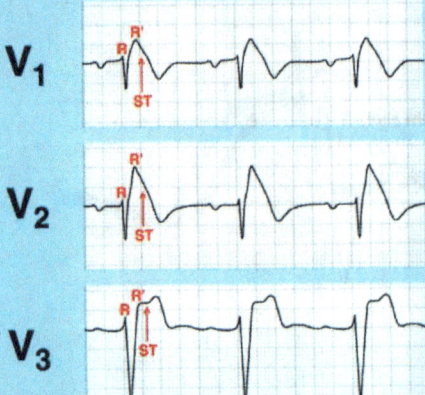

Brugada syndrome is a hereditary condition that can cause sudden death in individuals without heart disease. It is characterized by Right Bundle Branch Block with ST elevation in leads V_1 to V_3. Look for it; this malady is not rare.

Sudden cardiac death (cardiac arrest) can occur spontaneously in patients with Brugada _____.

syndrome

In Brugada syndrome there is RBBB and ST elevation in leads V_1 to V_3. The elevated ___ segments have a peculiar, peaked downsloping shape, particularly in V_1 and V_2.

ST

Note: Brugada syndrome is a familial condition caused by dysfunctional cardiac Na^+ (sodium) channels. Prophylaxis against the deadly arrhythmias requires ICD implantation in order to immediately treat cardiac arrest (usually ventricular fibrillation.)

Note: This syndrome is responsible for nearly one-half of the sudden deaths in healthy young individuals without structural heart disease.

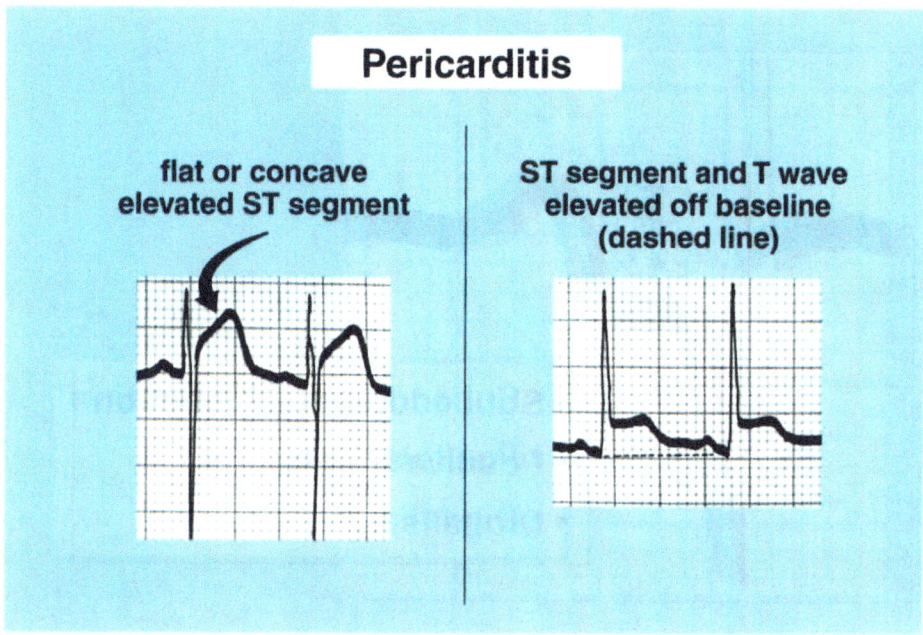

Pericarditis

flat or concave elevated ST segment

ST segment and T wave elevated off baseline (dashed line)

With *pericarditis,* the ST segment is elevated and usually flat or concave. The entire T wave may be elevated off the baseline.

Note: Pericarditis is inflammation of the membrane (*pericardium*) that surrounds the heart. Pericarditis may be caused by a virus, bacteria, cancer, or other sources of inflammation, including myocardial infarction.

Pericarditis can elevate the ___ segment. It usually produces an elevated ST segment that is flat or slightly concave (middle sags downward). This resolves with time.   ST

Pericarditis seems to elevate the entire __ wave off the baseline; that is, the baseline gradually angles back down (often including the P wave) all the way to the next QRS (illustration on right).   T

Note: The characteristics shown in the left illustration are found in leads in which the QRS is usually mainly negative (like the right chest leads). The pattern shown in the right illustration is seen in leads where the QRS is mainly positive (such as the lateral and inferior limb leads). Sometimes PVC's are produced.

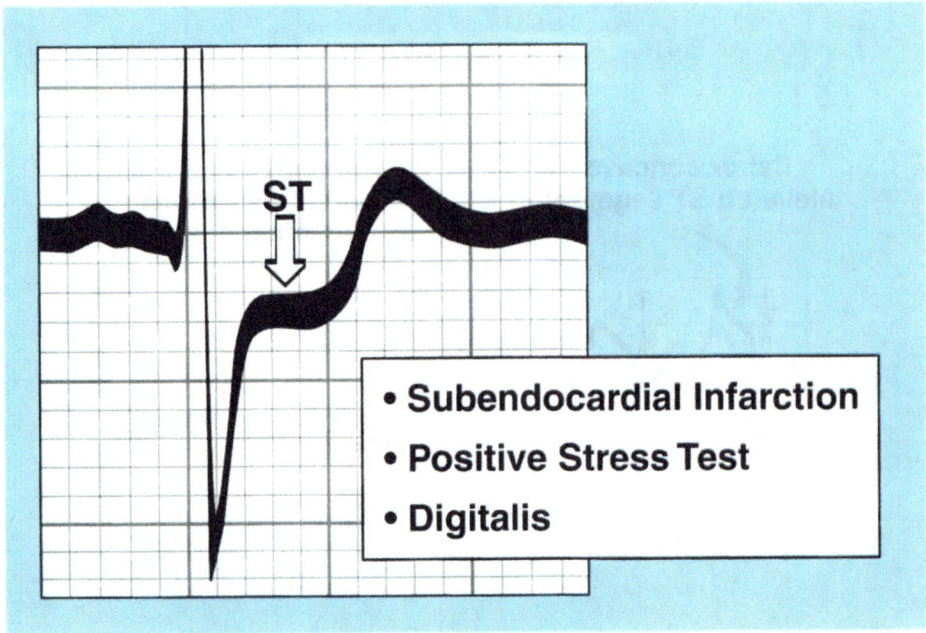

The ST segment may become depressed under certain circumstances or conditions.

Note: During an angina* attack, the ST segment may be temporarily depressed.

A subendocardial infarction, an infarct that does not extend
through the full thickness of the _____ ventricular wall,   left
will depress the ST segment.

When a patient with narrowed coronaries exercises, the
myocardium demands more blood flow than its arteries can
deliver. A *stress* (or "exercise") *test* will record depression
of the ___ segment on EKG when such a patient is exercised.   ST

Digitalis can cause _____ of the ST segment,   depression
however it has a unique, unforgettable appearance
(see page 317).

* Chest pain caused by diminished coronary blood flow (without infarction).

Subendocardial Infarction

(flat) ST depression

Subendocardial infarction causes flat depression of the ST segment; however, any significant ST depression (in leads where the QRS is upright) indicates compromised coronary blood flow until proven otherwise.

Subendocardial infarction (often referred to as subendocardial injury) is identified by flat ST _____ depression, which   segment may be either horizontal or down-sloping.

Note: Subendocardial infarction, a type of "non-Q wave infarction" involves only a small area of myocardium just beneath the endocardial lining. Classical myocardial infarction is said to be *transmural*; that is, the full thickness of the left ventricular wall is damaged in the infarcted area. Even though subendocardial infarction involves only a small area of the myocardium, it must be respected as a true M.I. that requires appropriate care. A subendocardial M.I. may enlarge or extend and become more life-threatening.

Note: Any patient with acute ST depression (or elevation), particularly if it persists, should have an immediate, complete workup including cardiac enzymes.

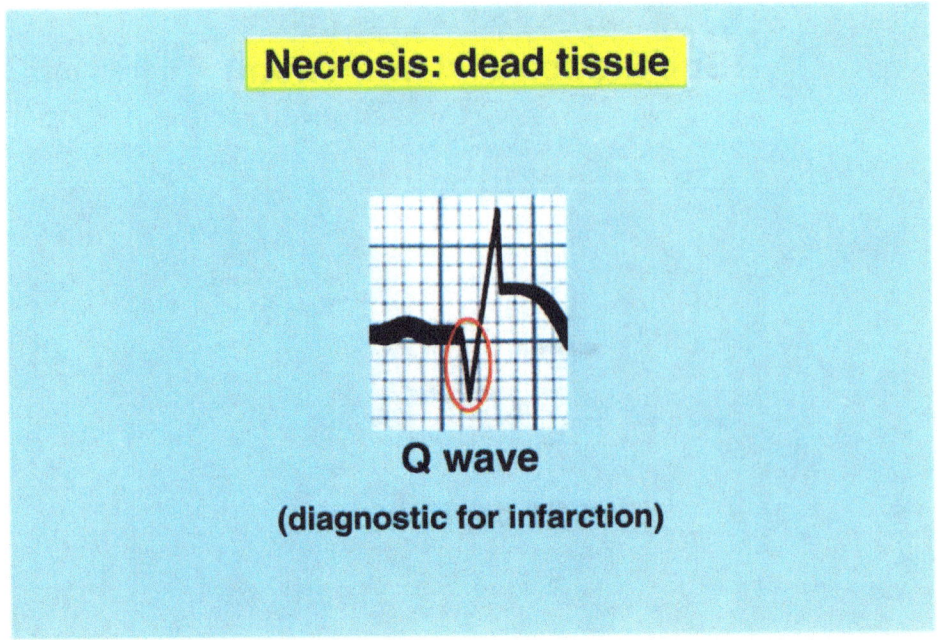

Q wave

(diagnostic for infarction)

The Q wave indicates **necrosis** (dead tissue) and makes the diagnosis of infarction.

The diagnosis of myocardial infarction is usually based on the
presence of significant ___ waves produced by an area of necrosis   Q
in the wall of the left ventricle.

Note: The Q wave is the first downward stroke of the QRS complex,
and it is never preceded by anything in the complex. In the QRS
complex, if there is any positive wave — even a tiny spike — before
the downward wave, the downward wave is an S wave (and the upward
wave preceding it is an R wave).

Significant Q _____ are absent in normal tracings.   waves
We use a capital "Q" to designate a significant Q wave,
however "q" (small, lower case q) waves are not significant
(see next page).

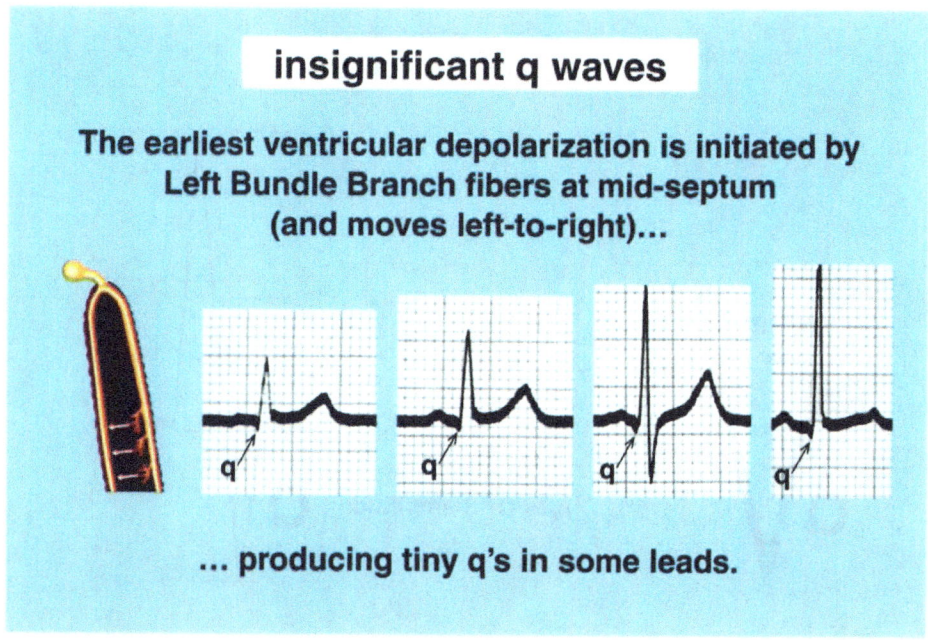

insignificant q waves

The earliest ventricular depolarization is initiated by Left Bundle Branch fibers at mid-septum (and moves left-to-right)...

... producing tiny q's in some leads.

Normally, ventricular depolarization begins midway down the interventricular septum. Septal depolarization (initiated at mid-septum by the Left Bundle Branch) is left-to-right, and this <u>initial</u> rightward ventricular activation may produce tiny, *insignificant q* (small q) *waves* in leads where the QRS is usually upright.

The Right Bundle Branch traverses the septum vertically without branching, however the _____ Bundle Branch gives off terminal Purkinje filaments at mid-septum.

Left

So this <u>initial</u> mid-septal depolarization moves left-to-right, <u>away from</u>:

- the positive left arm electrode of *lateral* leads I and AVL, and...

- the positive left foot electrode of *inferior* leads II, III, and AVF, and...

- the positive chest electrode of left chest leads V_5 and V_6...

... to occasionally record tiny, insignificant __ waves in those leads.

q

Note: This mid-septal depolarization is brief since the efficient ventricular conduction system quickly transmits depolarization to the endocardial surface of both ventricles. So brief is this mid-septal depolarization that only a tiny q wave of less than .04 second is recorded. Insignificant q waves are, by definition, less than one millimeter (.04 sec.) in duration.

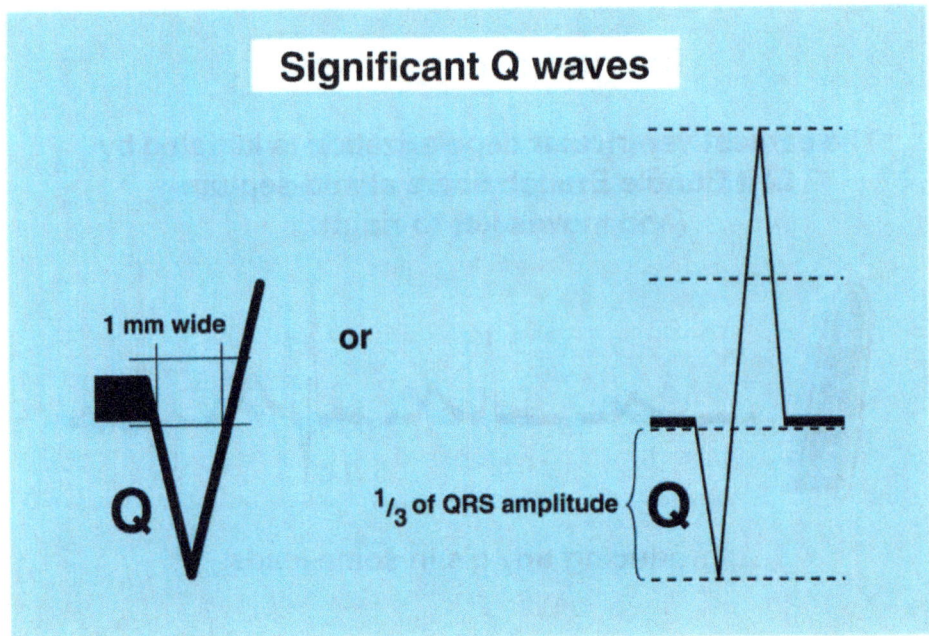

A *significant Q wave* is at least one small square wide (.04 sec.) or one-third of the entire QRS amplitude. Significant Q waves indicate the necrosis of a myocardial infarction.

Significant Q waves are indicative of the necrosis of a myocardial _____.

infarction

A significant Q wave is one small square (one millimeter) or more wide, and therefore is at least ___ second or more in duration.

.04

An old, but persistent, criterion of the significant Q wave is when the Q wave is _____ the amplitude (height and depth) of the entire QRS complex.

one-third

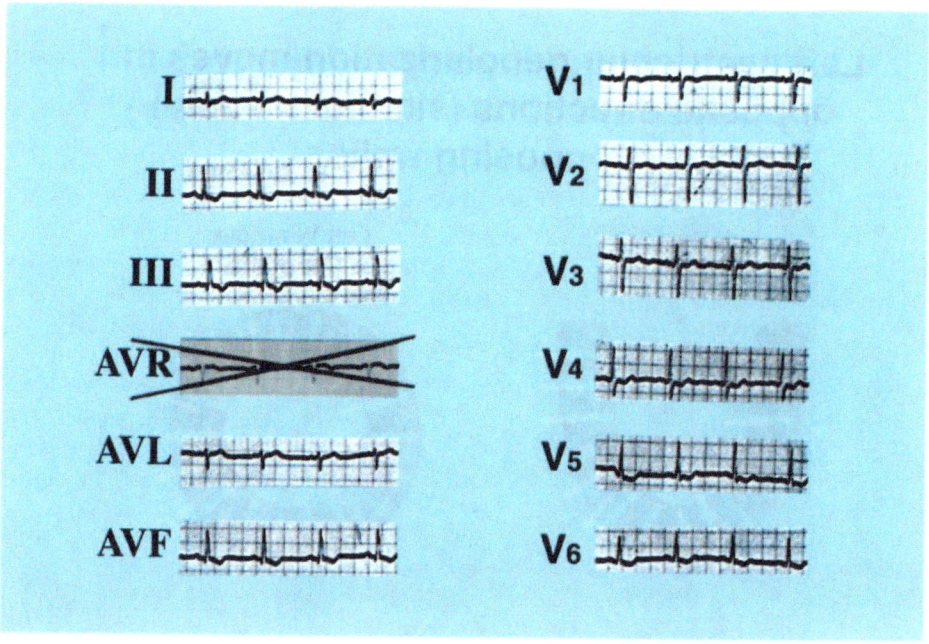

When looking at an EKG tracing, note which leads have significant Q waves.
Omit lead AVR. Keep in mind the leads that make up the *lateral*, *inferior*, and
chest lead designations.

To check for an infarction, we scan all leads (except AVR)
for the presence of _____ Q waves.   significant

Note: Forget about lead AVR, since this lead is positioned in such a
way that data regarding Q waves are unreliable. Lead AVR is like an
upside-down lead II, so the large Q waves that are commonly seen in
lead AVR are really the upside-down R waves from lead II. Even if you
don't understand the logic behind AVR's phony Q's, don't bother to
check it for signs of infarction.

When examining a tracing, either a long strip or mounted, write
down those _____ in which you find significant Q* waves,   leads
ST segment elevation (or depression), and inverted T waves.

* For proper documentation, insignificant q waves should be recorded as well.

Left ventricular depolarization moves in opposite directions (simultaneously) in opposing walls

**Left Ventricle
sagital section**

**Left Ventricle
top view**

Purkinje fibers conduct so rapidly that depolarization is initiated in all endocardial surfaces lining the left ventricle nearly simultaneously. So, depolarization passes from endocardium to epicardium in all left ventricular areas at once.

Note: Vectors describe the path of myocardial conduction (endocardium to epicardium), so left ventricular depolarization moves in opposite directions in opposing walls simultaneously.

In the left ventricle, depolarization of the lateral wall moves toward the patient's left, while depolarization of the medial (septal) wall moves toward the _____.   right

Depolarization of the anterior left ventricular wall moves anteriorly, while simultaneously, depolarization of the posterior left ventricular wall moves in a _____ direction.   posterior

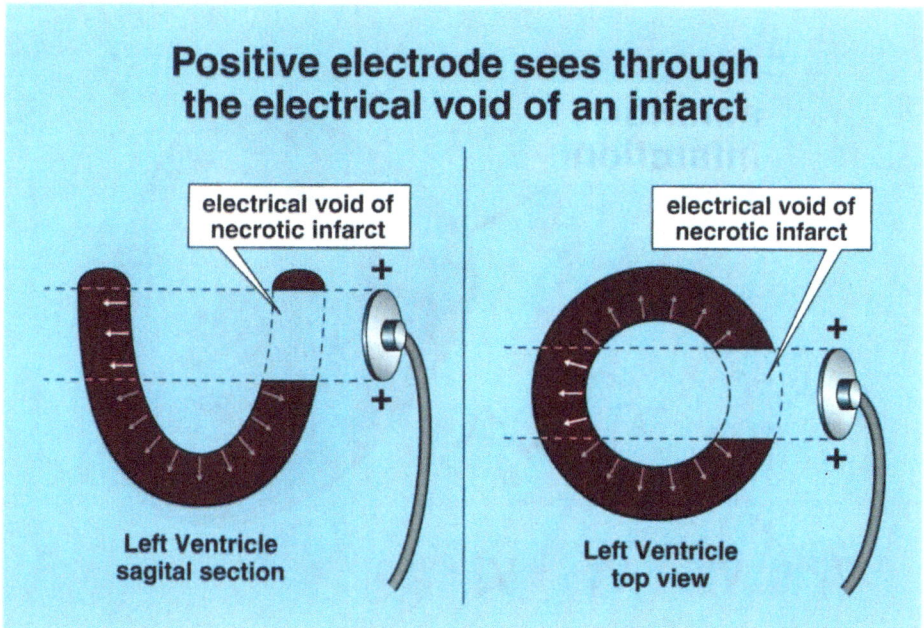

An infarct is necrotic; it cannot depolarize and has no vectors. So, the **positive** electrode nearest the infarct detects no "toward" vectors, it sees only the "away" vectors from the opposite wall (through the necrotic void). Therefore, a Q wave is inscribed on EKG in the leads which use that positive electrode for recording.

Note: Depolarization moving away from a positive electrode records a negative wave (in this case a Q wave) on EKG.

Note: Take your time and visualize each sentence as you read it.

In recording the initial left ventricular depolarization:

• with an *anterior* infarct, the positive (chest) electrode detects only the initial "away" vectors from the opposite side, so a Q is inscribed on EKG in leads V_1 - V_4 which use that positive electrode for recording.

• with a *lateral* infarct, the positive left arm electrode detects only the initial "away" vectors from the opposite side, so a Q is inscribed on EKG in leads I and AVL, which use that positive electrode for recording.

• with an *inferior* infarct, the positive left foot electrode detects only the initial "away" vectors from the opposite side, so a Q is inscribed on EKG in leads II, III, and AVF, which use that positive electrode for recording.

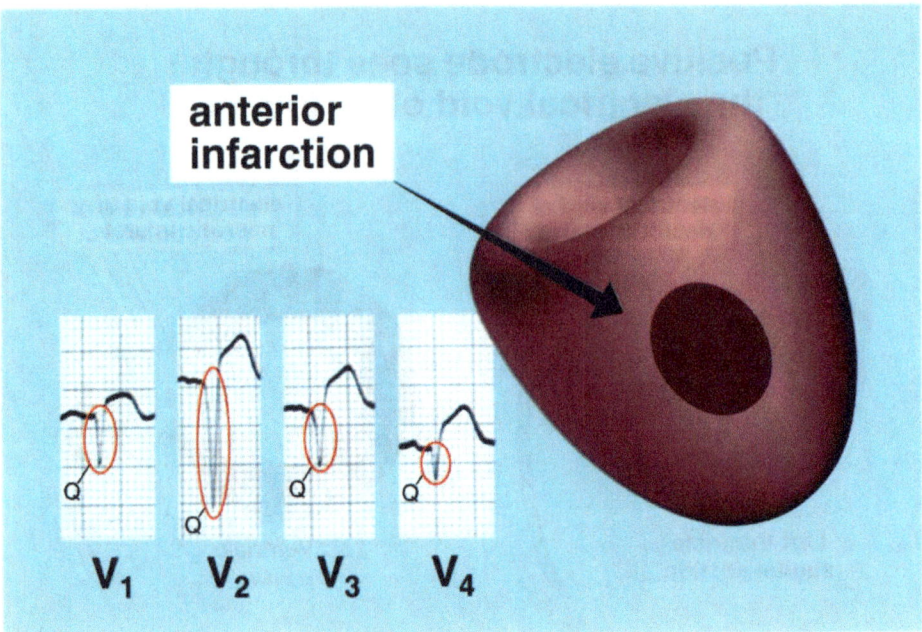

Q waves in V_1, V_2, V_3, or V_4 signify an *anterior infarction*. The infarction in the illustration is definitely acute, because of the ST elevation in all four leads.

Note: The chest lead electrodes are mainly positioned anteriorly, so this is a good way to remember the leads for anterior infarction.

The presence of Q waves in V_1, V_2, V_3, or V_4 indicates an infarction in the anterior wall of the _____ ventricle.   left

Note: The anterior portion of the left ventricle includes part of the interventricular septum. Some cardiologists say that when isolated Q waves appear in V_1 and V_2, the infarction includes the septum, so it is called an antero-*septal* infarction. Similarly, isolated Q waves in V_3 and V_4 (more laterally located chest leads) are said to represent an antero-*lateral* infarction. Remember that (insignificant) q waves are seen normally in V_5 and V_6.

Note: Statistically, anterior infarctions are very deadly, but fortunately, immediate treatment with intravenous thrombolytic medications or angioplasty with stenting has improved the survival rate substantially.

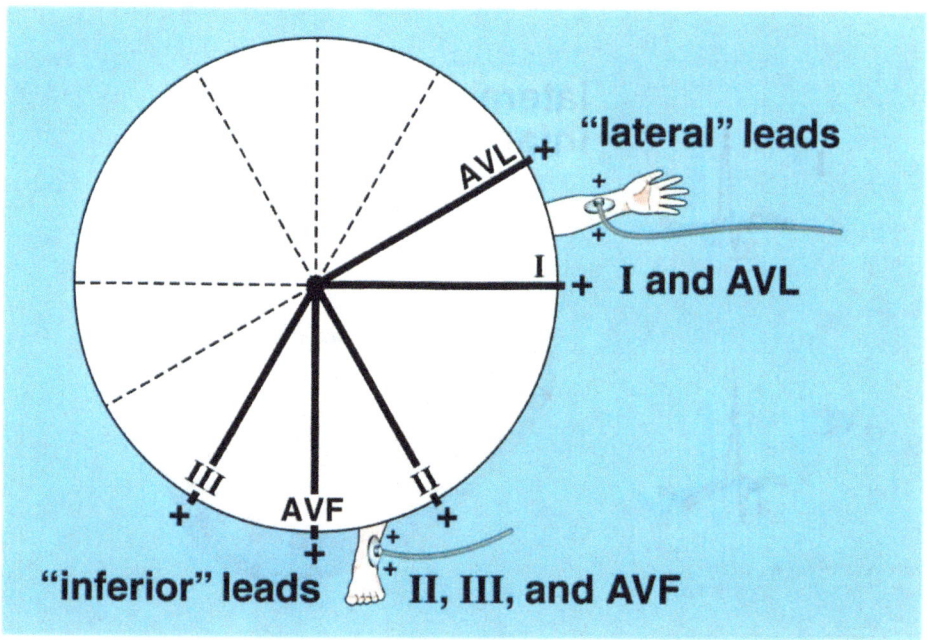

The positive electrode that is used to record the *lateral* limb leads, I and AVL, is on the left arm. The positive electrode used to record the *inferior* limb leads, II, III, and AVF, is on the left "foot."

The lateral limb leads are I and AVL; they are recorded by a positive left arm _____.

electrode

Yawn... excuse me.

The inferior leads are II, III, and AVF; they are recorded by a positive electrode on the left _____.

foot

Note: Yes, it is necessary to have this page here. You'll see why in just a few seconds.

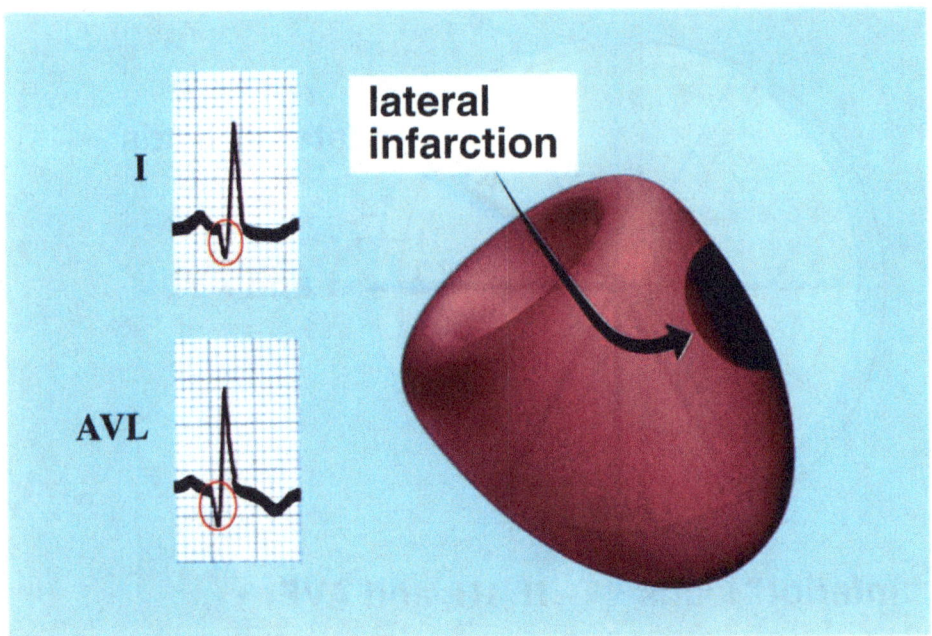

If there are Q waves in the *lateral* leads, I and AVL, there is a *lateral* infarction.

Note: Depolarization moving <u>away from</u> a positive electrode records
a <u>negative</u> wave (in this case a Q wave) on EKG.

A *lateral* infarction involves the *lateral* portion of the _____ ventricle.   left

In *lateral* infarction, the positive left arm electrode senses only
the initial "away" vectors from the opposite (septal) wall,
so it records a Q wave in the *lateral* _____, I and AVL.   leads

When a *lateral* infarction occurs, Q waves appear in the
lateral leads, which are leads I and ____; Q waves are   AVL
produced by the initial "away" vectors recorded by the
positive left arm electrode through the void of the necrotic
lateral infarct.

Note: One might abbreviate Lateral Infarction as L.I.,
which is diagnosed using leads AV<u>L</u> and <u>I</u>.

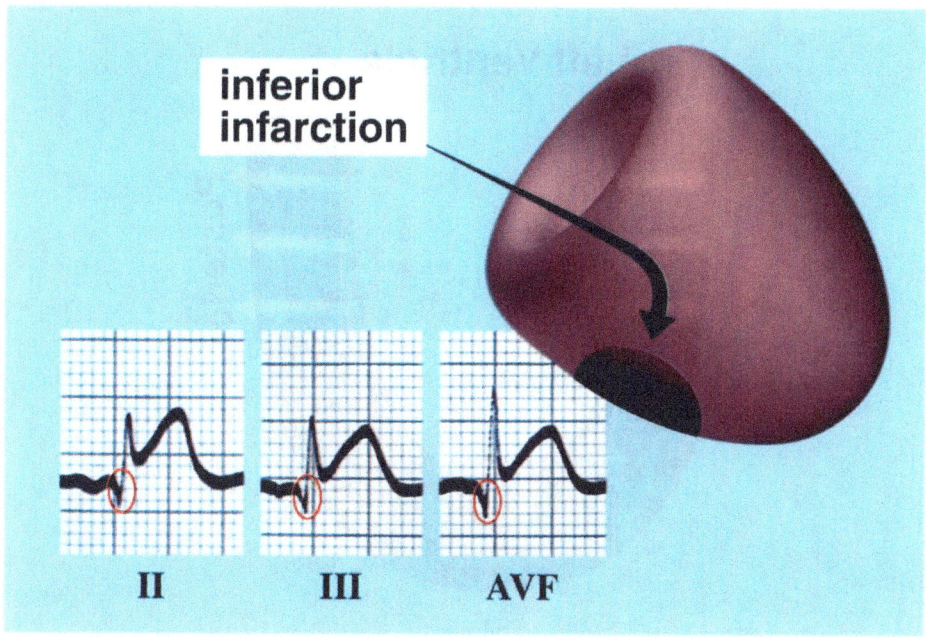

inferior infarction

II   **III**   **AVF**

Inferior infarction is diagnosed by the presence of Q waves in the *inferior* leads, II, III, and AVF. Check the ST segments to see if this infarction is acute.

Note: Depolarization moving <u>away from</u> a positive electrode records a <u>negative</u> wave (in this case a Q wave) on EKG.

The inferior wall of the left ventricle rests upon the diaphragm, so the alternate term "diaphragmatic" infarction is occasionally used instead of "inferior" _____.   infarction

In *inferior* infarction, absent the initial "toward" vectors, the positive left foot electrode senses only the initial "away" vectors from the opposite wall, so it records a Q wave in the *inferior* _____, II, III, and AVF.   leads

An *inferior* infarction is identified by significant Q waves in *inferior* leads II, III, and ____; Q waves are produced by   AVF the initial "away" vectors recorded by the positive left foot electrode through the void of the necrotic *inferior* infarct.

Note: Autopsy data show that about one-third of inferior infarctions also include portions of the right ventricle.

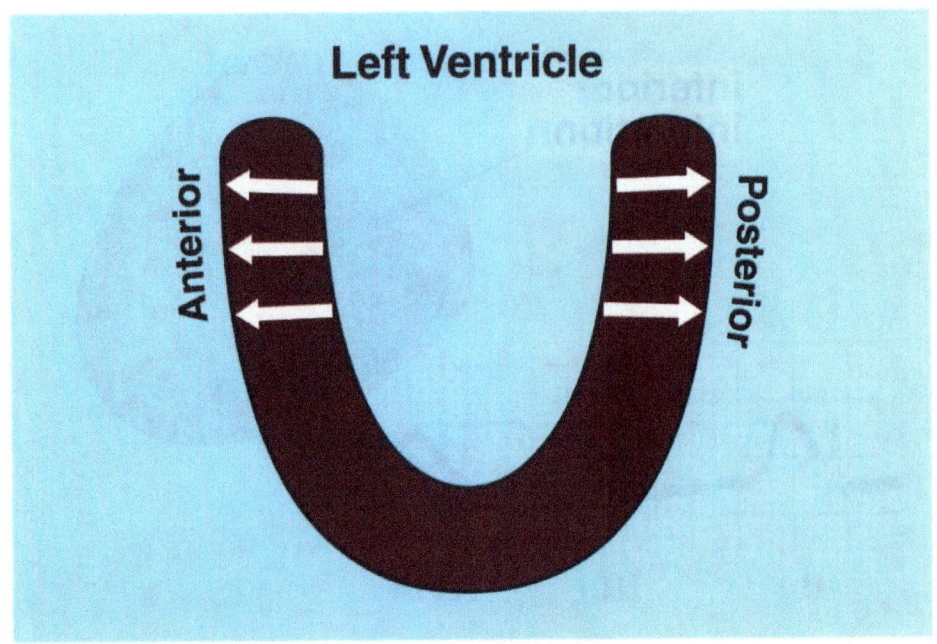

Depolarization of the anterior wall and depolarization of the posterior wall of the left ventricle are in opposite directions.

Note: Left ventricular depolarization may be said to proceed from the *endocardium* (inner lining) to the *epicardium* (outer surface).

Depolarization of the anterior wall of the left ventricle proceeds from the inner endocardium, which lines the ventricle, through the full thickness of the ventricular wall to the outer ventricular surface (_____).   epicardium

Similarly, depolarization of the posterior wall of the _____ ventricle proceeds from the endocardium   left
to the epicardium.

So, vectors representing depolarization of the anterior and the posterior portions of the left ventricle point in _____ directions.   opposite

Acute Anterior Infarction
(note ST elevation)

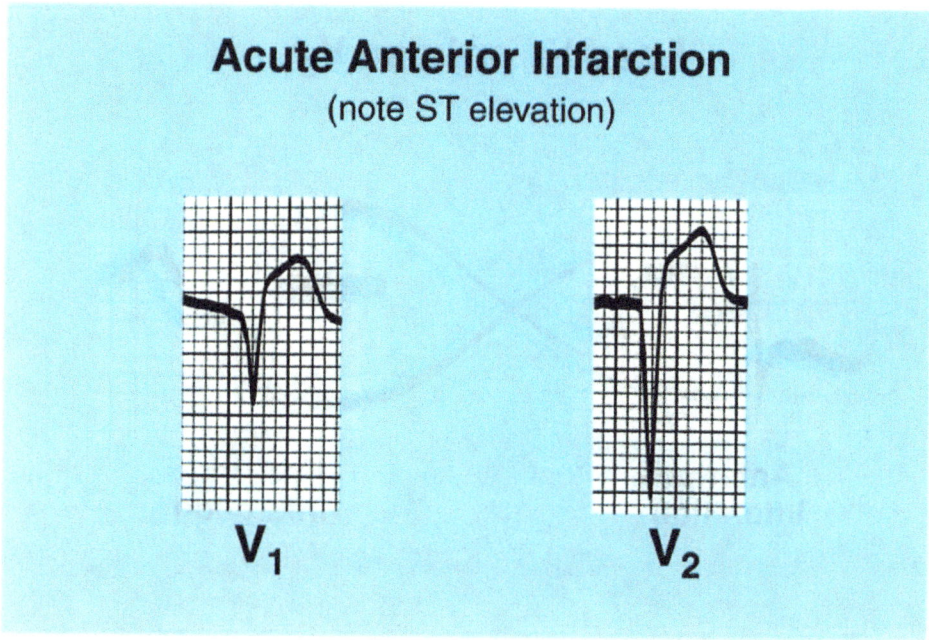

V_1 V_2

If an acute anterior infarction produces Q waves and ST elevation in V_1 and V_2 then a posterior infarction would appear the opposite.

An acute anterior infarction produces significant Q waves
with ST _____ in the first few chest leads.   elevation

Considering only V_1 and V_2 the appearance of
significant Q waves and ST elevation indicates
an acute _____ infarction.   anterior
                                                     (antero-septal)

Note: Acute posterior infarction of the left ventricle would
produce the exact opposite to the pattern of acute anterior
infarction, because the anterior and posterior walls of the
left ventricle depolarize in opposite directions. This will be
clarified on the next page.

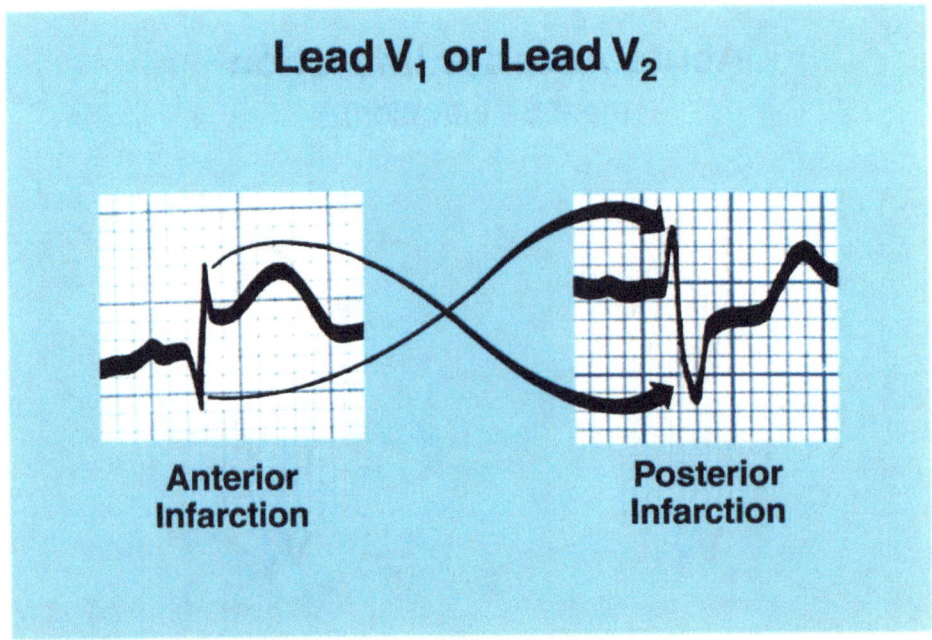

In acute *Posterior Infarction* there is a large R wave (the opposite of a Q wave) in
V_1 and V_2.

Note: In lead V_1 a Q wave turned upside-down would look like an R
wave (and as you recall, R waves in lead V_1 are normally very tiny).

A significant "Q wave" from an infarction in the posterior portion
of the _____ ventricle will cause a large R (positive deflection)   left
wave to appear in lead V_1.

Suspect a true posterior infarction when you see a large ___ wave   R
in V_1 or V_2 — even though Right Ventricular Hypertrophy can
also produce a large R in V_1.

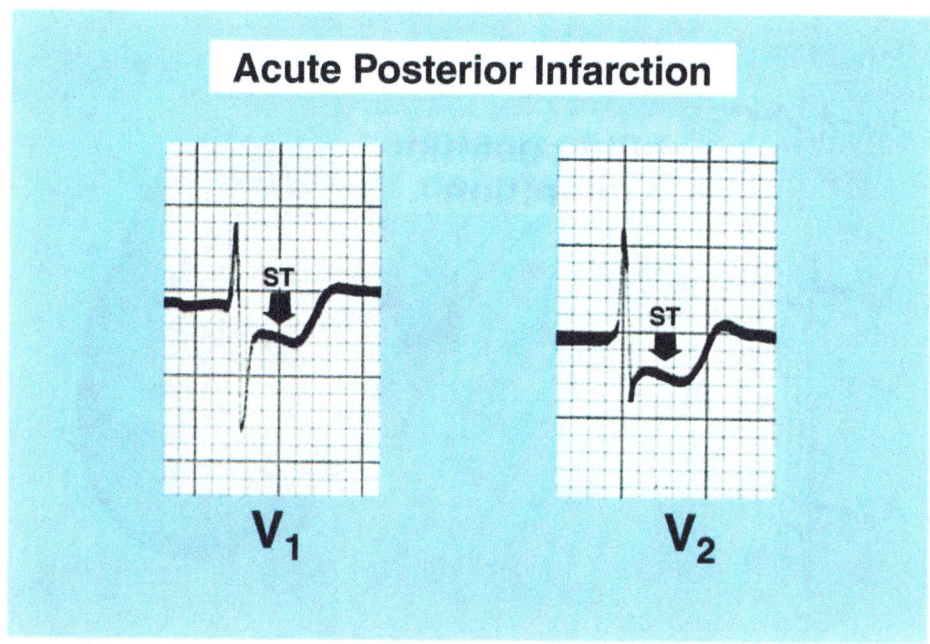

Acute Posterior Infarction

V_1

V_2

In acute posterior infarction, there is ST <u>depression</u> (the opposite of the usual ST elevation of Injury) in V_1 or V_2.

Acute anterior infarction produces Q waves in the chest leads and the ST segments are _____.

elevated

Note: Since the posterior wall of the left ventricle depolarizes in a direction opposite to that of the anterior wall, an acute infarction of the posterior wall causes ST *depression* in V_1 or V_2.

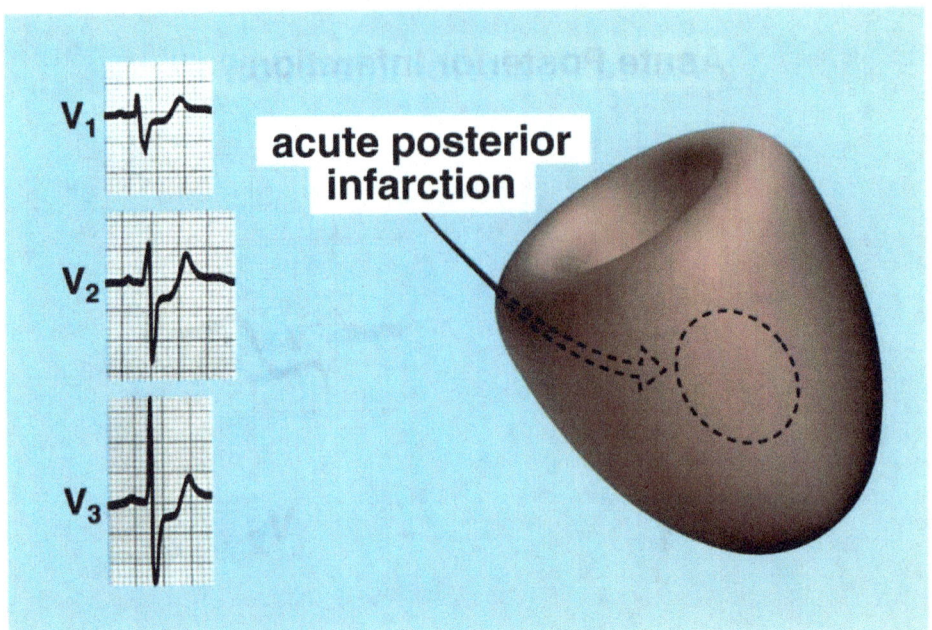

In summary, acute posterior infarction is characterized by a large R wave and ST depression in V_1 or V_2 (sometimes even in V_3).

Note: Always be suspicious of ST segment depression in the right chest leads, for it could indicate an acute posterior infarction. If you do not remember those things that can cause ST depression, look back at page 270. For instance, the diagnosis of an "anterior subendocardial infarction" (because of depressed ST segments in chest leads, see page 271) should be made only with extreme caution, because this ST depression may actually represent an acute true posterior infarct.

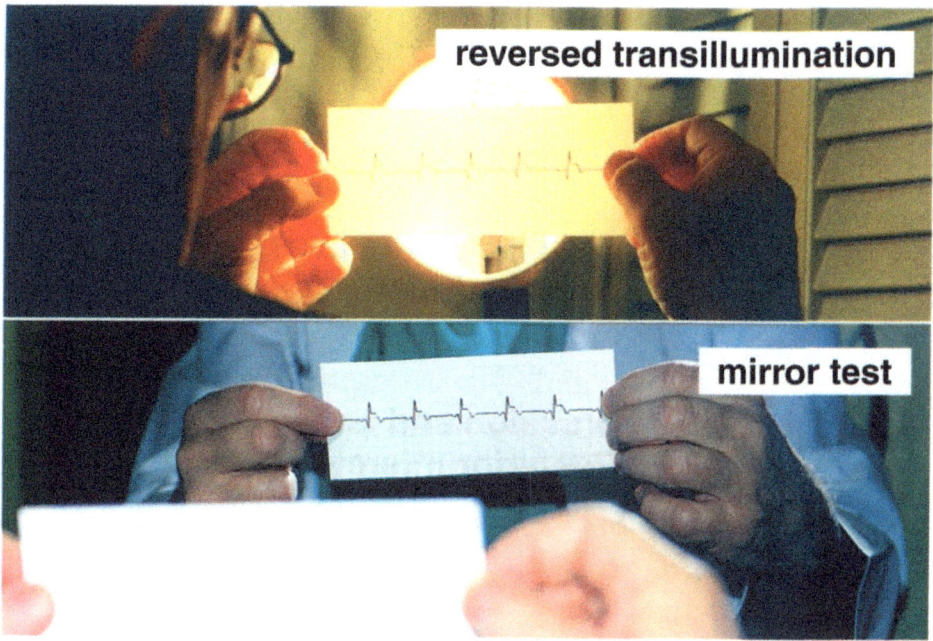

If you suspect an acute posterior infarction (large R wave and ST depression in V_1 or V_2), then try "reversed trans-illumination" or the "mirror test." You must follow the instructions for each test precisely.

Note: If acute posterior infarction is suspected because of tall R waves and ST depression in V_1 or V_2 — try *reversed trans-illumination* or the *mirror test*. Both of these tests require that you <u>invert the tracing first, then hold the blank (unprinted) back side towards your face.</u>

• <u>Reversed trans-illumination</u>: First, *invert the EKG tracing*, then hold the inverted tracing so that it faces a strong light. Observe the back side of the tracing to check for "Q waves and ST elevation" in the inverted V_1 and V_2 leads.

• <u>Mirror Test</u>: First, *invert the EKG tracing*, then observe it in a mirror. If there is an acute posterior infarction, you will see the classic signs of "Q waves and ST elevation" in the reflection of the inverted V_1 and V_2 leads.

Note: With either test, remember to first *invert the tracing*. Then face the tracing toward a mirror for the mirror test; or for reversed trans-illumination, place the tracing in front of a strong light, viewing the EKG through its back side.

Always Check V₁ and V₂ for:

1. ST elevation and Q waves (Anterior Infarct)

2. ST depression and large R waves (Posterior Infarct)

Although posterior infarctions are severe, they are easy to overlook.

When making your routine reading of an EKG, pay special attention
to leads V_1 and ___ while looking for signs of infarction. V_2

Note: ST changes in V_1 and V_2 are always significant and important…
both depression <u>and</u> elevation.

Check for Q waves in V_1 and V_2 and be sure to observe the
height of the __ waves.   R

Note: And remember how important T wave inversion can be in all leads.

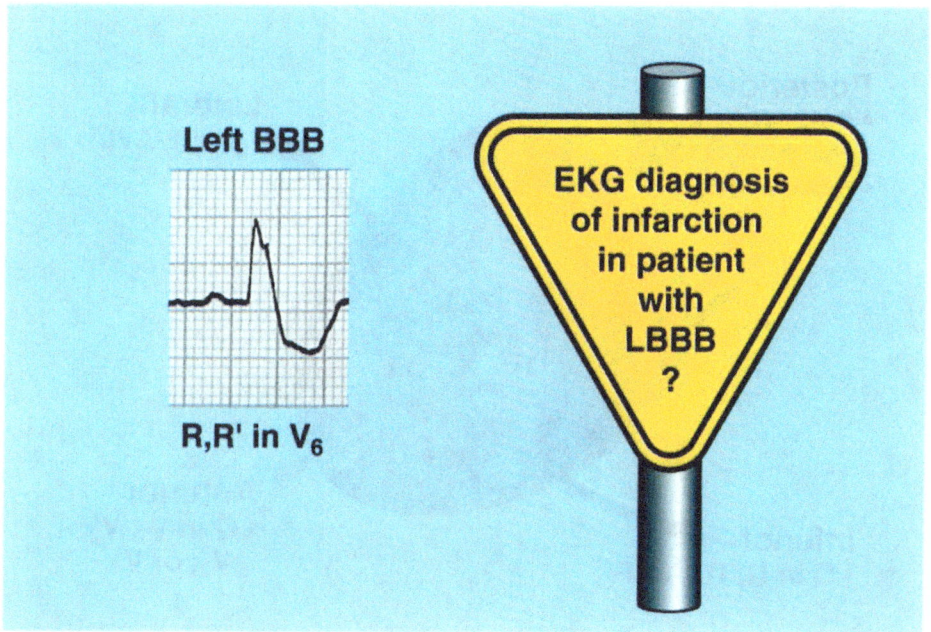

The EKG diagnosis of infarction is generally not valid in the presence of Left Bundle Branch Block.

In Left Bundle Branch Block, the left ventricle (generally, the main chamber to suffer infarction) depolarizes after the _____ ventricle depolarizes.   right

So any Q wave originating in the left ventricle could not appear at the beginning of the QRS _____ (with Left BBB); rather,   complex it would fall somewhere in the middle of the QRS complex. In this instance it would be difficult to detect significant Q waves.

Note: One special exception is possible. The right and left ventricles share the interventricular septum in common. So an infarct in the septal area would be shared by the right ventricle, which depolarizes first in Left BBB. This would produce Q waves at the beginning of the wide QRS. Therefore, even in the presence of Left BBB, Q waves in the chest leads might suggest (but not confirm) septal (anterior) infarction.

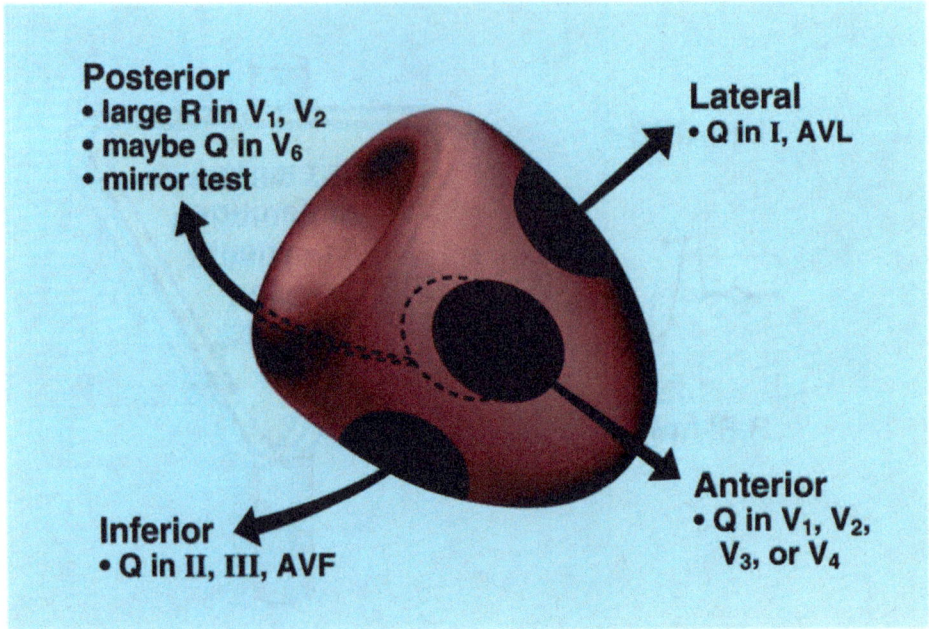

Posterior
- large R in V₁, V₂
- maybe Q in V₆
- mirror test

Lateral
- Q in I, AVL

Inferior
- Q in II, III, AVF

Anterior
- Q in V₁, V₂, V₃, or V₄

Locating an infarct is important because treatment modalities and prognosis depend on the location of the infarction.

There are four general locations within the _____ ventricle
where infarctions commonly occur.   left

Note: More than one area of the left ventricle may infarct. One
infarction may be very old, while another is very recent (acute). So
correlate the ST elevation with the appropriate leads both to locate, and
to determine the acuteness of each infarct. If ST elevation is present in
leads *without* Q waves, "non-Q wave infarction" must be ruled out.

Be careful about diagnosing an infarction in the
presence of _____ Bundle Branch Block.   Left

Note: Isolated areas of Ischemia (T wave inversion) or ST elevation
without Q's (for non-Q wave infarction) can also be "located" by using
the same location criteria.

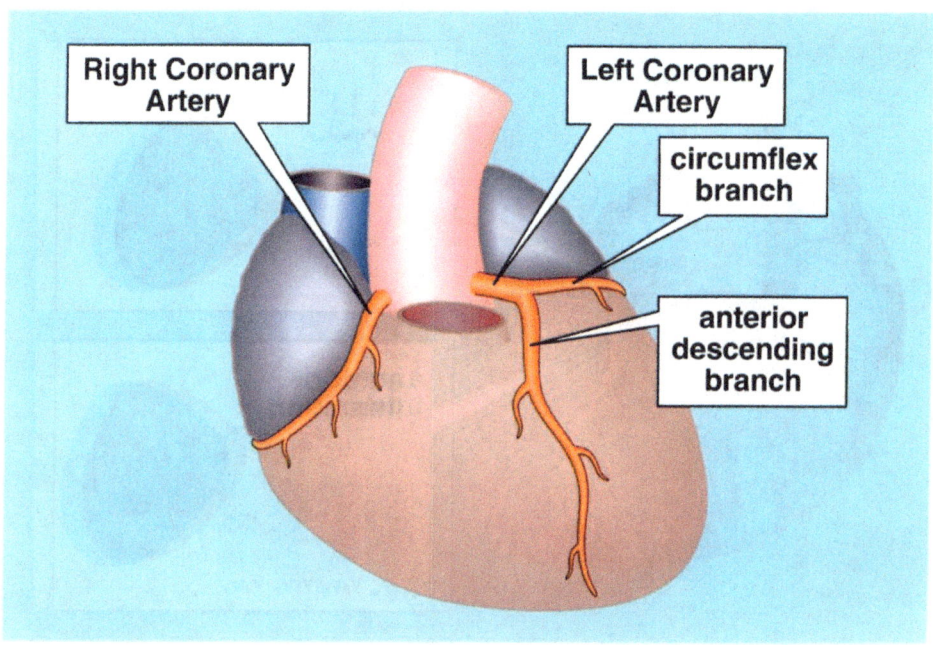

It is common practice to determine the location of an infarction, but with a little anatomical knowledge of the heart's coronary blood supply*, we can make a far more sophisticated diagnosis.

There are two coronary arteries that provide the heart with a continuous supply of oxygenated _____.   blood

Quickly review the illustration.
The *Left Coronary Artery* has two major branches; they are the *Circumflex* branch and the _____ *Descending* branch.   *Anterior*

The *Right Coronary Artery* curves around the right
_____.   ventricle

* The pulmonary artery has been "surgically" removed in this illustration to show the origin of the coronary arteries at the base of the aorta.

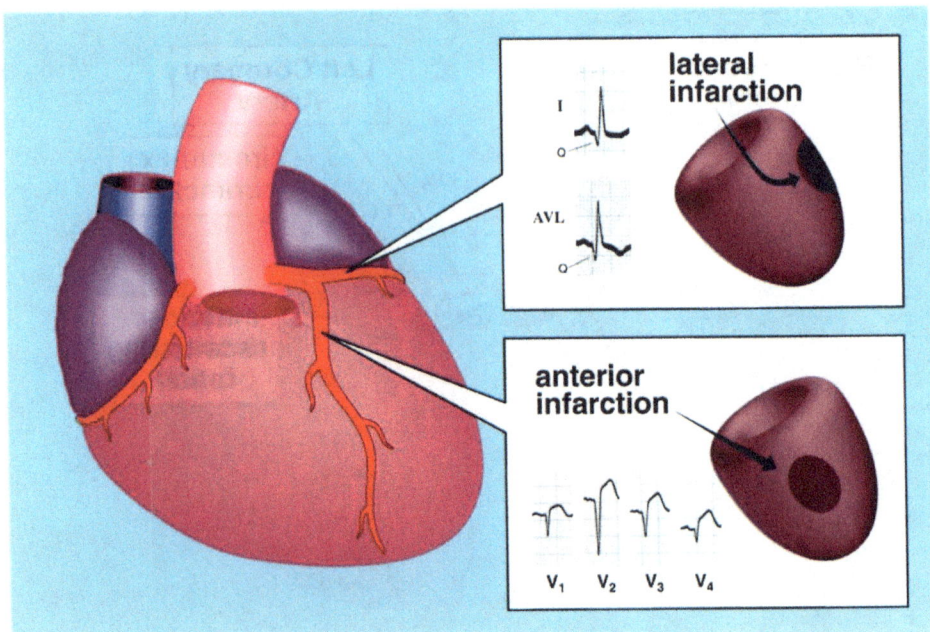

A *lateral infarction* is caused by an occlusion of the Circumflex branch of the Left Coronary Artery. An anterior infarction is due to an occlusion of the Anterior Descending branch of the Left Coronary Artery.

The Circumflex branch of the Left Coronary Artery distributes blood to the _____ portion of the left ventricle.   lateral

The Anterior Descending branch of the Left Coronary Artery supplies blood to the anterior portion of the _____ ventricle.   left

The Circumflex and the Anterior Descending are the two main branches of the _____ Coronary Artery.   Left

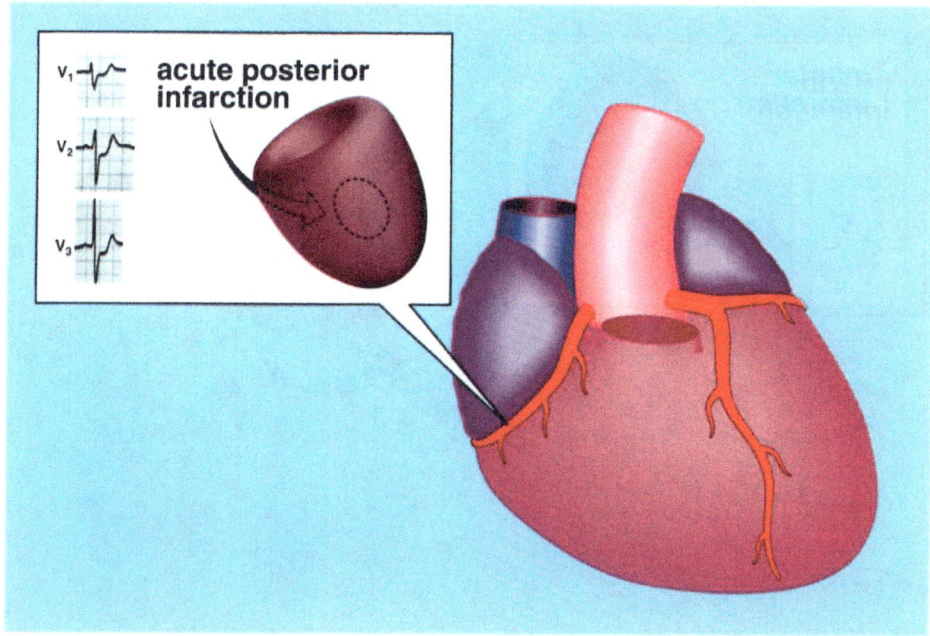

True posterior infarctions are generally caused by an occlusion of the Right Coronary Artery or one of its branches.

The Right Coronary Artery wraps around the right ventricle posteriorly to supply the _____ portion of the left ventricle.   posterior

So, a posterior infarction usually is caused by an occlusion of a branch of the _____ Coronary Artery.   Right

Note: For a long time the Right Coronary Artery was thought to play only a minor role in supplying blood to the heart. Sophisticated techniques of cardiac catheterization and coronary angiography have shown that the Right Coronary Artery usually provides the blood supply to the SA Node, the AV Node, and the His Bundle. It is no wonder that acute posterior infarction is often associated with serious arrhythmias. Wise health care providers treat posterior infarction with concern and respect.

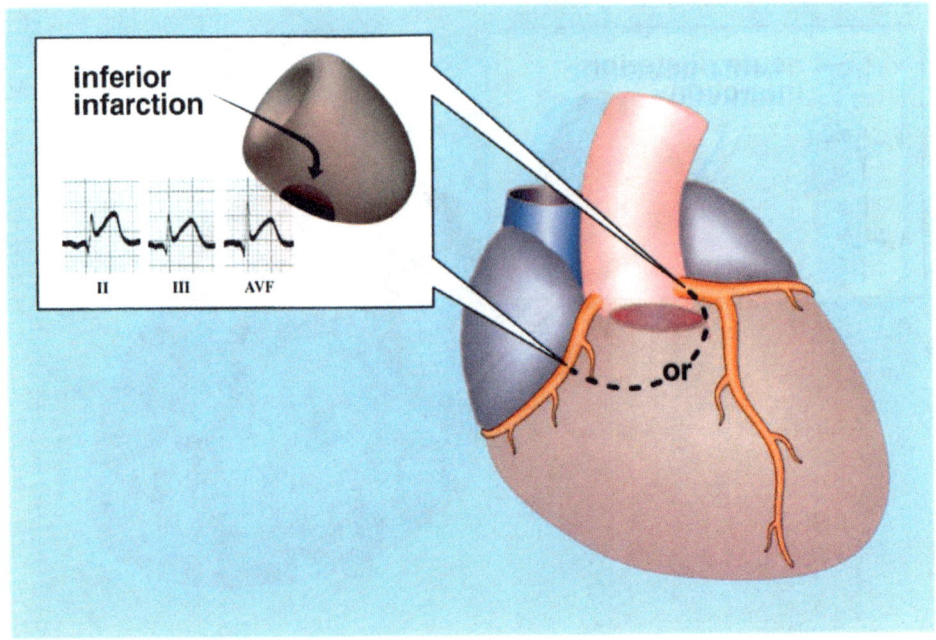

The base of the left ventricle receives its blood supply from branches of either the Right or the Left Coronary Artery, depending on which artery is "dominant."

Inferior ("diaphragmatic") infarctions are caused by an occluded terminal branch of either the Right or the _____ Coronary Artery.   Left

So the diagnosis of inferior infarction does not necessarily identify the artery branch that is occluded, unless you have a previous coronary arteriogram (an x-ray highlighting the coronary arteries) to identify which _____ artery supplies the inferior portion   coronary of that patient's left ventricle.

Note: Left or Right Coronary "dominance" denotes which coronary artery is the major source of blood supply to the base of the left ventricle. Right Coronary dominance is by far most common in humans.

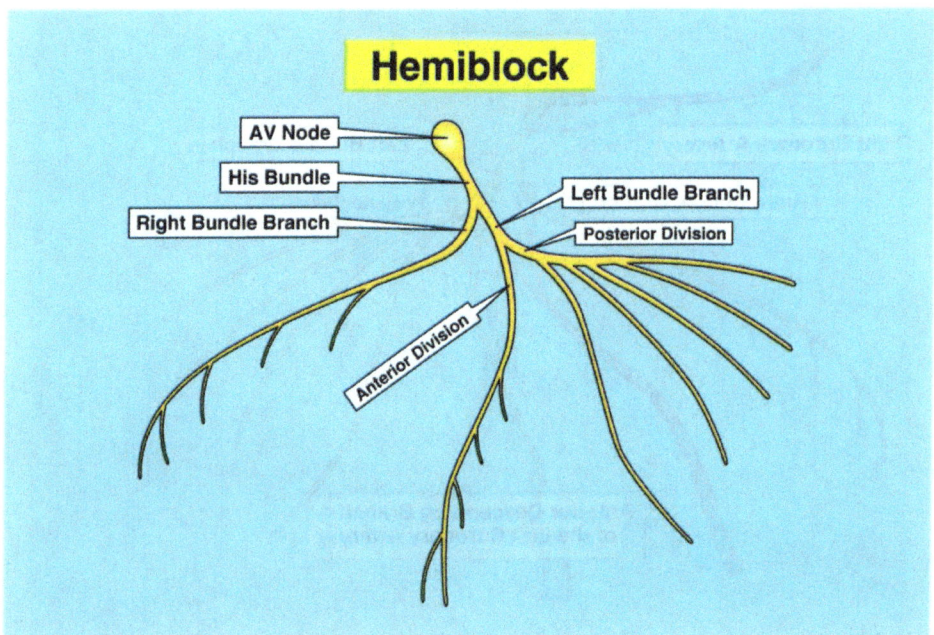

Hemiblocks are presented in this section (Infarction) because they commonly occur with infarction and an associated diminished blood supply to one of the two divisions of the Left Bundle Branch.

Note: The Left Bundle Branch subdivides into two divisions.

The hemiblocks are blocks of either the Anterior or the
Posterior Division of the _____ Bundle Branch.   Left

Hemiblocks are commonly due to loss of blood supply to
either the Anterior or the Posterior _____ of the Left   Division
Bundle Branch.

Note: The Right Bundle Branch does not have consistent, named
subdivisions of either clinical or electrocardiographic importance (yet).

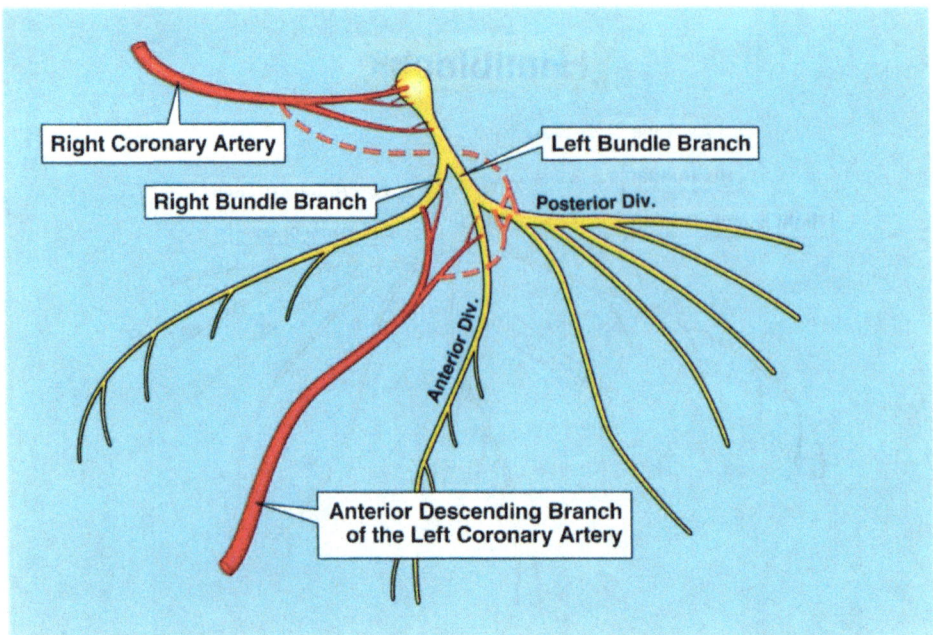

To understand hemiblocks, you should be familiar with the blood supply to the AV Node and the ventricular conduction system. Follow text and illustration closely.

The Right Coronary Artery usually renders a blood supply*
to the AV Node, Bundle of His and a variable twig to the
Posterior Division of the Left _____ Branch.   Bundle

The Left Coronary Artery also sends a variable twig to
the Posterior Division of the Left Bundle _____.   Branch

A total occlusion of the Anterior Descending branch of the
Left Coronary Artery may cause a subsequent Right Bundle Branch
_____ with an Anterior Hemiblock (a block of the Anterior   Block
Division of the Left Bundle Branch). Study the illustration carefully.

Note: The key to knowing hemiblocks is understanding that an infarction
may be due to an occlusion of a vessel at any of numerous locations, and
therefore may cause a variety of blocks of the Bundle Branch system.
There can be single blocks of a bundle or division, or combinations of
these blocks, that spare one or more branches. A coronary obstruction that
is not quite complete may cause an *intermittent* block.

* Let's not forget that the SA Node is usually dependent on the Right Coronary Artery.

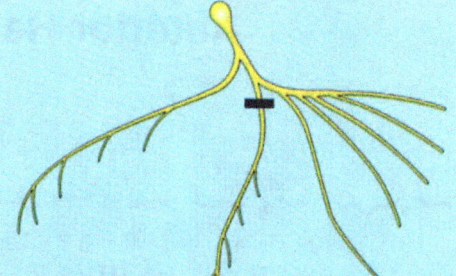

Anterior Hemiblock

- **LAD - usually assoc. with an M.I. (or other heart disease)**

- **Normal or slightly widened QRS**

- Q_1S_3

Anterior Hemiblock refers to a block of the Anterior Division of the Left Bundle Branch, and the above criteria are used in the diagnosis.

The slight delay of conduction to the antero-lateral and superior area of the left ventricle causes (late) unopposed depolarization upward and leftward, recognized on EKG as Left _____ Deviation. Acute LAD is usually what makes you suspect Anterior Hemiblock.   Axis

With pure Anterior Hemiblock, the QRS is widened only .10 to .12 sec., but association with other blocks of the Bundle _____ system will widen the QRS more.   Branch

Anterior Hemiblock is a block of the Anterior Division of the Left Bundle Branch. Finding a Q in I and a wide and/or deep __ in III ("Q_1S_3") helps to confirm the diagnosis of Anterior Hemiblock.   S

Note: The patient's previous EKG's are essential in making a diagnosis of Anterior (or any) Hemiblock. You *must* always rule out pre-existing sources of Left Axis Deviation, e.g., Left Ventricular Hypertrophy, "horizontal heart," or Inferior Infarction.

Anterior Hemiblock

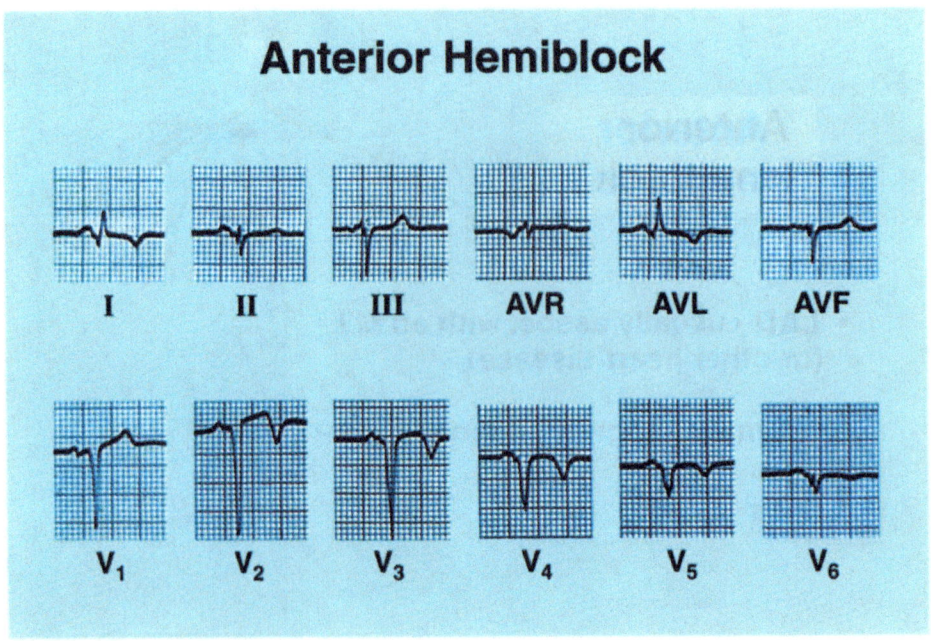

An occlusion of the Anterior Descending coronary artery produces an Anterior Infarction, and about one-half of these patients develop Anterior Hemiblock. Study the illustration on page 296.

Anterior Hemiblock is a block of the Anterior Division
of the Left Bundle Branch, which produces unopposed, late
superior-leftward depolarization in the left ventricle,
resulting in Left Axis _____.   Deviation

An occlusion of the *Anterior* Descending coronary artery
will produce an *Anterior* Infarction, which often causes
Anterior _____. (That's easy to remember.)   Hemiblock

If a patient with an acute Anterior Infarction has an associated
Axis change from normal to -60°, you should suspect
Anterior _____ (and look for Q_1S_3).   Hemiblock

But if a patient with an Inferior Infarction develops Left Axis
Deviation, don't jump to hasty conclusions! Inferior Infarction
can cause LAD, so _____ Hemiblock may not be the   Anterior
culprit.

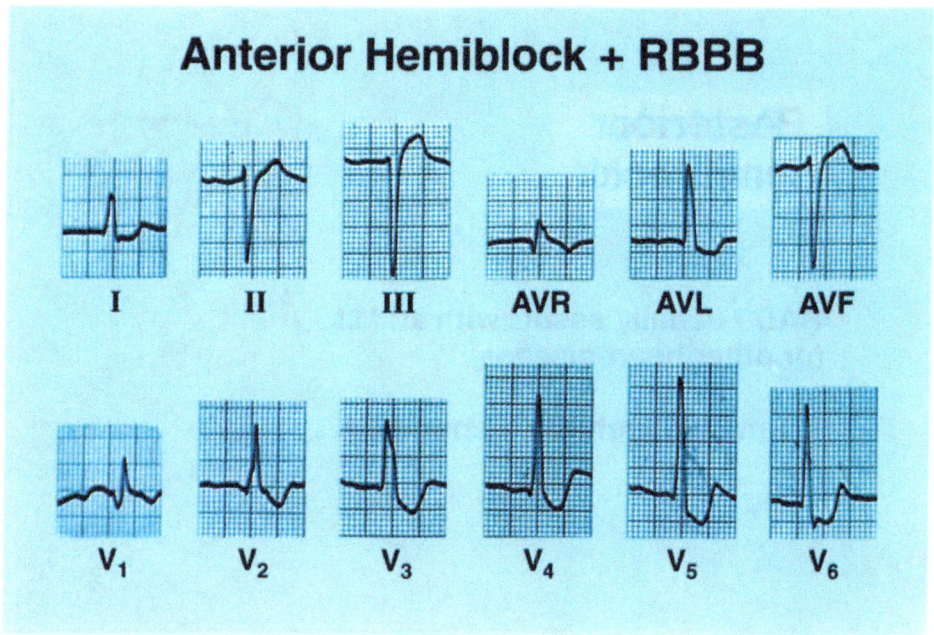

Anterior Hemiblock + RBBB

I   II   III   AVR   AVL   AVF

V_1 V_2 V_3 V_4 V_5 V_6

An infarction of the anterior wall of the left ventricle (due to an occluded Anterior Descending branch of the Left Coronary Artery) may cause Anterior Hemiblock <u>and</u> Right Bundle Branch Block. Review the illustration on page 296.

Note: Don't forget that the Anterior Descending also renders blood supply to the Right Bundle Branch, so Anterior Infarction may have an associated Right Bundle Branch Block, depending on the location of occlusion.

With Right Bundle Branch Block, the Mean QRS Vector is within the normal range or shows minimal Right Axis _____.   Deviation

However, when a patient develops a Right Bundle Branch Block with Left Axis Deviation as well, this is probably caused by Anterior Hemiblock, particularly if there is an acute Anterior _____.   Infarction

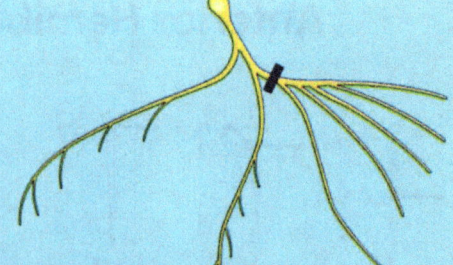

Posterior Hemiblock

- **RAD - usually assoc. with an M.I. (or other heart disease)**

- **Normal or slightly widened QRS**

- **S_1Q_3**

Pure, isolated *Posterior Hemiblock* is rare because the posterior division is short, thick, and commonly has a dual blood supply. See the illustration on page 296.

An inferior infarction may impair the blood supply to the Posterior division of the Left Bundle _____.   Branch

Posterior Hemiblocks cause Right Axis _____ due to the late, unopposed depolarization forces toward the right.   Deviation

When Posterior Hemiblock is suspected, look for a deep or unusually wide S in I and Q in III (known as S_1Q_3) to help confirm the _____ of Posterior Hemiblock.   diagnosis

Posterior Hemiblock

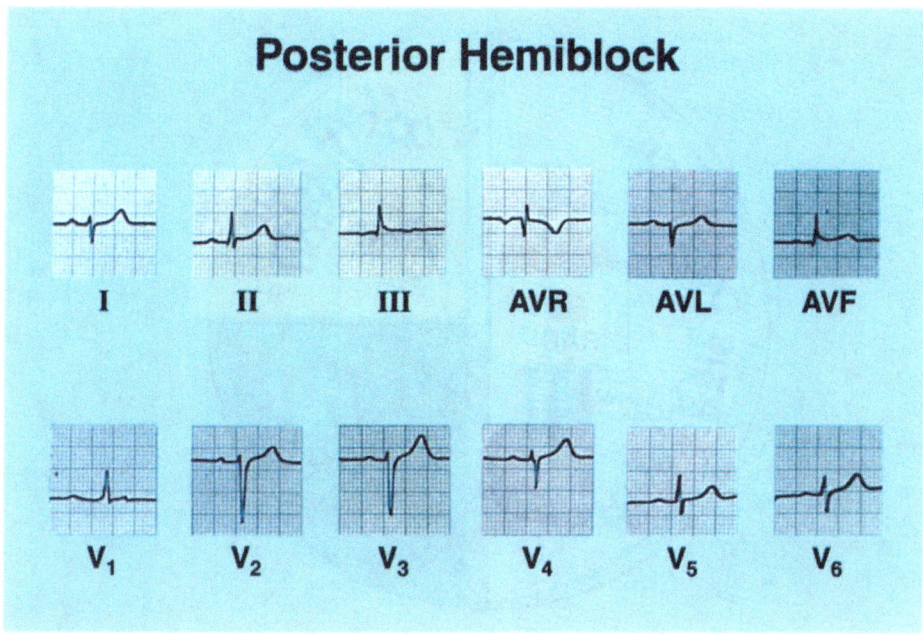

I   II   III   AVR   AVL   AVF

V₁   V₂   V₃   V₄   V₅   V₆

Posterior Hemiblock is always to be respected, and all Inferior Infarctions should be scrutinized to rule it out.

A lateral infarction, either recent or old, can cause
Right Axis Deviation, which can be confused with
Posterior Hemiblock. In the presence of a _____ M.I.,   lateral
the EKG diagnosis of Posterior Hemiblock is equivocal.

Make certain that by history and previous EKG's,
chronic Right Axis Deviation due to slender body build
("vertical heart"), _____ Ventricular Hypertrophy,   Right
and pulmonary disease, etc. are ruled out.

Note: Posterior Hemiblock is serious, and when associated with Right
Bundle Branch Block, this combination is considered very dangerous
because of the tendency to progress into AV Blocks.

Important!: AV Block refers to "atrio-ventricular block", that is, a
block between atrial depolarization and ventricular depolarization, so
we commonly think of a block in the AV Node or in the His Bundle.
However, simultaneous blocks of both Bundle Branches can block AV
conduction. Also, RBBB in association with the simultaneous blocks
of *both* divisions of the Left Bundle Branch can produce a block of AV
conduction. Please contemplate that for a while.

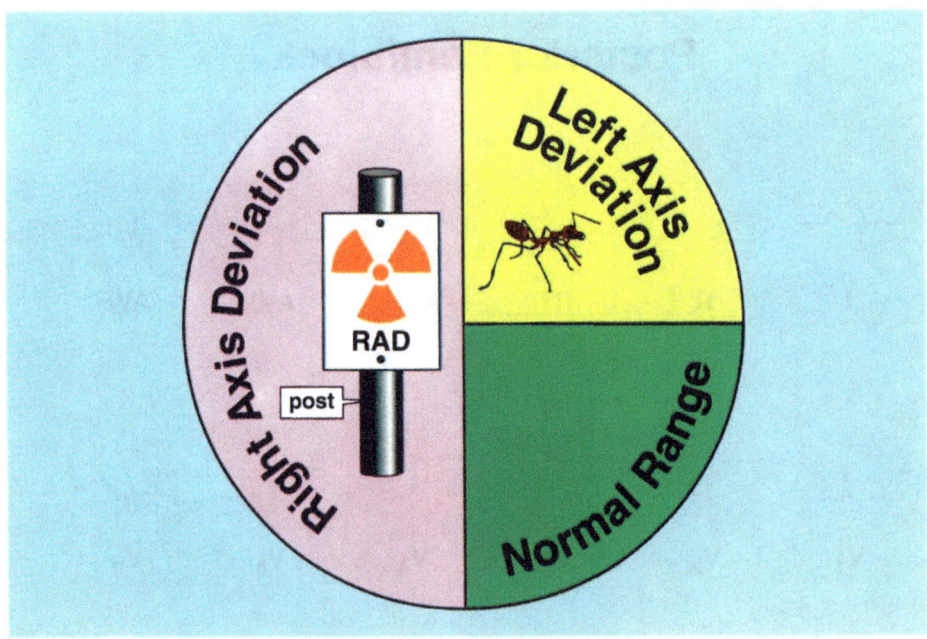

Yes, you see an *ant* in the Left Axis Deviation quadrant, a memory tool for <u>Left</u> axis shift suggests <u>Ant</u>erior Hemiblock. And, that's a *"rad"* (short for "radiation") sign on a *post* that represents a shift to <u>R</u>ight <u>A</u>xis <u>D</u>eviation suggesting <u>Post</u>erior Hemiblock. For some reason this silly illustration will stick in your mind.

When a patient with a normal axis shifts into an abnormal axis, particularly when associated with a serious cardiac event, we suspect _____.   hemiblock

A shift from normal axis to <u>R</u>ight <u>A</u>xis <u>D</u>eviation is characteristic of <u>Post</u>erior _____.   Hemiblock

A shift from normal axis to <u>L</u>eft <u>A</u>xis <u>D</u>eviation is characteristic of <u>Ant</u>erior _____.   Hemiblock

 * I wonder how the Japanese translators will deal with that?

Bifascicular Blocks

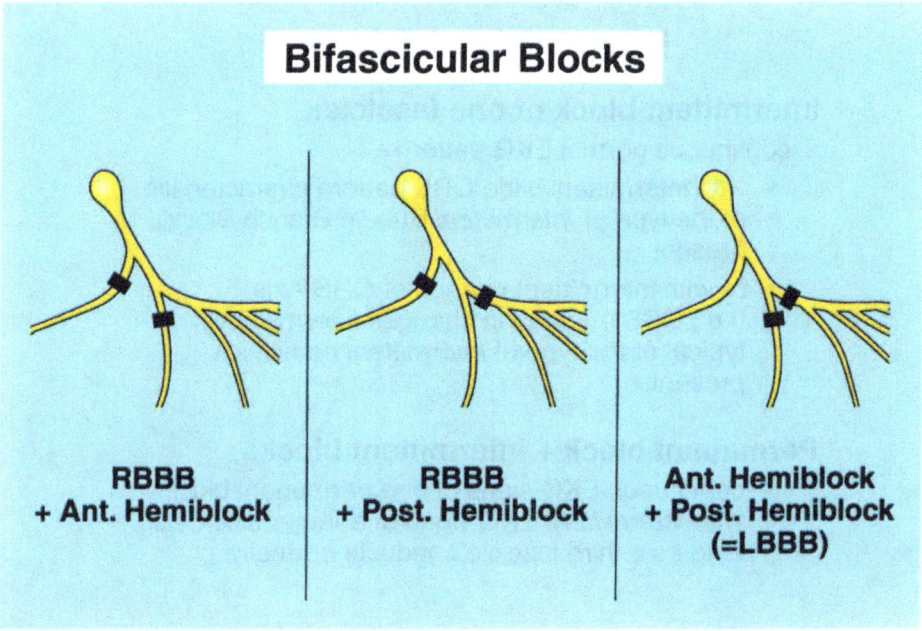

**RBBB
+ Ant. Hemiblock**

**RBBB
+ Post. Hemiblock**

**Ant. Hemiblock
+ Post. Hemiblock
(=LBBB)**

The word "fascicle" means bundle (bundle of Purkinje fibers), so any main division of the ventricular conduction system is a fascicle. *Both* Bundle Branches as well as both divisions of the Left Bundle Branch are fascicles.

Note: Previously, "Bundle" implied only the Right or the Left Bundle Branch. But now, to avoid confusion for combinations of blocks (e.g., Hemiblock + Bundle Branch Block) we use a more inclusive term, "fascicular" block, to denote a Bundle Branch Block with a Hemiblock.

Note: "Bifascicular" block means that two fascicles are blocked. Anterior Hemiblock plus Posterior Hemiblock is clinically the same as Left Bundle Branch Block. So Bifascicular Block generally refers to Right Bundle Branch Block together with a block of either the Anterior Division or the Posterior Division (of the Left Bundle Branch).

Note: A block of both the Right and the Left Bundle Branch is a Complete AV Block. Right BBB plus a block of both the Anterior and Posterior Divisions (of the Left Bundle Branch) is also a Complete AV Block. Complete AV Block is very serious since only a ventricular focus remains to *s l o w l y* pace the ventricles... so slowly that syncope often occurs (airway!), and a patient's life is at stake.

Note: When Bundle Branch Blocks or fascicular blocks are *intermittent*, we don't see them continuously on monitor or EKG tracing; just occasionally.

Intermittent Block

Intermittent block of one fascicle:

continuous normal EKG pattern –

- with intermittent wide QRS pattern characteristic of the type of *intermittent* Bundle Branch Block present.
- or with intermittent change of QRS Axis (i.e., QRS orientation changes intermittently) typical of the type of *intermittent* hemiblock present.

Permanent block + Intermittent block:

- continuous EKG signs of one permanent block with *intermittent* EKG signs of another block, as long as a third fascicle conducts normally.

Fortunately, combinations of (fascicular) blocks are often *intermittent*, making them quite obvious. Intermittent change in QRS axis (e.g., upright QRS's that transiently change to downward QRS's) usually indicates *intermittent* hemiblock, and a steady rhythm with transiently widened QRS's suggests *intermittent* BBB.

Intermittent block may exist in more than one fascicle in the same patient, producing a variety of transient changes of ____ Axis (intermittent [anterior or posterior] hemiblock) or...   QRS

...transiently widened QRS's typical of intermittent (left or right) ____ on EKG or cardiac monitor*. Don't ignore these intermittent changes; document them and give proper notification.   BBB

Note: Like a failing light bulb that occasionally flickers, sick fascicles may suffer intermittent block. As a failing, flickering light bulb eventually burns out, similarly, intermittent fascicular blocks often warn of impending permanent block of the fascicle. With a pre-existing permanent block of another fascicle, intermittent fascicular block can be a timely warning (the only warning!) of an imminent complete block (that's why the first word on this page is "fortunately"). In most cases, permanent block plus intermittent block is an indication for an artificial pacemaker.

* It is important and challenging to differentiate between intermittent anterior and posterior hemiblock, as well as intermittent right and left Bundle Branch Block. You know how already, but a little review wouldn't hurt.

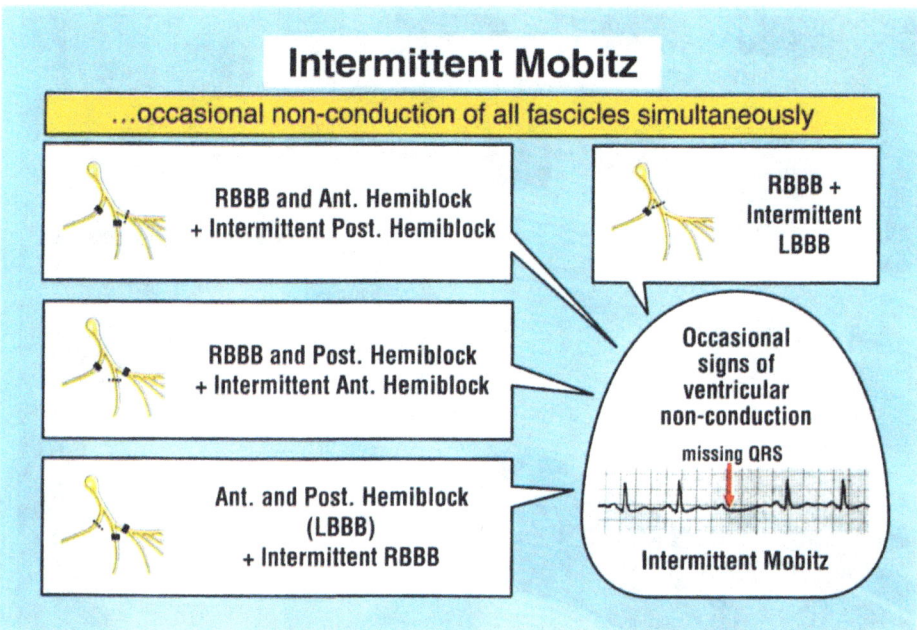

Considering the three pathways of ventricular depolarization, it becomes apparent that one fascicle must remain functional at least intermittently to provide AV conduction. Early detection allows for early intervention (see page 199).

"Trifascicular" blocks are diagnosed only when one or more of the fascicular blocks is _____,   intermittent otherwise there would be no AV conduction.

Also, the diagnosis of "bilateral" (Left and Right) Bundle Branch _____ is made only if one of the Bundles has an   Block intermittent block (or there would be no AV conduction).

Note: If all fascicles are permanently blocked except one that has an intermittent block, then an intermittent Mobitz pattern (occasional non-conduction to the ventricles) will emerge. If that Mobitz pattern becomes more frequent in the tracing, or if a continuous Mobitz 2:1 pattern begins, or worse yet, if there is a continuous high ratio Mobitz block, there is a strong likelihood that complete AV block is imminent and an implantable pacemaker is needed. Knowledge plus vigilance saves lives.

Warning! With Mobitz, every cycle missing its QRS has a regular, punctual P wave — but *never* a premature P' wave (see Note, page 128). This distinction is critical!

Note: Quickly review from page 295 to this page.

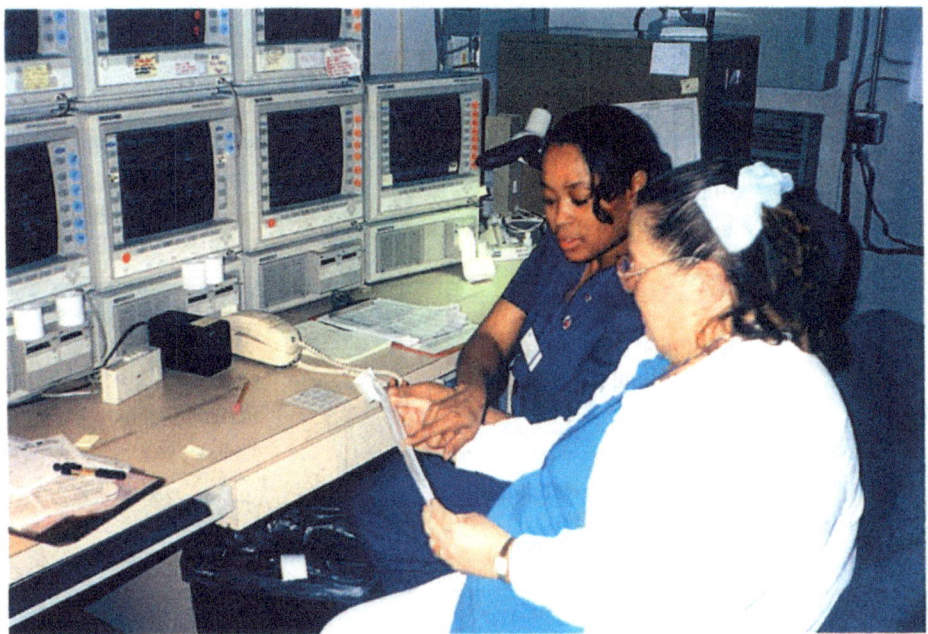

Patients with acute myocardial infarctions are placed in coronary care units and monitored continuously. In most hospitals patients with symptoms (only) of myocardial infarction receive the same cautious care. Patients with no physical symptoms of infarction but with definite EKG criteria of acute infarction ("silent infarction") require admission and monitoring also.

Note: Just as medical treatment of arrhythmias changes with the times, so do the attitudes toward indications for artificial pacemakers, angioplasty with stenting, coronary bypass procedures, and thrombolytic treatment. Keep up with the changing standards in your local medical community, read the current literature, and *always know the basics*.

You should always know how to determine the location of an infarction and the vessel(s) involved, as well as their association with _____.   Hemiblocks

In patients with myocardial infarction, be alert for subtle changes of Axis (change of QRS orientation in the same lead), and also rhythm changes that may indicate impending _____ AV block. Vigilance is critical.   complete

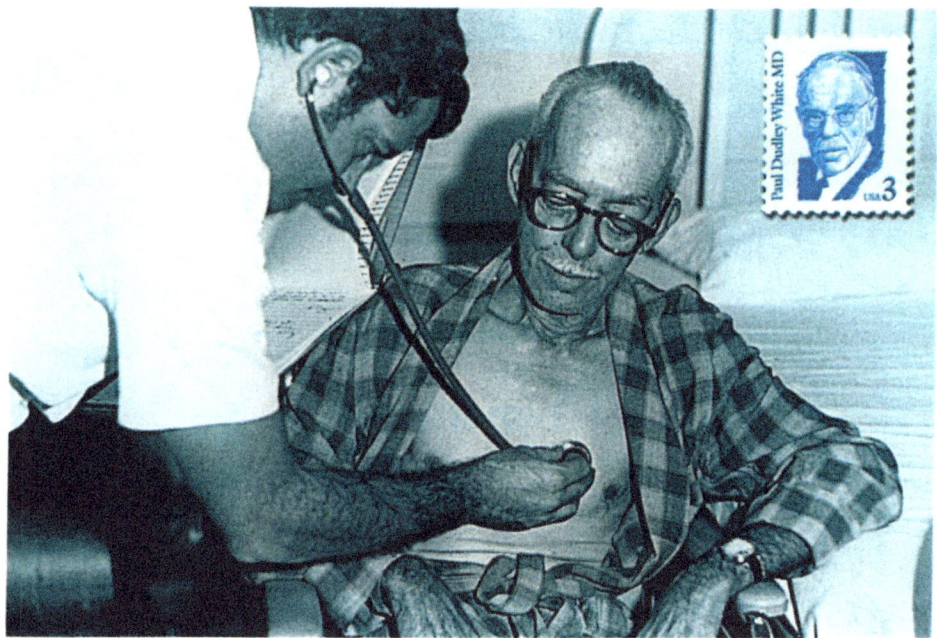

Remember that the patient's history and clinical diagnosis are still the most valuable tools you have (using your knowledge and judgment) in determining infarction and infarction-related problems.

The EKG has never become obsolete because it provides more
_____ information than any other diagnostic modality.   cardiac

There is no substitute for obtaining an accurate _____,   history
even if it is volunteered by witnesses to an event.

Although the laboratory provides much useful information,
the ____ is an <u>immediate</u> diagnostic gift for those skilled   EKG
in its interpretation.

Note: The value of an EKG increases multifold when it is compared
to a patient's previous tracings — get them as soon as possible!
Incidentally, is this a photo of Dr. Paul Dudley White, and who
is his examining physician with the Elvis sideburns?

Note: Review Infarction by turning to the **P**ersonal **Q**uick **R**eference
Sheets on pages 342 and 343, and again, look at your simplified
methodology (page 334).

1. Rate

2. Rhythm

3. Axis

4. Hypertrophy

5. Infarction

You now have the knowledge and certainly the interest and enthusiasm to interpret EKG's, but always do it methodically. Begin with Rate, then Rhythm, Axis, Hypertrophy, and Infarction. Get accustomed to this routine.

Note: In the excitement of an emergency you may be tempted to hunt for Q waves. By breaking the routine you will inevitable miss important diagnostic information - valuable information necessary for the proper treatment of the patient. Keep a cool head and read every EKG properly. Your patients will benefit from your thoroughness.

Note: Take one final look at page 334 and review each step of the entire methodology. Then (please) slowly review all of the PQRS pages from 334 to 343. But before you close this book there is some very helpful information in the Miscellaneous chapter. It is next. No, you aren't done yet.

Before you begin, look at this chapter's summary on pages 344 to 346.

Miscellaneous Effects

Pulmonary

Electrolytes

Medications

Artificial Pacemakers

Heart Transplants

The above effects are common to, but not necessarily diagnostic of, certain conditions or situations that can produce recognizable changes on the EKG.

Note: Certain effects may be recognized by their characteristic appearance on the electrocardiogram or on cardiac monitor. For most of the conditions to be discussed in this section, the electrocardiographic signs merely alert us to be aware of existing conditions, certain pathology, or drug or electrolyte effects. But to confirm your suspicion, you should review the medical history, carry out a detailed physical exam, and obtain proper diagnostic tests. Rarely is a diagnosis based entirely on any of the following EKG findings, however they are exceptionally helpful.

Three Important Syndromes
detection can save a life

Brugada Syndrome
- RBBB with ST elevation in V_1, V_2, and V_3 (see page 268)
- susceptible to deadly arrhythmias

Wellens Syndrome
- marked T wave inversion in V_2 and V_3
- Ant. Descending Coronary stenosis

Long QT Syndrome
- QT interval longer than $\frac{1}{2}$ of the cardiac cycle
- predisposed to ventricular arrhythmias

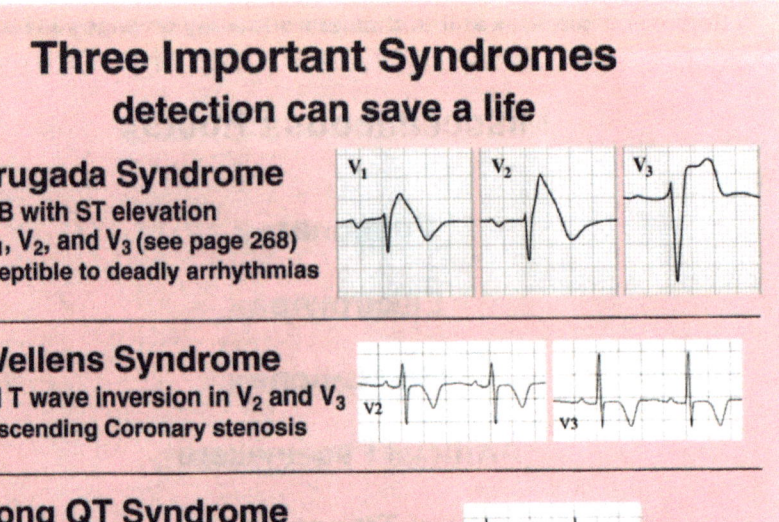

Each of these perilous syndromes are easily detected in relatively asymptomatic patients. Routine examination of all EKG's for these innocuous-looking hallmarks can avoid an inevitable demise. Conventional treatment offers the patient reasonable longevity. The satisfaction of saving a human life is your reward for your vigilance.

Patients with *Brugada Syndrome*, a familial condition, may succumb to deadly arrhythmias; implantation with an ICD can prevent sudden _____.

death

Wellens Syndrome, caused by a stenosed anterior descending coronary artery, is easily recognized. Angioplasty with stenting or a coronary bypass graft can remove the imminent peril of impending myocardial _____.

infarction

There are six known forms of (hereditary) *Long QT Syndrome*; these patients are predisposed to dangerous ventricular arrhythmias. A long QT interval exceeds one-half of the _____ cycle.

cardiac

Note: If everyone who reads this book becomes familiar with, and routinely looks for, these important diagnostic signs, it will serve humanity immensely. A glance at the right chest leads and observing the QT interval is sufficient.

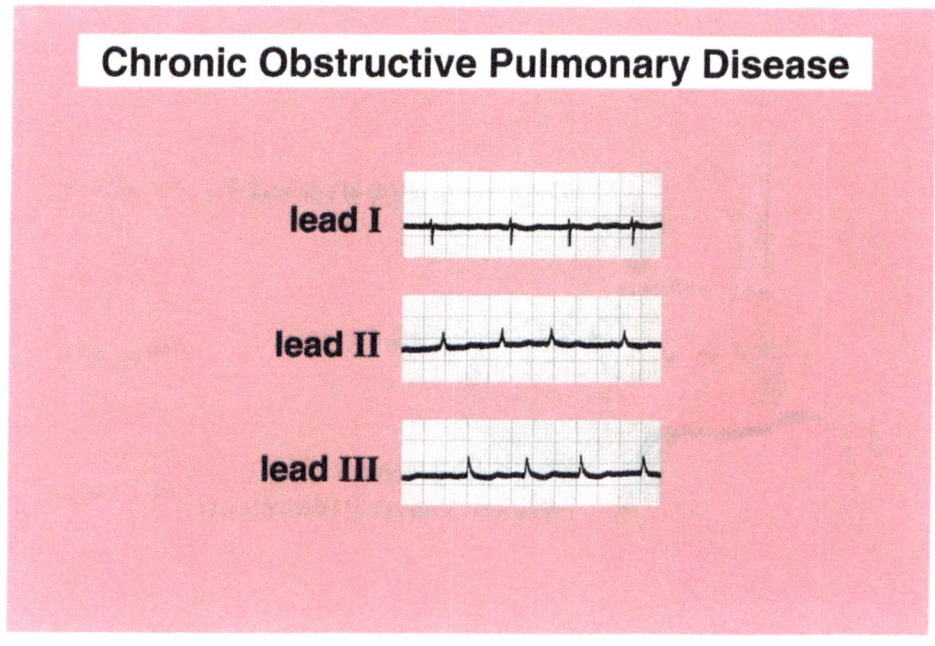

Chronic Obstructive Pulmonary Disease (COPD) often produces low voltage amplitude in all leads, and there is usually Right Axis Deviation.

Chronic Obstructive Pulmonary Disease (COPD) commonly produces QRS complexes of small amplitude* in all leads. In fact, all waves in the EKG are minimized in _____.   COPD

With COPD, the right ventricle works against considerable resistance, so there is usually some degree of Right Ventricular Hypertrophy and therefore associated _____ Axis Deviation   Right (notice negative QRS's in lead I).

Note: Multifocal Atrial Tachycardia (MAT) is also seen with COPD.

* Low voltage in all leads also appears with hypothyroidism and chronic constrictive pericarditis.

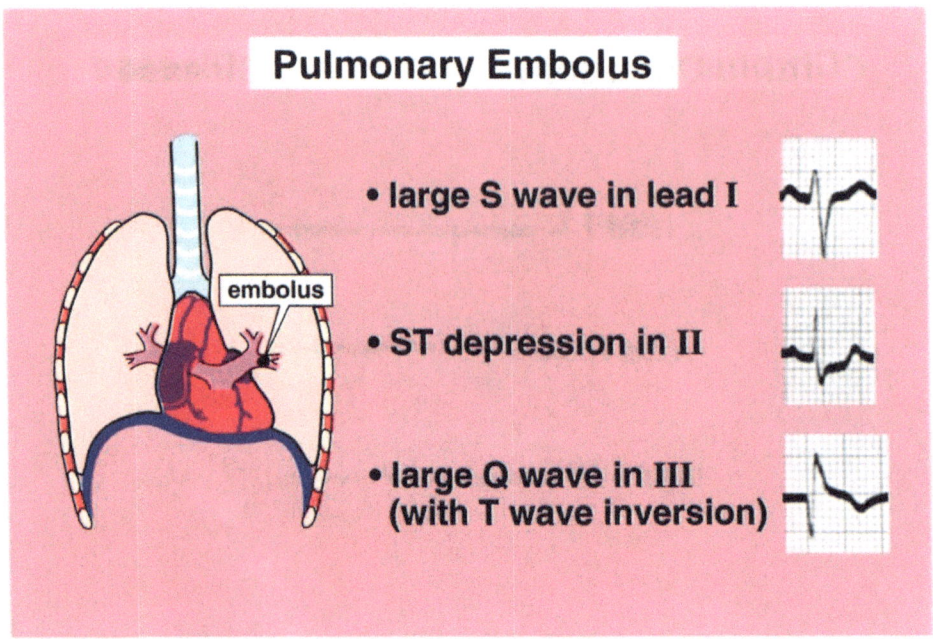

With *Pulmonary Embolus* we usually see a large S wave in lead I, and a Q wave and an inverted T wave in lead III ($S_1Q_3 \bot_3$)*.

$S_1Q_3 \bot_3$ syndrome characterizes acute *cor pulmonale* resulting from pulmonary embolus. It is called $S_1Q_3 \bot_3$ because of the large S wave in lead I, and there is a Q wave and an inverted T wave in lead ___.   III

Note: Notice the typical tendency toward Right Axis Deviation (lead I).

There is usually ST segment _____ in lead II.   depression

* Don't be confused by the inverted T in the printed text. It's a great memory tool, even if the publisher dislikes it.

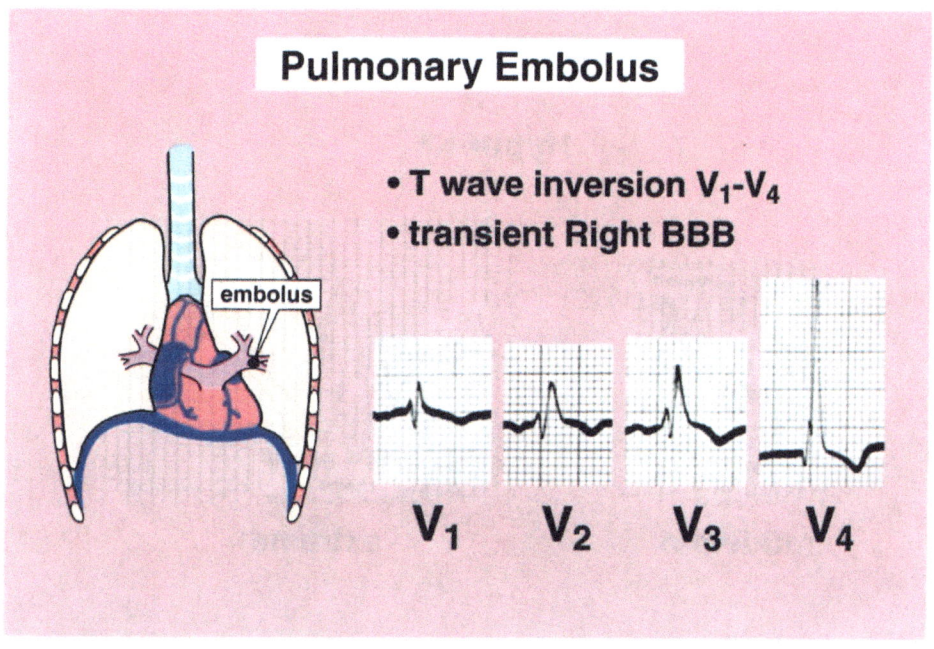

Pulmonary Embolus

• **T wave inversion V₁-V₄**
• **transient Right BBB**

embolus

V₁   V₂   V₃   V₄

Also with pulmonary embolus, there is usually T wave inversion in V_1 through V_4. Often there is Right Bundle Branch Block.

T wave inversion in the chest leads (particularly in leads V_1 through V_4) is a very important diagnostic sign of pulmonary _____.   embolus

Pulmonary embolus may cause _____ Bundle Branch Block.   Right
This block often subsides after the patient improves.

We can recognize the presence of Right Bundle Branch Block by the R,R' in the right _____ leads.   chest

Note: Occasionally the Right Bundle Branch Block may be "incomplete" (QRS of normal width, but R,R' is present).

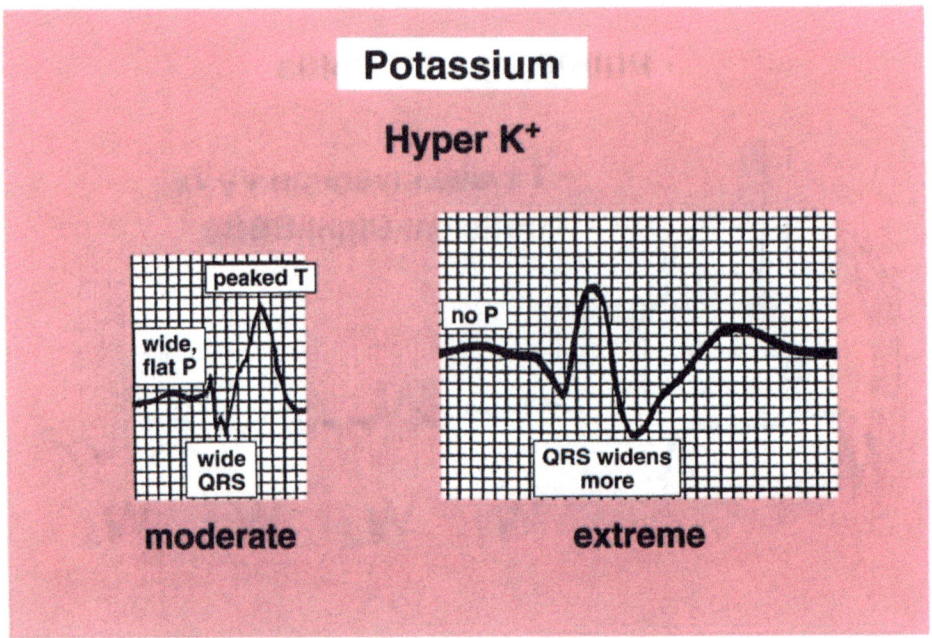

With elevated serum potassium the P wave flattens down, the QRS complex widens, and the T wave becomes peaked.

Note: The potassium ion (K^+) plays an extremely important role in cardiac electrophysiology. The range of normal serum K^+ concentration is very narrow. In medical parlance we add the suffix "-emia" to the end of the ion name to denote its presence in the blood... but it sounds funny with "potassium." So its chemical symbol, K, is pronounced verbally, and the prefix "hyper" for increased, or the prefix "hypo" for decreased, is added to communicate deviations from normal. Now you'll understand both *hyper-* and *hypo-* kalemia* (pronounced "kay-LEE-mia"). And that's right, it's written "kalemia." That should help you and also your friends who might be perplexed...

The most striking and classic feature of elevated
serum potassium is the _____ T wave.   peaked

The P wave widens and flattens with increased serum
potassium, and with extreme hyperkalemia the __ wave   P
nearly disappears.

When a patient has hyperkalemia, ventricular depolarization
takes longer, so the QRS complex _____.   widens

* The "l" is added to enhance the phonics, so you don't have to get the "l" out of there
  (chuckle!).

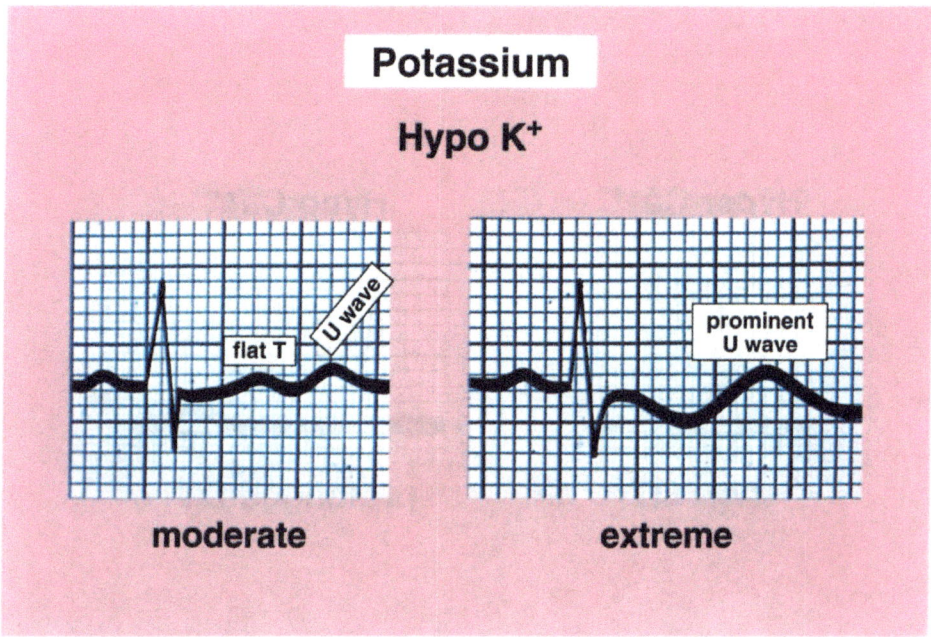

As the serum potassium drops below normal levels, the T wave becomes flat
(or inverted) and a U wave appears.

With hypokalemia, as the serum potassium concentration drops,
the __ wave flattens out, and if the K⁺ concentration drops lower,   T
the T wave inverts.

Note: I always think of the T wave as a tent housing potassium ions.
When there is an increase in potassium ions, the tent peaks up, but
lowering of potassium ions lowers the height of the tent.

With hypokalemia a __ wave appears. This wave becomes more   U
pronounced as the loss of potassium becomes more severe.

Note: Potassium is not just "one of those serum electrolytes."
Potassium plays a critical role in repolarization and also in maintaining
a precise resting potential. A decrease in potassium makes ventricular
automaticity foci extremely irritable. In fact, low potassium can initiate
Torsades de Pointes, and it can also evoke dangerous ventricular tachy-
arrhythmias. Hypokalemia also enhances the toxic effects of digitalis
excess.

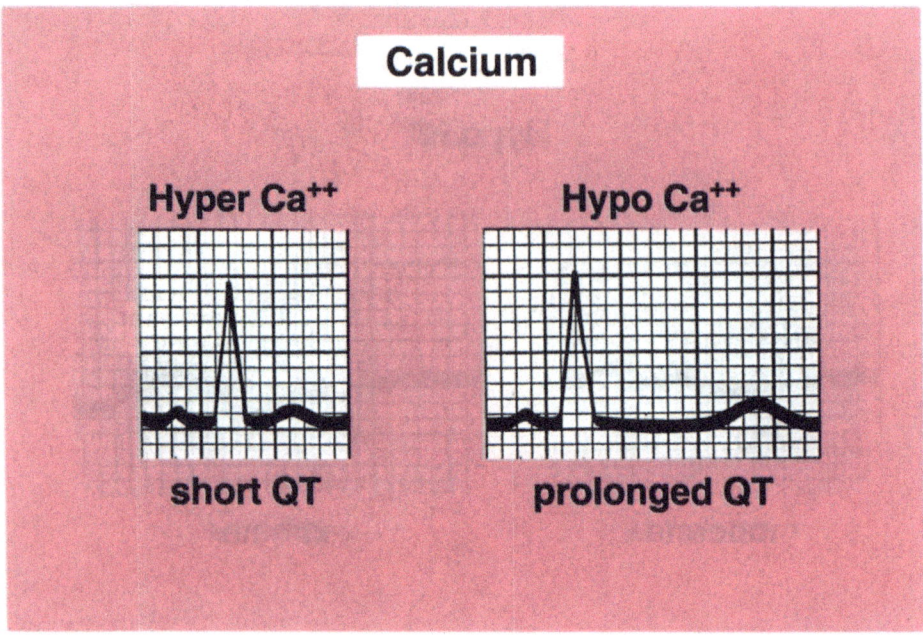

With *hypercalcemia,* the QT interval shortens; however *hypocalcemia* prolongs the QT interval.

Note: Since you already understand "hyper-" and "hypo-", I only need mention that "-calcemia" is pronounced "cal-SEE-mia".

Hypocalcemia will prolong the ___ interval.   QT

Note: The QT interval is measured from the beginning of the QRS complex to the end of the T wave. Normally, the QT interval should be less than half of the cycle length.

An increase in calcium (Ca^{++}) ions accelerates both ventricular depolarization and ventricular repolarization. This is manifested as a short QT _____.   interval

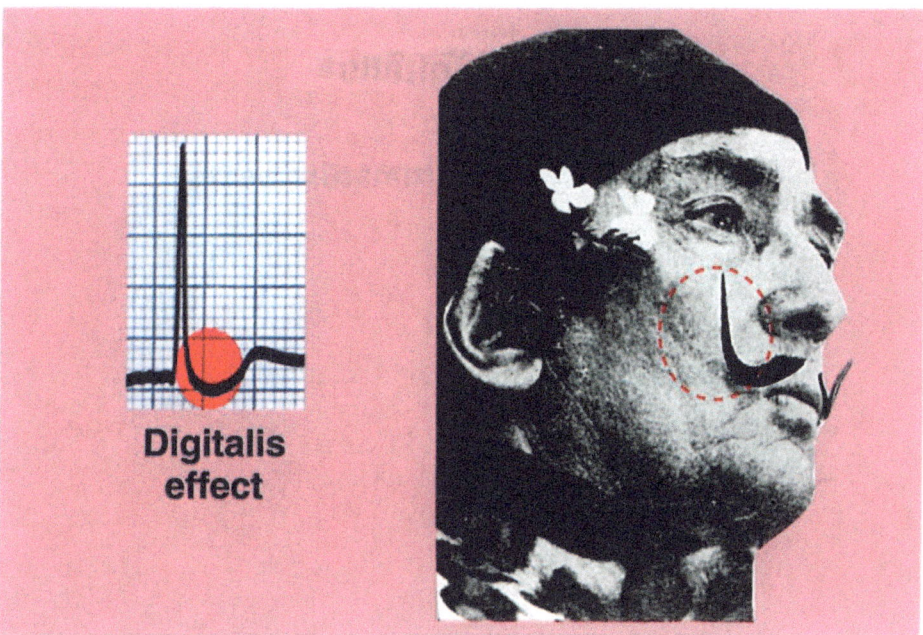

Digitalis causes a gradual downward curve of the ST segment, to give it the appearance of Salvador Dali's mustache. Notice that the lowest portion of the ST segment is depressed below the baseline.

Digitalis produces a unique, gradual downward curve of the ___ segment; this is the classical "digitalis effect."

ST

Note: To identify the classical pattern of digitalis effect, you should observe a lead with no demonstrable S wave. The downward portion of the R wave gradually thickens as it curves down into the ST segment, which is usually depressed. The downward limb of the R wave has a gentle, curving slope that gradually blends into the depressed ST segment. Look for it the next time you have a patient on a digitalis preparation.

Note: Digitalis in therapeutic doses has a parasympathetic effect. With a Sinus Rhythm, digitalis slows the SA Node pacing rate. Conduction through the AV Node is slowed, and digitalis also inhibits the AV Node's receptiveness to multiple stimuli, allowing fewer stimuli to reach the ventricles (necessary with Atrial Flutter and Atrial Fibrillation) to permit a more physiological and more efficient ventricular response rate. Digitalis has a very narrow range of therapeutic effectiveness, and should this therapeutic range be exceeded, a multitude of undesirable effects can result. See the next two pages...

Excess Digitalis

- **atrial & Junctional premature beats**

- **PAT with block**

- **Sinus block**

- **AV blocks**

Excess digitalis tends to cause AV Blocks of many varieties, and may even induce Sinus (SA) Block.

Note: Supraventricular (particularly atrial) foci are exceptionally sensitive to digitalis, so premature atrial beats (PAB's) are often the earliest warning sign that your patient has elevated levels of digitalis. Atrial automaticity foci are very effective digitalis sensors.

Digitalis in excess may cause transient Sinus _____.   Block

Digitalis retards conduction of depolarization through the AV Node; and in excess, it can cause various types of ___ Block, particularly rate-dependent AV Block.   AV

Automaticity foci of the atria and the AV Junction can become irritable when _____ preparations are present in excessive concentrations in your patient.   digitalis

Note: Low serum potassium can enhance the toxicity of digitalis, so that digitalis, even in therapeutic concentrations, can produce undesirable signs of toxicity if the serum potassium is low.

Digitalis Toxicity

- **atrial & Junctional tachy-arrhythmias**

- **PVC's**

- **Ventricular Bigeminy, Trigeminy**

- **Ventricular Tachycardia**

- **Ventricular Fibrillation**

Atrial and Junctional automaticity foci are very likely to become irritable in the presence of excessive digitalis. In fact, marked *digitalis toxicity* can even provoke ventricular foci into rapid and dangerous rhythms.

The foci of the atria and AV Junction are most sensitive to excessive digitalis, but with marked digitalis _____, even ventricular foci may become so irritable that they spontaneously emit PVC's.

toxicity

Marked digitalis toxicity can make ventricular foci so irritable that they may suddenly fire multiple discharges that initiate dangerous _____ tachy-arrhythmias.

ventricular

Note: Digitalis preparations have been used medicinally by civilized people since the thirteenth century. But like most other cardiac medications, in certain circumstances or in high concentrations, digitalis can induce deadly arrhythmias.

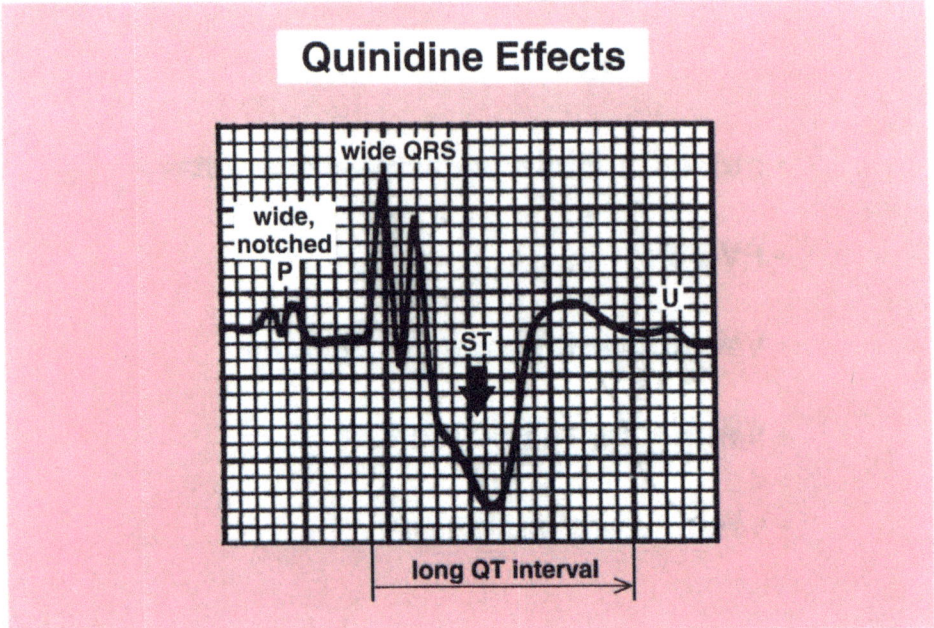

Quinidine causes widening of the P wave and widening of the QRS complex. There is often ST depression with a prolonged QT. The presence of U waves is typical as well.

Note: Quinidine retards depolarization and repolarization through both the atrial and the ventricular myocardium. Most of the effects of quinidine that we see on EKG relate to its pharmacological effects on sodium and potassium ion channels.

Quinidine causes a wide, notched ___ wave on EKG, and the   P
QRS complex is also widened.

Quinidine prolongs the ___ interval, and depresses the   QT
ST segment. Look for U waves (which represent delayed
repolarization of the ventricular conduction system).

Note: Episodes of Torsades de Pointes – a rapid and dangerous
ventricular rhythm can result from quinidine toxicity (see page 158).

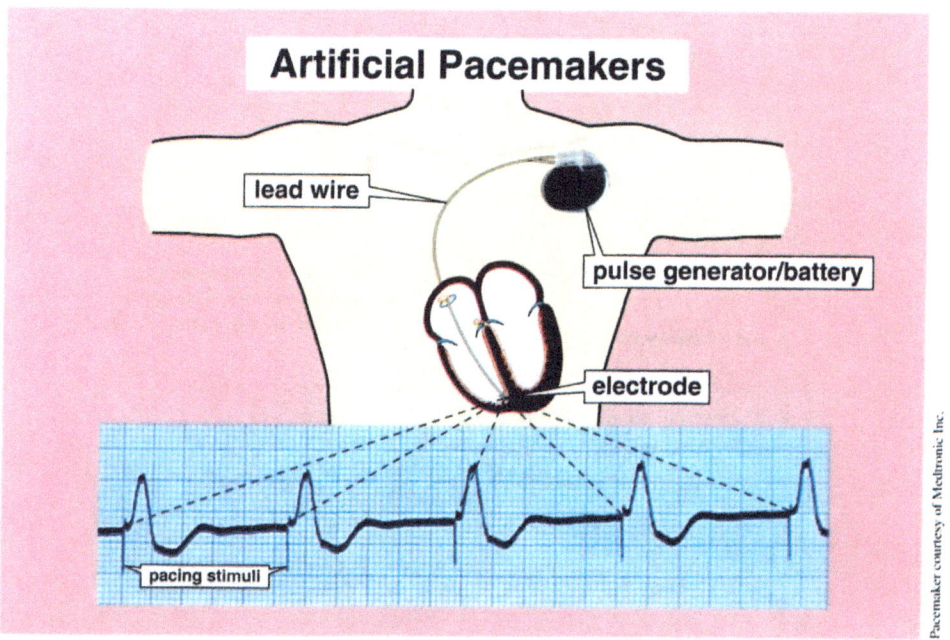

Artificial pacemakers have a pulse generator with a long-lasting lithium battery. The pacemaking stimuli are designed for ventricular or atrial (or both) pacing modalities, and a wide variety of sensing features are available.

Note: Artificial pacemakers are surgically implanted as a permanent pacemaking source. Originally, they were designed to counter the bradycardia that attends Complete AV Block and Sick Sinus Syndrome. Now, the uses and variety of pacemaker types is well beyond the scope of this book, so we will review only basic principles of artificial cardiac pacing. In most cases the electrode lead wire is passed transvenously into the right side of the heart; however, sometimes the stimulating electrode is surgically attached to the epicardial surface of the heart.

The pacemaker generator emits regular pacing stimuli, which record on the _____ as a narrow vertical spike.

EKG

The pacemaker emits regular, paced electrical _____, and each stimulus should "capture" (i.e., depolarize) the myocardial tissue in contact with the electrode. The depolarization stimulus then conducts through the myocardium.

stimuli

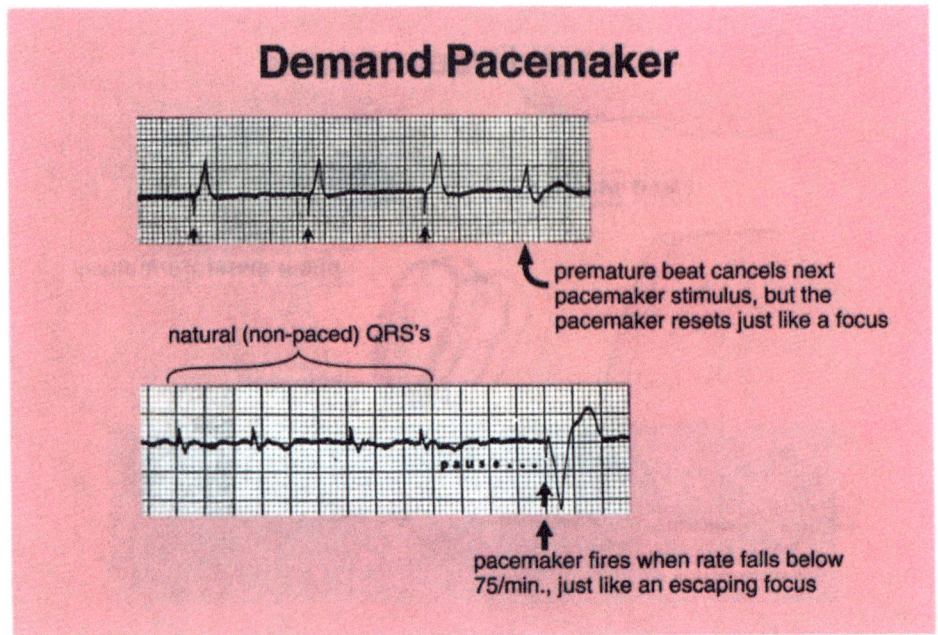

Demand Pacemaker

premature beat cancels next pacemaker stimulus, but the pacemaker resets just like a focus

natural (non-paced) QRS's

pause...

pacemaker fires when rate falls below 75/min., just like an escaping focus

The *demand* feature of many artificial pacemakers is designed to imitate the physiological mechanisms of an automaticity focus (great idea!). The demand pacemaker is programmed with an "inherent rate" that is overdrive-suppressed by normal Sinus pacing.

Note: The illustration depicts the EKG of a demand pacemaker with a ventricular sensing electrode and a ventricular pacing electrode.

A demand pacemaker is *overdrive-suppressed* by normal Sinus pacing, but should the Sinus rate drop below the pacemaker's programmed inherent rate, the pacemaker, no longer overdrive-suppressed, escapes to assume pacemaking responsibility at its inherent _____.

rate

But if the SA Node resumes pacing at a normal rate (which is faster than the _____ rate of the demand pacemaker) the demand pacemaker is overdrive-suppressed and stops pacing.

inherent

The demand pacemaker is designed to *reset* just like an automaticity focus. When the demand pacemaker senses a PVC, it resets its pacing (at the cycle length of its inherent rate) in step with the ____ . This provides for uninterrupted cardiac function (clever engineers design to imitate Nature).

PVC

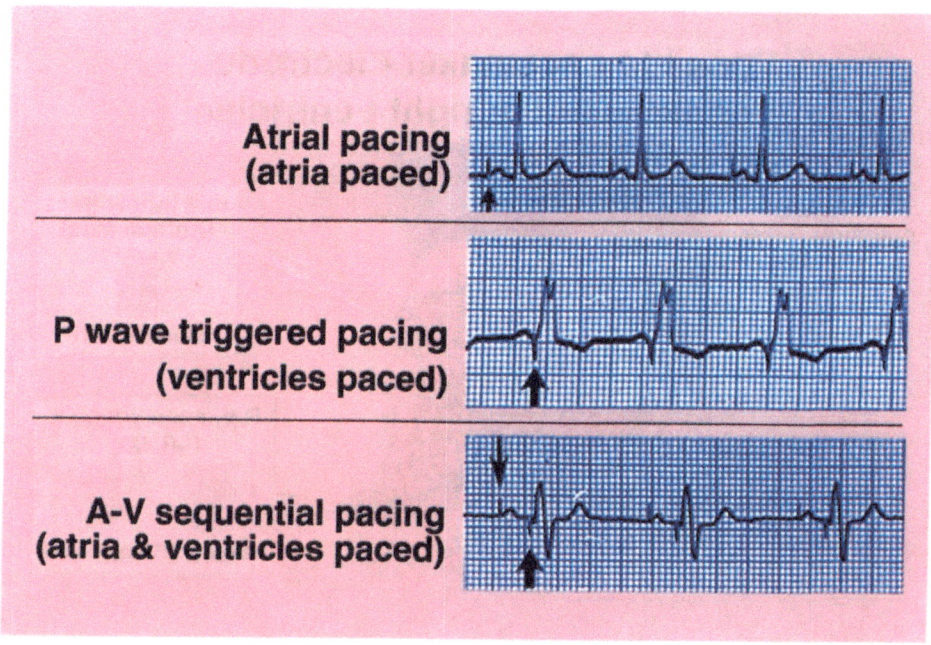

Contemporary pacemakers offer many features that can be used to treat many types of cardiac dysfunction and pathology.

With failure of the SA Node, *Atrial Pacing* can be used when the AV Node and ventricular conduction system function normally, so the artificially paced atrial stimuli are properly conducted from the atria to the _____.

ventricles

A complete AV block prevents normal Sinus pacing from conducting to the ventricles and may require *P wave triggered pacing**, which senses the patient's ___ wave, then after a brief pause (imitating normal AV conduction) it generates a stimulus for ventricular depolarization.

P

SA Node malfunction combined with complete AV block sometimes necessitates *A-V sequential pacing,* which provides a stimulus for atrial depolarization followed by a brief pause, then the ventricles are _____.

depolarized

Note: Modern pacemakers are computerized wonders that can detect and respond to physiological needs such as decreased rate during sleep and increased rate during exercise.

* Also called "atrial synchronous" or "atrial tracking" pacing.

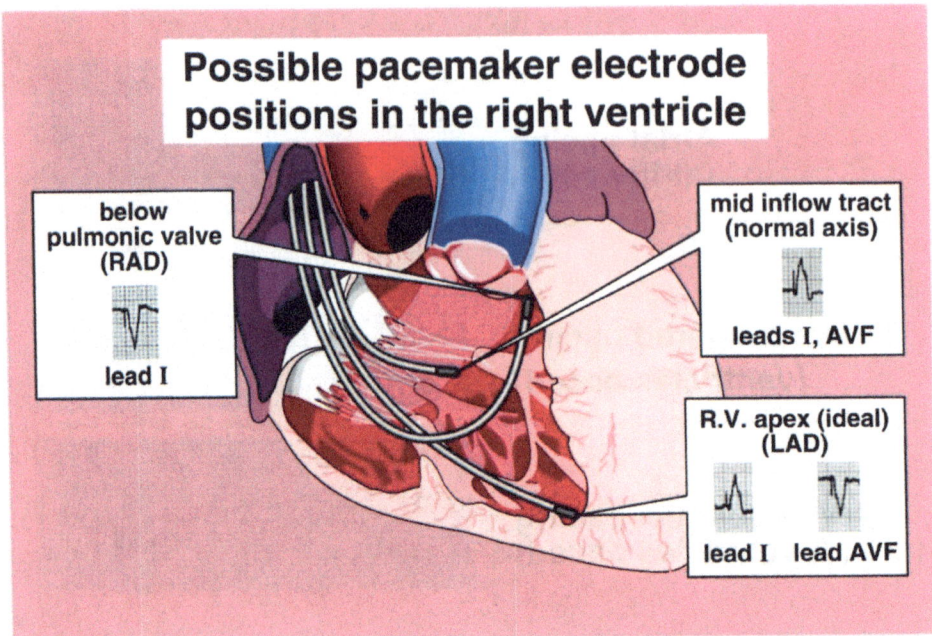

Usually a right ventricular electrode is used for cardiac pacemaking; the electrode tip of the lead is positioned within the cavity of the right ventricle. Three possible catheter lead positions are shown with the way they record on EKG.

Note: The ideal location of the tip electrode of a right ventricular pacemaker, is in the apex of the right ventricle. The resultant QRS complex has a Left Bundle Branch Block pattern with Left Axis Deviation.

When a paced QRS shows a LBBB pattern with a normal axis, the electrode tip is in the mid-inflow tract of the right _____.   ventricle

But if you notice a paced QRS with a LBBB pattern and Right Axis Deviation, the tip of the _____ is just   electrode below the pulmonic valves.

Note: Certain cardiac patients may have a surgically implanted "pacemaker", called an *Implantable Cardioverter Defibrillator* (ICD, see next page) that can pace, detect and interpret rhythm disturbances, and treat tachyarrhythmias by overdrive pacing or cardioversion, even defibrillate in the event of ventricular fibrillation. Oh, Brave New World!

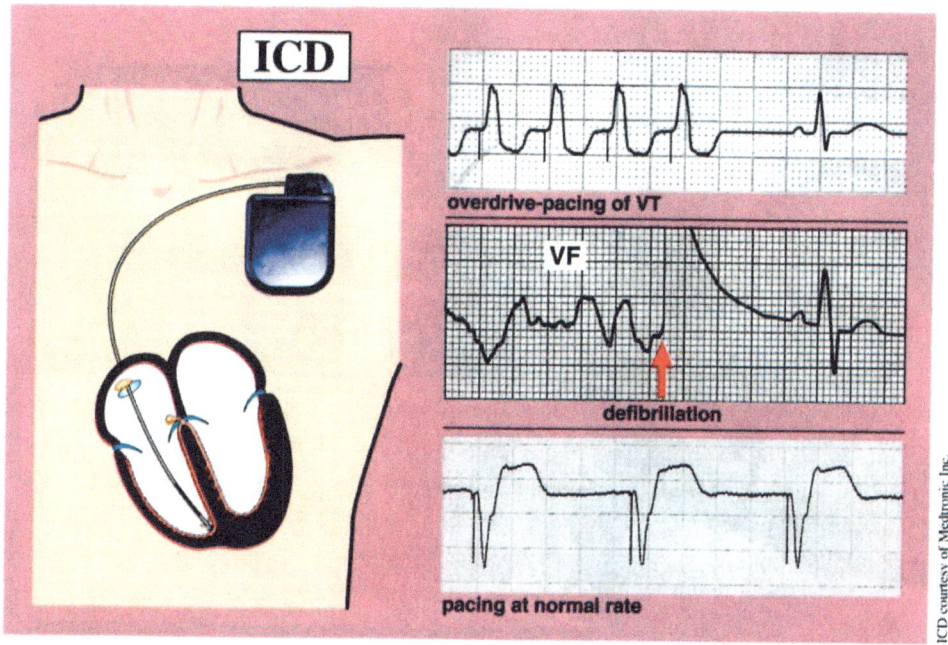

ICD

overdrive-pacing of VT

VF

defibrillation

pacing at normal rate

ICD courtesy of Medtronic Inc.

The Implantable Cardioverter Defibrillator (ICD) is a self-contained, computerized device that can instantly analyze and treat most dangerous cardiac arrhythmias. It can simulate normal sinus pacing, institute overdrive (suppression) pacing to treat ventricular tachycardia, provide cardioversion, and even defibrillate VF.

The ICD can detect and treat certain arrhythmias with cardioversion (a precisely timed electrical shock), and...

it can diagnose ventricular tachycardia and respond with overdrive pacing to suppress the causative ventricular _____.   focus

The ICD can detect ventricular fibrillation and instantly defibrillate the heart, and...

should the SA Node perform sluggishly after defibrillation, the ICD will provide pacemaking stimuli at a physiological _____.   rate

Note: The ICD is a technological masterpiece!

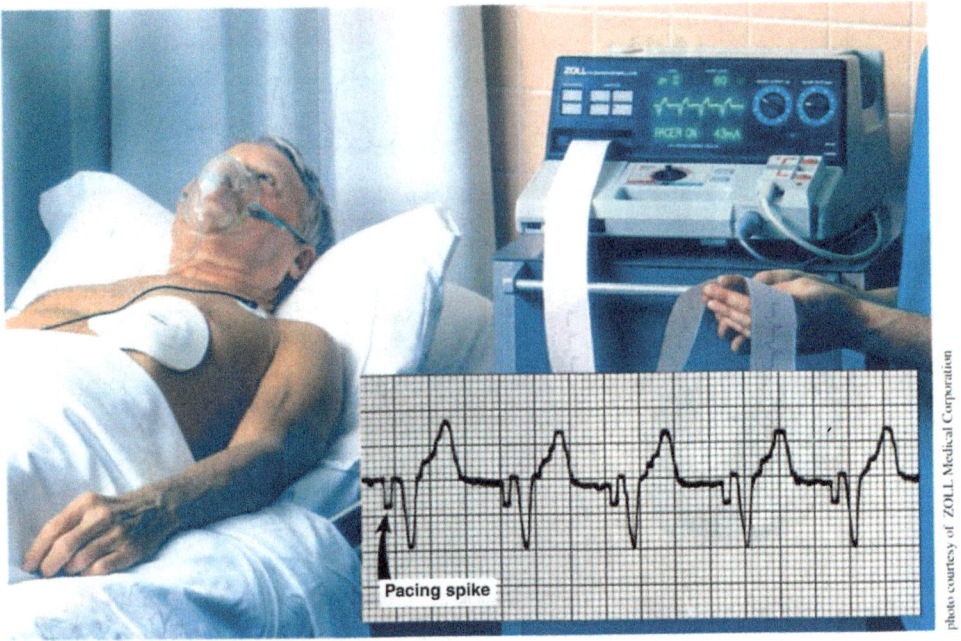

There is an *external non-invasive* pacemaking device that effectively delivers pacing stimuli to the heart through intact skin in emergency situations.

Sophisticated pacemakers are available that can painlessly pace the heart through the intact _____. These external, non-invasive pacemakers are ideal for temporary pacing.

skin

Pacing the heart through the body surface requires an impulse of longer duration than that of intracardiac pacemakers so each pacing spike is wide with a _____ end.

flat

Note: Another externally applied emergency device, the *Automated External Defibrillator* (AED), records and analyses the patient's EKG, and then automatically defibrillates the patient if a deadly arrhythmia is detected. The AED is very accurate in its computerized recognition of Ventricular Fibrillation and high rate Ventricular Tachycardia; it is easily operated by moderately trained personnel. Numerous trials and studies have proven the AED to be a very effective method of defibrillation in a non-hospital setting. See page 170.

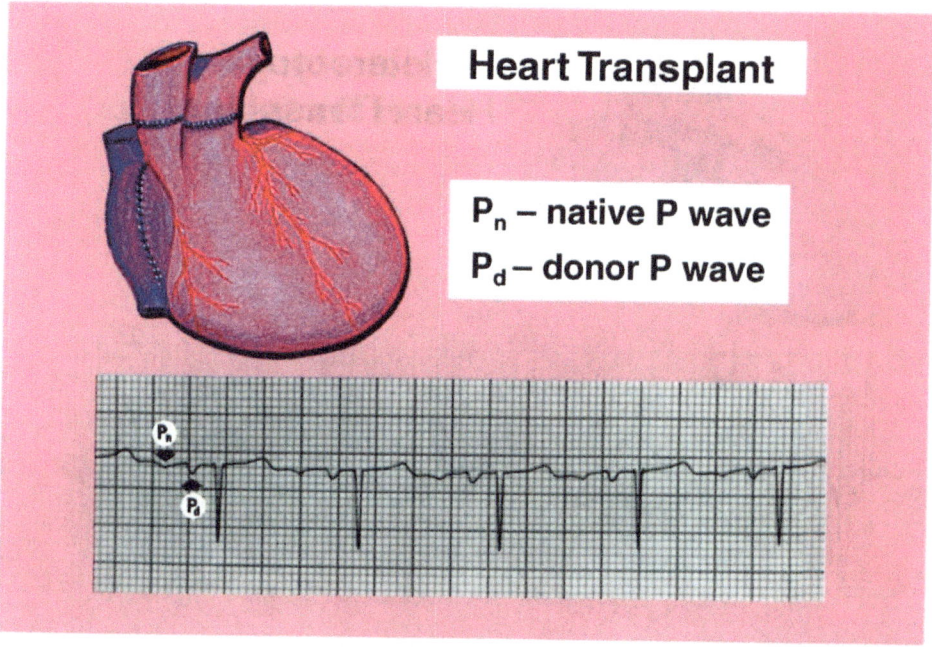

Heart Transplant

P_n – native P wave

P_d – donor P wave

A *heart transplant* procedure leaves portions of the recipient patient's "native" atria in place. These portions of atria contain the patient's own SA Node, so the transplant patient has his native SA Node, plus the SA Node of the donor heart.

Note: To expedite these procedures, the portions of the native atria that contain the large vessel orifices are left behind to be sutured to the atria of the transplanted heart. So the recipient patient retains the native SA Node, and the donor heart that the patient receives also has a functioning SA Node.

Transplant patients therefore have two SA Nodes, each producing ____ waves.

P

The native SA Node produces depolarizations (P_n) that do not pass beyond the suture line, so they do not depolarize the donor _____.

atria

The transplanted "donor" heart has its own functional SA Node that remains the dominant pacemaker, so all of its P waves (P_d) are followed by ____ complexes.

QRS

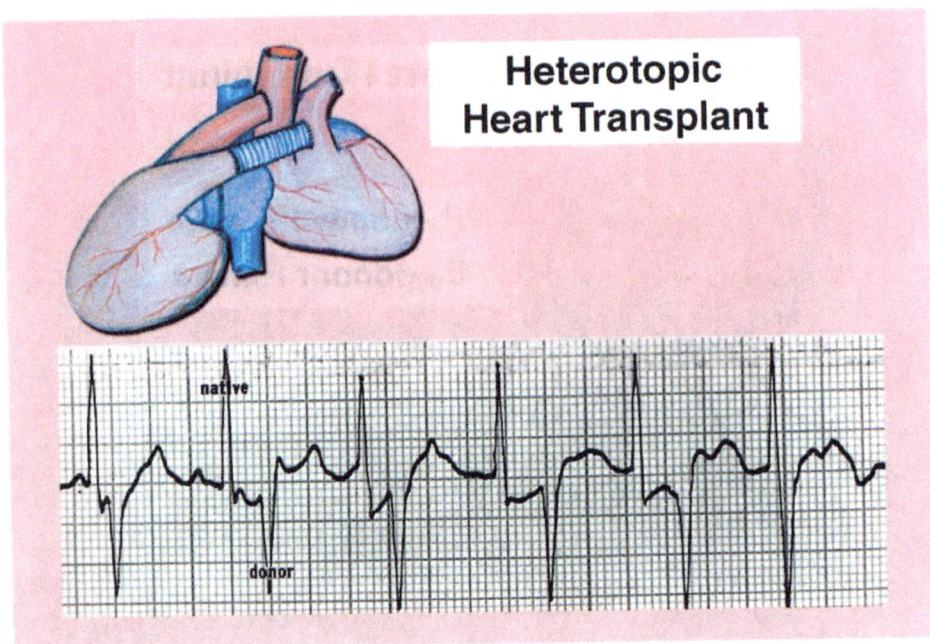

A *heterotopic* heart transplant is a procedure that leaves the native heart in place, while a temporary, donor heart is surgically attached to assist the pumping effort.

In order to assist in pumping, a heterotopic heart transplant gives the patient (temporarily) two _____.

hearts

So the EKG in this temporary, emergency situation displays the simultaneous recording of the electrical activity of two separate _____.

hearts

Note: With great advances in medical technology and increasing sophistication of biomechanical engineering, attempts are constantly being made to devise an efficient artificial heart. It is unlikely that a totally artificial heart will ever approach the efficacy and safety of that Designed by Nature.

Let me know if your understanding was a kind of ecstacy. (It has been for me.) –DD

Cardiac Monitor Displays

Cardiac monitors display the same information as recorded on a standard 12 lead EKG. Some initial apprehension may arise because of lack of familiarity with the display. The EKG tracing is in bright green on a black background, and the amplitude of waves (height and depth) is increased. Because the "leads" of a cardiac monitor are modifications of standard leads with exaggerated amplitudes to aid in visualization at a distance, voltage (height and depth) criteria can not be utilized. But don't despair, this is just another method of displaying the heart's electrical activity… and familiarity eventually breeds content.

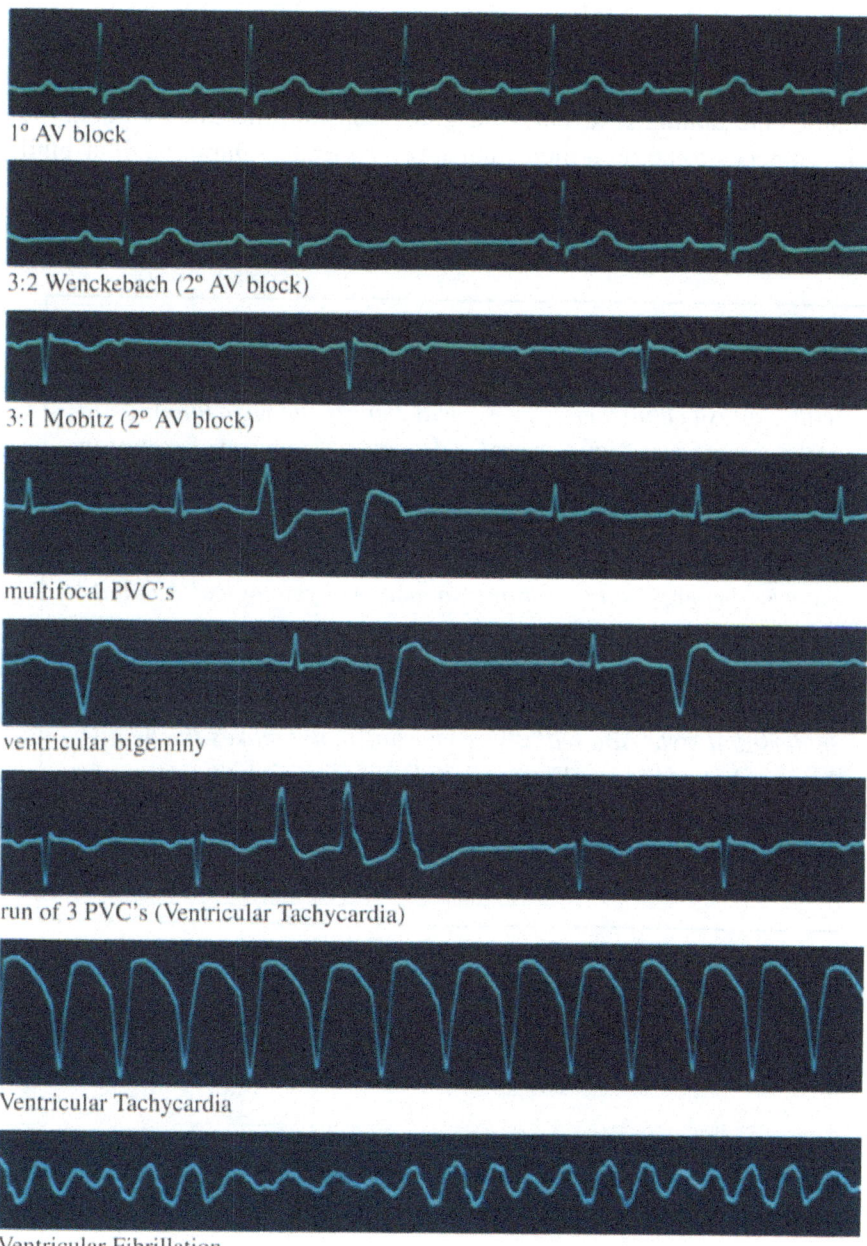

1° AV block

3:2 Wenckebach (2° AV block)

3:1 Mobitz (2° AV block)

multifocal PVC's

ventricular bigeminy

run of 3 PVC's (Ventricular Tachycardia)

Ventricular Tachycardia

Ventricular Fibrillation

> ## Electrocardiography was your challenge; knowledge, your achievement.

Now that you are certainly pleased with your understanding of basic electrocardiography, and proud of your ability to interpret the information on EKG's and cardiac monitors, you realize how logical and marvelously Designed is the heart.

You're probably ready for *Ion Adventure in the Heartland*, Dr. Dubin's highly-acclaimed, entertaining text. For your giant leap into the 21st century, your knowledge needs to be on a molecular level, so let Dr. Dubin be your guide and simplify your understanding.

*Ion Adventure in the Heartland is an exciting full-color expedition deep into the secret molecular wonderland of cardiac physiology with a splash of biochemistry. We will explore the vivid inner world of the magnificent "ion movers," a dynamic microcosm of exotic **ion channels**, **ion pumps**, **ion exchangers**, the mysterious **connexons**, and the fast moving ions that they control. You will be immersed in this never-before-seen, living wonderland that generates the heart's electrical energy and power in responce to physiological demands. What a performance to behold, as we expose the private activities of these ion movers, exquisitely orchestrated by the autonomic nervous system. The book is narrated in Dr. Dubin's entertaining, easy to understand style. You will discover what really makes the healthy heart tick, yet falter with stress and disease. Though this adventure is not likely to become a great movie, it is an easy to understand, illustrated story of the intimate lifestyles of the ions and their movers as recorded by the surface EKG.*

To learn more:

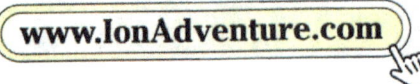

www.IonAdventure.com

COVER Publishing Company
P.O. Box 07037, Fort Myers, FL 33919
U. S. A.
Telephone: 1-800-441-8398

***Ion Adventure in the Heartland,* is an exciting adventure in living color, providing vital knowledge for the medical profession in millennium 2000.**

Scientists and researchers in the twentieth century found the micro-structure of the cells of the heart to be an engineering wonder. Research continues to reveal intriguing information, while raising many new questions. Current concepts may seem complex–even intimidating–to medical professionals, although, in reality, they are easy to understand.

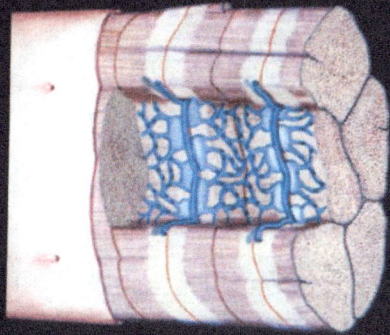

The key to cardiac function is at the ionic-molecular level, where autonomic control occurs, and where medications work. All the electrical and mechanical properties of the heart are due to the movement of only three types of ions...yes, three little ions!

Let me have them come forward to introduce them by name:

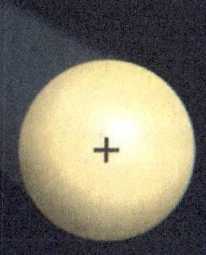
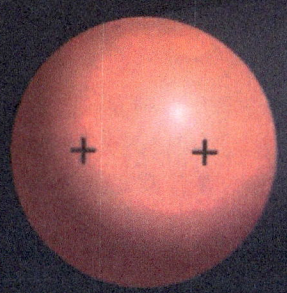
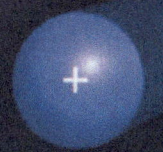

Sodium ion (Na⁺)   Calcium ion (Ca⁺⁺)   Potassium ion (K⁺)

Ion-moving ("ion-kinetic") structures of the cell membrane (and cell interior) produce ion movement. Most of these structures are sophisticated molecular portals that employ precision mechanisms to control and regulate the movement of Na^+, Ca^{++}, and K^+ ions. Each variety of ion-kinetic structure has its own unique behavior.

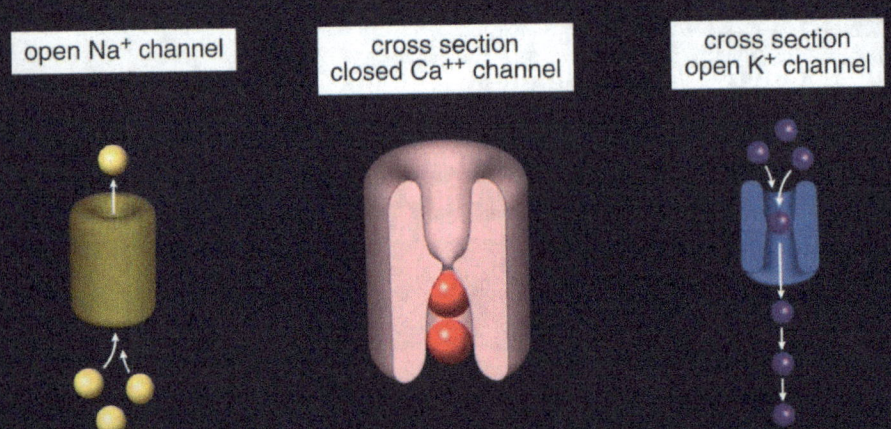

open Na^+ channel

cross section
closed Ca^{++} channel

cross section
open K^+ channel

We are launching an expedition to explore this incredible ionic-molecular microcosm to learn just how these mechanisms move Na^+, Ca^{++}, and K^+ ions to govern the heart's function. We would love to have you join us on this fascinating adventure.

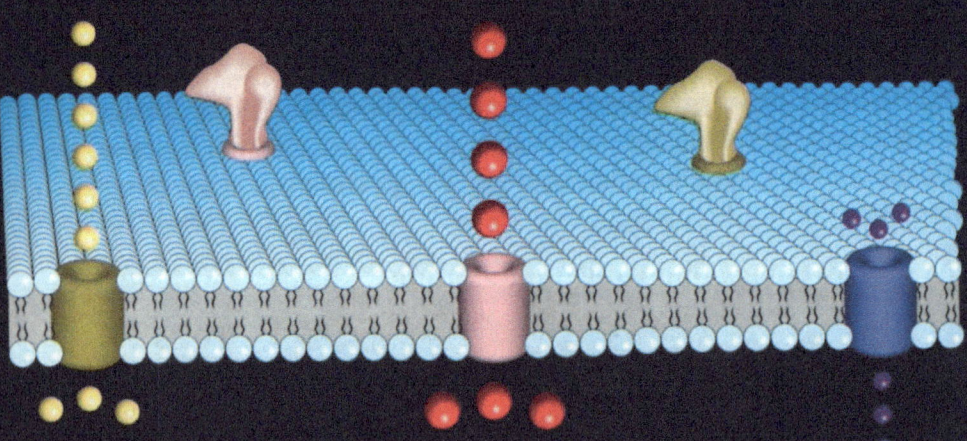

Our fantastic journey is narrated by a five year old boy named Dale, so certainly anyone who has read Rapid Interpretation of EKG's can easily master this vital medical knowledge, which is so useful and necessary in millennium 2000.

Hurry… your knowledge is needed!

www.IonAdventure.com

Telephone: 1-800-441-8398

Personal Quick Reference Sheets

(pages 333 to 346)

from: ***Rapid Interpretation of EKG's***
by Dale Dubin, MD
www.theMDsite.com

There is no need to remove these reference pages from your book. To download and print them in full color, go to:

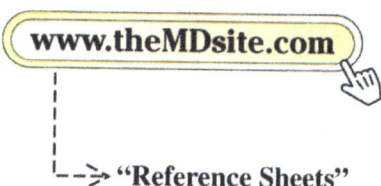

- - -> **"Reference Sheets"**

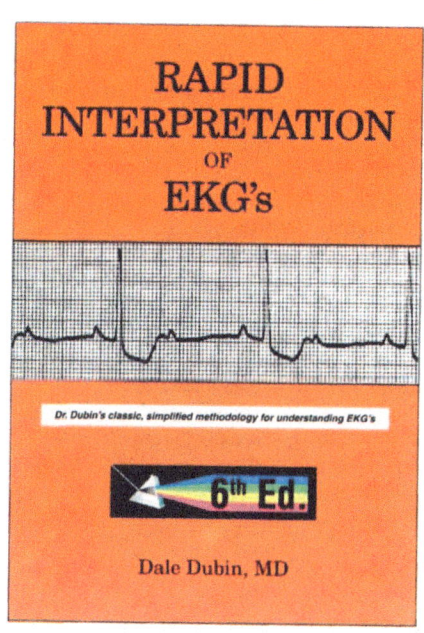

May humanity benefit from your knowledge,

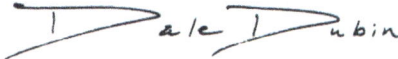

Learning Web Sites:

Physicians and medical students: **www.theMDsite.com**

Nurses and nurses in training: **www.CardiacMonitors.com**

Emergency medical personnel: **www.EmergencyEKG.com**

Dubin's Method
for
Reading EKG's

from: *Rapid Interpretation of EKG's*
by Dale Dubin, MD
www.theMDsite.com

1. RATE (pages 65-96)
Say "300, 150, 100" ..."75, 60, 50"

- but for bradycardia:
  rate = cycles/6 sec. strip $\times$ 10

2. RHYTHM (pages 97-202)
Identify the basic rhythm, then scan tracing for prematurity,
pauses, irregularity, and abnormal waves.

- Check for: P before each QRS.
  QRS after each P.
- Check: PR intervals (for AV Blocks).
  QRS interval (for BBB).
- If Axis Deviation, rule out Hemiblock.

3. AXIS (pages 203-242)
- QRS above or below baseline for Axis Quadrant
  (for Normal vs. R. or L. Axis Deviation).
  For Axis in degrees, find isoelectric QRS in a limb lead
  of Axis Quadrant using the "Axis in Degrees" chart.
- Axis rotation in the horizontal plane: (chest leads)
  find "transitional" (isoelectric) QRS.

4. HYPERTROPHY (pages 243-258)
P wave for atrial hypertrophy.
Check V_1 { R wave for Right Ventricular Hypertrophy.
S wave depth in V_1...
+ R wave height in V_5 for Left Ventricular Hypertrophy.

5. INFARCTION (pages 259-308)
Scan all leads for:

- Q waves
- Inverted T waves
- ST segment elevation or depression

Find the location of the pathology (in the Left ventricle),
and then identify the occluded coronary artery.

Personal Quick Reference Sheets

Rate (pages 65 to 96)

from: *Rapid Interpretation of EKG's*
by Dale Dubin, MD
www.theMDsite.com

Determine Rate by Observation (pages 78-88)

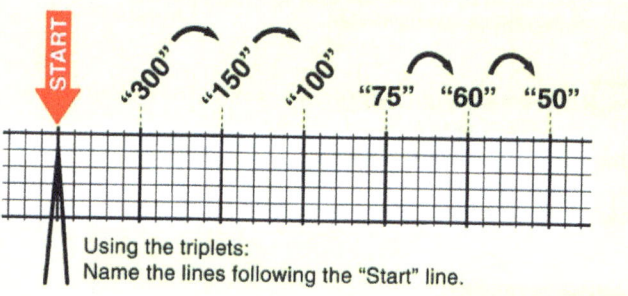

Using the triplets:
Name the lines following the "Start" line.

Fine division/rate association: reference (page 89)

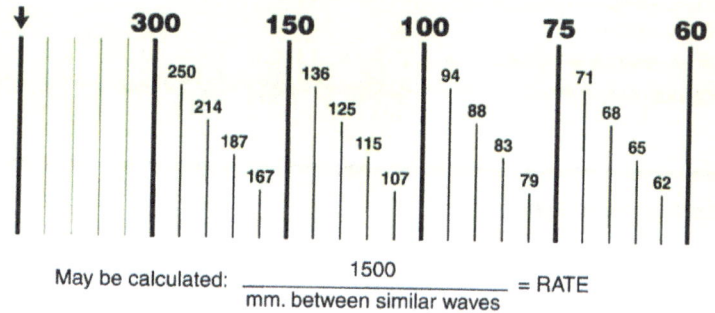

May be calculated: $\dfrac{1500}{\text{mm. between similar waves}}$ = RATE

Bradycardia (slow rates) (pages 90-96)

- Cycles/6 second strip × 10 = Rate
- When there are 10 large squares between similar waves, the rate is 30/minute.

Sinus Rhythm: origin is the SA Node ("Sinus Node"), normal sinus rate is 60 to 100/minute.

- Rate more than 100/min. = *Sinus Tachycardia* (page 68).
- Rate less than 60/min. = *Sinus Bradycardia* (page 67).

Determine any co-existing, independent (atrial/ventricular) rates:

- Dissociated Rhythms: (pages 155, 157, 186-189)
  A Sinus Rhythm (or atrial rhythms) may co-exist with an independent rhythm from an automaticity focus of a lower level. Determine rate of each.

Irregular Rhythms: (pages 107-111)

- With Irregular Rhythms (such as Atrial Fibrillation) always note the general (average) ventricular rate (QRS's per 6-sec. strip × 10) or take the patient's pulse.

Rhythm (pages 97 to 111)

from: ***Rapid Interpretation of EKG's***
by Dale Dubin, MD
www.theMDsite.com

★ **Identify basic rhythm...**
  ...then scan entire tracing for pauses, premature beats, irregularity, and abnormal waves.

★ **Always:**
  • Check for: P before each QRS.
    QRS after each P.
  • Check: PR intervals (for AV Blocks).
    QRS interval (for BBB).
  • Has QRS vector shifted outside normal range? (to rule out Hemiblock).

Irregular Rhythms (pages 107-111)

Sinus Arrhythmia (page 100)

Irregular rhythm that varies with respiration.
All P waves are identical.
Considered normal.

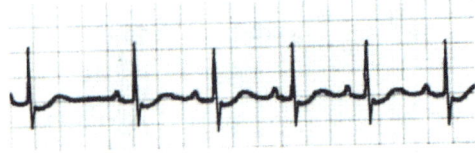

Wandering Pacemaker (page 108)

Irregular rhythm. P waves change shape as pacemaker location varies.
Rate under 100/minute...

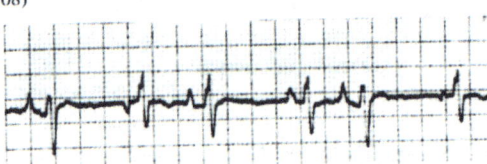

...but if the rate exceeds 100/minute, then it is called

Multifocal Atrial Tachycardia
(page 109)

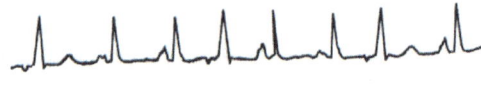

Atrial Fibrillation (pages 110, 164-166)

Irregular ventricular rhythm.
Erratic atrial spikes
(no P waves) from
multiple atrial automaticity
foci. Atrial discharges
may be difficult to see.

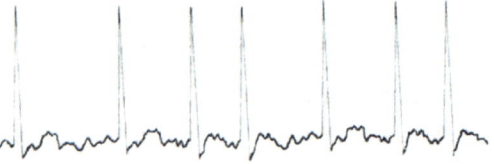

Rhythm continued (pages 112 to 145)

from: *Rapid Interpretation of EKG's*
by Dale Dubin, MD
www.theMDsite.com

Escape (pages 112-121) – the heart's response to a pause in pacing

- An unhealty Sinus (SA) Node may fail to emit a pacing stimulus ("Sinus Block"); this pause may evoke an escape beat from an automaticity focus.

pause

Atrial Escape Beat
(page 119)

or

Junctional Escape Beat
(page 120)

or

Ventricular Escape Beat
(page 121)

Then...

the SA Node usally resumes pacing.

- But a sick Sinus (SA) Node may cease pacing ("Sinus Arrest"), causing an automaticity focus to "escape" to assume pacemaker status.

Atrial Escape Rhythm Rate 60-80/min.

(page 114)

or

Junctional Escape Rhythm Rate 40-60/min.

("idiojunctional rhythm")
(pages 115-116)

or

Ventricular Escape Rhythm Rate 20-40/min.

(page 117)

("idioventricular rhythm")

Premature Beats (pages 122-145) – from an irritable automaticity focus

- An irritable automaticity focus may suddenly discharge, producing a:

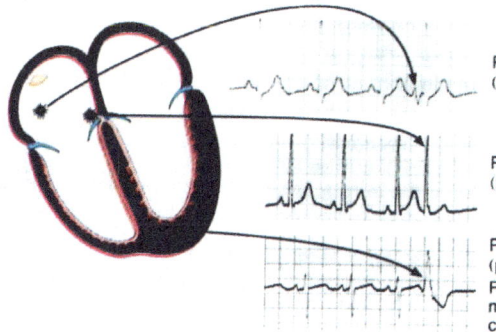

Premature Atrial Beat
(pages 124-130)

Premature Junctional Beat
(pages 131-133)

Premature Ventricular Contraction
(pages 135-141)
PVC's may be:
multiple, multifocal, in runs, or coupled with normal cycles.

Rhythm continued (pages 146 to 172)

from: *Rapid Interpretation of EKG's*
by Dale Dubin, MD
www.theMDsite.com

Tachyarrhythmias (pages 146-172), "focus" = automaticity focus

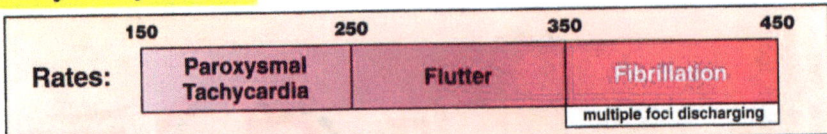

Rates:	150	250	350	450
	Paroxysmal Tachycardia	Flutter	Fibrillation *multiple foci discharging*	

Paroxysmal (sudden) Tachycardia ...rate: 150-250/min. (pages 146-163)

"Supraventricular Tachycardia" (page 153)

Paroxysmal Atrial Tachycardia
An irritable atrial focus discharging at
150-250/min. produces a normal wave
sequence, if P' waves are visible. (page 149)

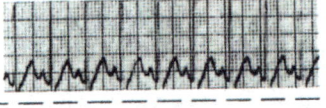

• P.A.T. with block
Same as P.A.T. but only every
second (or more) P' wave
produces a QRS. (page 150)

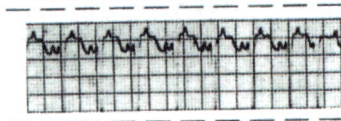

Paroxysmal Junctional Tachycardia
AV Junctional focus produces a rapid
sequence of QRS-T cycles at 150-250/min.
QRS may be slightly widened. (pages 151-153)

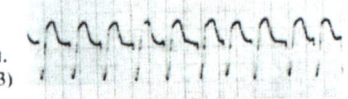

Paroxysmal Ventricular Tachycardia
Ventricular focus produces a rapid
(150-250/min.) sequence of (PVC-like)
wide ventricular complexes. (pages 154-158)

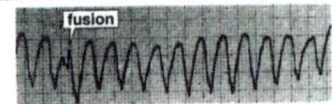
fusion

Flutter ...rate: 250-350/min.

Atrial Flutter
A continuous ("saw tooth") rapid sequence
of atrial complexes from a single rapid-firing
atrial focus. Many flutter waves needed to
produce a ventricular response. (pages 159, 160)

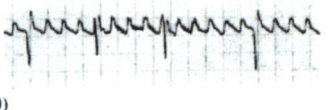

Ventricular Flutter (pages 161, 162) also see "Torsades de Pointes" (pages 158, 345)
A rapid series of smooth sine waves from a
single rapid-firing ventricular focus; usually in
a short burst leading to Ventricular Fibrillation.

Fibrillation ...erratic (multifocal) rapid discharges at 350 to 450/min. (pages 167-170)

Atrial Fibrillation (pages 110, 164-166)
Multiple atrial foci rapidly discharging
produce a jagged baseline of tiny spikes.
Ventricular (QRS) response is irregular.

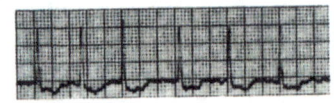

Ventricular Fibrillation (pages 167-170)
Multiple ventricular foci rapidly discharging produce a totally erratic ventricular rhythm
without identifiable waves. Needs **immediate**
treatment.

Personal Quick Reference Sheets

Rhythm: ("heart") blocks (pages 173 to 202)

from: ***Rapid Interpretation of EKG's***
by Dale Dubin, MD
www.theMDsite.com

Sinus (SA) Block (page 174)

An unhealthy Sinus (SA) Node misses one or more cycles (sinus pause)...

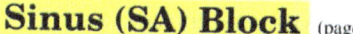 pause — the Sinus Node usually resumes pacing, but the pause may evoke an "escape" response from an automaticity focus. (pages 119-121)

AV Block (pages 176-189)

Blocks that delay or prevent atrial impulses from reaching the ventricles.

(left margin, rotated) ★ Always Check: • Is every P wave followed by a QRS? • PR intervals less than one large square?

1° AV Block ...prolonged PR interval (pages 176-178).
PR interval is prolonged to greater than .2 sec (one large square).

2° AV Block ... some P waves without QRS response (pages 179-185)

Wenckebach ...PR gradually lengthens with each cycle until the last P wave in the series does not produce a QRS.
(pages 180-182, 183)

Mobitz ...some P waves don't produce a QRS response. If "intermittent," an occasional QRS is dropped.
(pages 181-183)

More advanced Mobitz block may produce a 3:1 (AV) pattern or even higher AV ratio (page 181).

2:1 AV Block ...may be Mobitz or Wenckebach. PR length and QRS width or vagal maneuvers help differentiate.
(pages 182, 183)

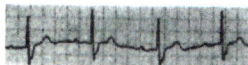

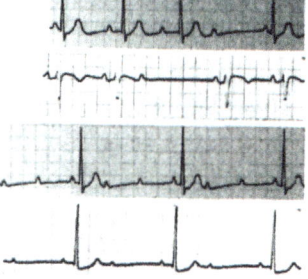

3° ("complete") AV Block ...no P wave produces a QRS response (pages 186-190)

3° Block: (page 188) — P waves—SA Node origin. QRS's—if narrow, and if the ventricular rate is 40 to 60 per min., then origin is a Junctional focus.

3° Block: (page 189) — P waves—SA Node origin. QRS's—if PVC-like, and if the ventricular rate is 20 to 40 per min., then origin is a Ventricular focus.

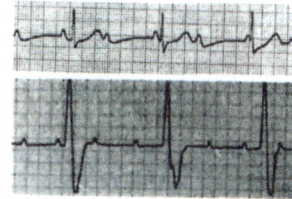

Bundle Branch Block ...find R,R' in right or left chest leads (pages 191-202)

Right BBB (pages 194-196)   **Left BBB** (pages 194-197)

★ Always Check: • is QRS within 3 tiny squares?

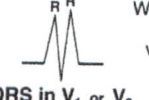
QRS in V₁ or V₂

With Bundle Branch Block the criteria for ventricular hypertrophy are unreliable.

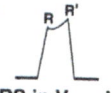
QRS in V₅ or V₆

Caution: With Left BBB infarction is difficult to determine on EKG.

Hemiblock ...block of Anterior or Posterior fascicle of the Left Bundle Branch.
(pages 295-305)

★ Always Check: • has Axis shifted outside Normal range?

Anterior Hemiblock
Axis shifts Leftward → L.A.D.
look for $Q_1 S_3$
(pages 297-299)

Posterior Hemiblock
Axis shifts Rightward → R.A.D.
look for $S_1 Q_3$
(pages 300-302)

Personal Quick Reference Sheets

Axis (pages 203 to 242)

from: *Rapid Interpretation of EKG's*
by Dale Dubin, MD
www.theMDsite.com

General Determination of Electrical Axis (pages 203-242)

Is QRS positive (⌐⌐) or negative (⌐⌐) in leads I and AVF?

Is Axis Normal? (page 227)

QRS in lead I (pages 215-222)
…if the QRS is Positive (mainly above baseline), then the Vector points to positive (patient's left) side.

Normal: { QRS upright in I and AVF
"two thumbs-up" sign

QRS in lead AVF (pages 223-226)
…if the QRS is mainly Positive, then the Vector must point downward to positive half of the sphere.

First Determine Axis Quadrant
(pages 214-231)

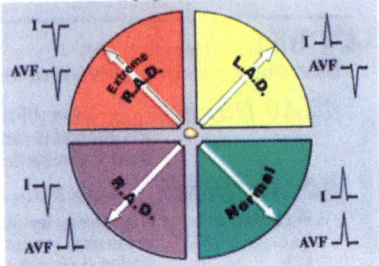

Axis in Degrees (pages 233, 234) (Frontal Plane)

After locating Axis Quadrant, find **limb** lead where QRS is most isoelectric:

Extreme Right Axis Deviation

lead		Axis
I	→	−90
AVL	→	−120
III	→	−150
AVF	→	−180

Left Axis Deviation

lead		Axis
I	→	−90
AVR	→	−60
II	→	−30
AVF	→	0

Right Axis Deviation

lead		Axis
AVF	→	+180
II	→	+150
AVR	→	+120
I	→	+90

Normal Range

lead		Axis
AVF	→	0
III	→	+30
AVL	→	+60
I	→	+90

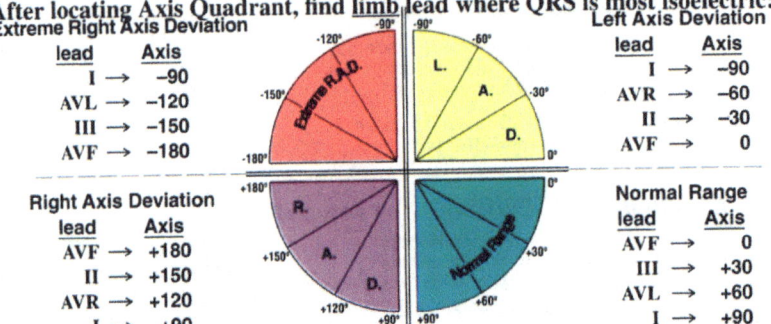

Axis Rotation (left/right) in the Horizontal Plane (pages 236-242)

Find transitional (isoelectric) QRS in a <u>chest</u> lead.

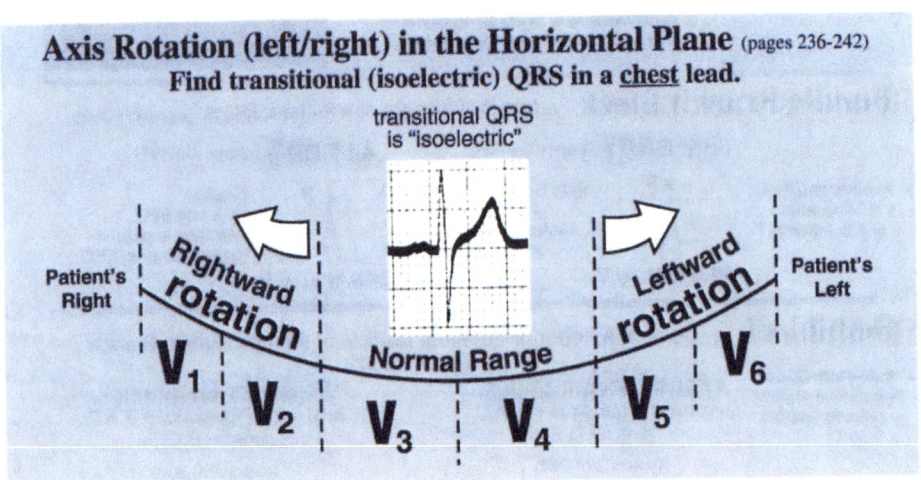

transitional QRS
is "isoelectric"

Patient's Right · **Rightward rotation** · Normal Range · **Leftward rotation** · Patient's Left

V_1 V_2 V_3 V_4 V_5 V_6

Hypertrophy (pages 243 to 258)

from: *Rapid Interpretation of EKG's*
by Dale Dubin, MD
www.theMDsite.com

Atrial Hypertrophy (pages 245-249)

Right Atrial Hypertrophy (page 248)

- large, diphasic P wave with tall initial component

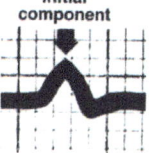

Left Atrial Hypertrophy (page 249)

- large, diphasic P wave with wide terminal component

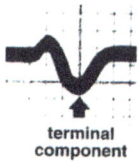

Ventricular Hypertrophy (pages 250-258)

Right Ventricular Hypertrophy (pages 250-252)

- R wave greater than S in V_1, but R wave gets progressively smaller from V_1 - V_6.
- S wave persists in V_5 and V_6.
- R.A.D. with slightly widened QRS.
- Rightward rotation in the horizontal plane.

Left Ventricular Hypertrophy (pages 253-257)

$$\begin{array}{l} \text{S wave in } V_1 \text{ (in mm.)} \\ + \ \text{R wave in } V_5 \text{ (in mm.)} \\ \hline \text{Sum in mm. is more than 35 mm. with L.V.H.} \end{array}$$

- L.A.D. with slightly widened QRS.
- Leftward rotation in the horizontal plane.

Inverted T wave:
slants downward
gradually,
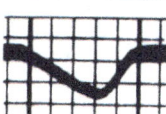
but up rapidly.

Infarction (pages 259 to 308)

from: ***Rapid Interpretation of EKG's***
by Dale Dubin, MD
www.theMDsite.com

Q wave = Necrosis (significant Q's only) (pages 272-284)

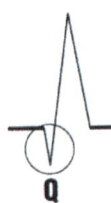

Q

- Significant Q wave is one millimeter (one small square) wide, which is .04 sec. in duration…
  … or is a Q wave 1/3 the amplitude (or more) of the QRS complex.

- Note those leads (omit AVR) where significant Q's are present … see next page to determine infarct location, and to identify the coronary vessel involved.

- Old infarcts: significant Q waves (like infarct damage) remain for a lifetime. To determine if an infarct is acute, see below.

ST (segment) elevation = (acute) Injury (pages 266-271) (also Depression)

elevation

- Signifies an acute process, ST segment returns to baseline with time.

- ST elevation associated with significant Q waves indicates an acute (or recent) infarct.

- A tiny "non-Q wave infarction" appears as significant ST segment elevation without associated Q's. Locate by identifying leads in which ST elevation occurs (next page).

- ST depression (persistent) may represent "subendocardial infarction," which involves a small, shallow area just beneath the endocardium lining the left ventricle. This is also a variety of "non-Q wave infarction." Locate in the same manner as for infarction location (next page).

T wave inversion = Ischemia (pages 264, 265)

T

inversion

- Inverted T wave (of ischemia) is symmetrical (left half and right half are mirror images). Normally T wave is upright when QRS is upright, and vice versa.

- Usually in the same leads that demonstrate signs of acute infarction (Q waves and ST elevation).

- Isolated (non-infarction) ischemia may also be located; note those leads where T wave inversion occurs, then identify which coronary vessel is narrowed (next page).

NOTE: Always obtain patient's previous EKG's for comparison!

Personal Quick Reference Sheets

Infarction Location
— and —
Coronary Vessel Involvement
(pages 259 to 308)

from: *Rapid Interpretation of EKG's*
by Dale Dubin, MD
www.theMDsite.com

Coronary Artery Anatomy (page 291)

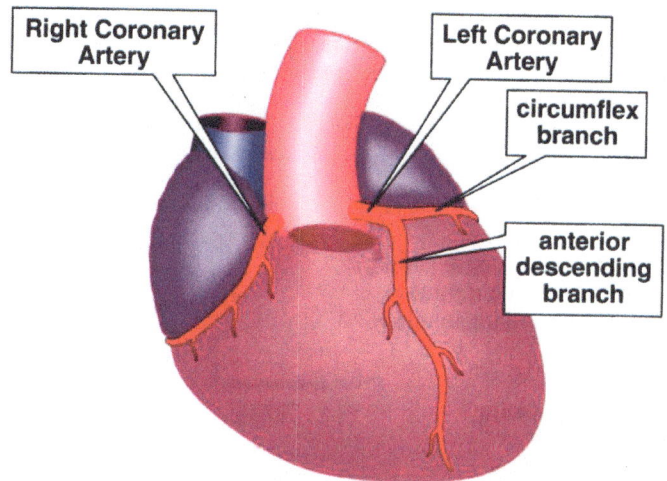

Right Coronary Artery

Left Coronary Artery

circumflex branch

anterior descending branch

Infarction Location/Coronary Vessel Involvement (pages 278-294)

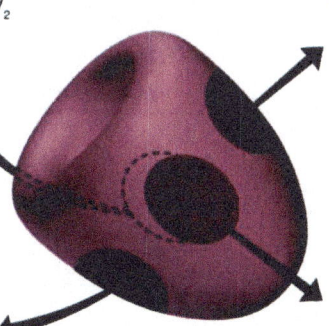

Posterior
• large R with ST depression in V_1 & V_2
• *mirror test* or *reversed transillumination test*
(Right Coronary Artery)
(pages 282-286)

Lateral
Q's in lateral leads I and AVL
(Circumflex Coronary Artery)
(pages 280, 292)

Inferior
(diaphragmatic)
Q's in inferior leads
II, III, and AVF
(R. or L. Coronary Artery)
(pages 281, 294)

Anterior
Q's in V_1, V_2, V_3, and V_4
(Anterior Descending Coronary Artery)
(pages 278, 292)

Personal Quick Reference Sheets

Miscellaneous (pages 309 to 328)

from: ***Rapid Interpretation of EKG's***
by Dale Dubin, MD
www.theMDsite.com

Pulmonary Embolism (pages 312, 313)

- $S_1Q_3L_3$ – wide S in I, large Q and inverted T in III
- acute Right BBB (transient, often incomplete)
- R.A.D. and rightward rotation (horizontal plane)
- inverted T waves $V_1 \rightarrow V_4$ and ST depression in II

Artificial Pacemakers (pages 321-326)

Modern artificial pacemakers have sensing capabilities and also provide a regular pacing stimulus. This electrical stimulus records on EKG as a tiny vertical spike that appears just before the "captured" cardiac response.

Demand Pacemakers: (page 322)

- are "triggered" (activated) when the patient's own rhythm ceases or slows markedly.

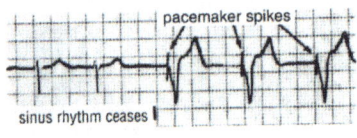
pacemaker spikes
sinus rhythm ceases

- are "inhibited" (cease pacing) if the patient's own rhythm resumes at a reasonable rate.

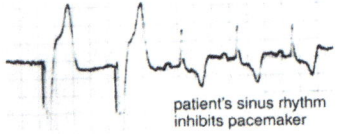
patient's sinus rhythm inhibits pacemaker

- will "reset" pacing (at same rate) to synchronize with a premature beat.

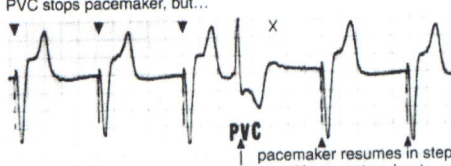
PVC stops pacemaker, but...
PVC
pacemaker resumes in step with premature beat.

Pacemaker Impulse (delivery modes)

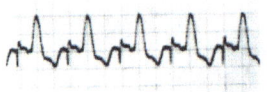

Ventricular Pacemaker (page 323)
(electrode in Right Ventricle)

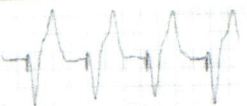

(Asynchronous) Epicardial Pacemaker
Ventricular impulse not linked to atrial activity.

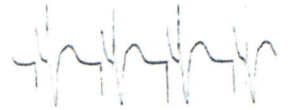

Atrial pacemaker (page 323)

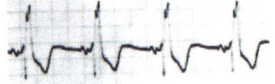

Atrial Synchronous Pacemaker (page 323)
P wave sensed, then after a brief delay, ventricular impulse is delivered.

Dual Chamber (AV sequential) Pacemaker
(page 323)

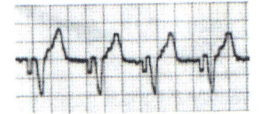

External Non-invasive Pacemaker
(page 326)

Personal Quick Reference Sheets

Miscellaneous continued

from: *Rapid Interpretation of EKG's*
by Dale Dubin, MD
www.theMDsite.com

Electrolytes

Potassium (pages 314, 315)

Increased K⁺ (page 314)
(hyperkalemia)

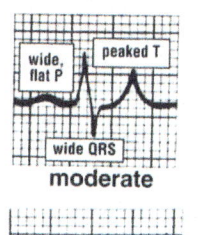

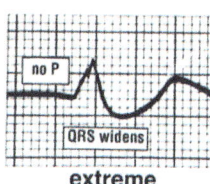

moderate   **extreme**

Decreased K⁺ (pages 315)
(hypokalemia)

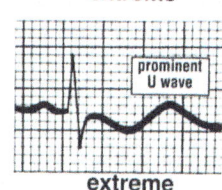

moderate   **extreme**

Calcium (page 316)

Hyper Ca⁺⁺   **Hypo Ca⁺⁺**

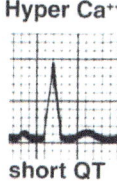

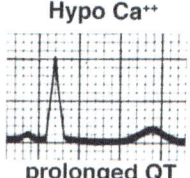

short QT   **prolonged QT**

Digitalis (pages 317-319)

EKG appearance with digitalis ("digitalis effect")
- remember Salvador Dali.
- T waves depressed or inverted.
- QT interval shortened.

⇨ ST gradually slopes below baseline

Digitalis Excess ———→ Digitalis Toxicity
(blocks)   (irritable foci firing rapidly)
- SA Block   - Atrial Fibrillation
- P.A.T. with Block   - Junctional or Ventricular Tachycardia
- AV Blocks   - multiple P.V.C.'s
- AV Dissociation   - Ventricular Fibrillation

Quinidine (page 320)

Quinidine Effects

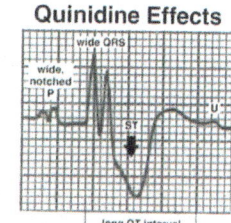

- EKG appearance with quinidine (page 320)

- Excess quinidine or other medications
that block potassium channels (or even
low serum potassium) may initiate
Torsades de Pointes (page 158)

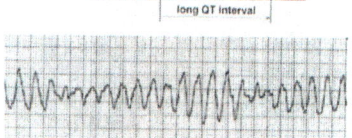

Torsades de Pointes

Personal Quick Reference Sheets

Practical Tips

from: ***Rapid Interpretation of EKG's***
by Dale Dubin, MD
www.theMDsite.com

Dubin's Quickie Conversion
—for—
Patient's Weight from Pounds to Kilograms

Patient wt. in kg. = Half of patient's wt. (in lb.) *minus* 1/10 of that value.

Examples:

180 lb. patient	160 lb. patient	140 lb. patient
(becomes 90 *minus* 9)	(becomes 80 *minus* 8)	(becomes 70 *minus* 7)
is 81 kg	is 72 kg	is 63 kg.

Modified Leads
—for—
Cardiac Monitoring

Locations are approximate. Some minor adjustment of electrode positions may be necessary to obtain the best tracing. Identify the specific lead on each strip placed in the patient's record.

	Identification	
Sensor Electrode	Letter	Color (inconsistent)
+	R (or RA)	red
–	L (or LA)	white
G˚	G (or RL)	variable

* Ground, Neutral or Reference

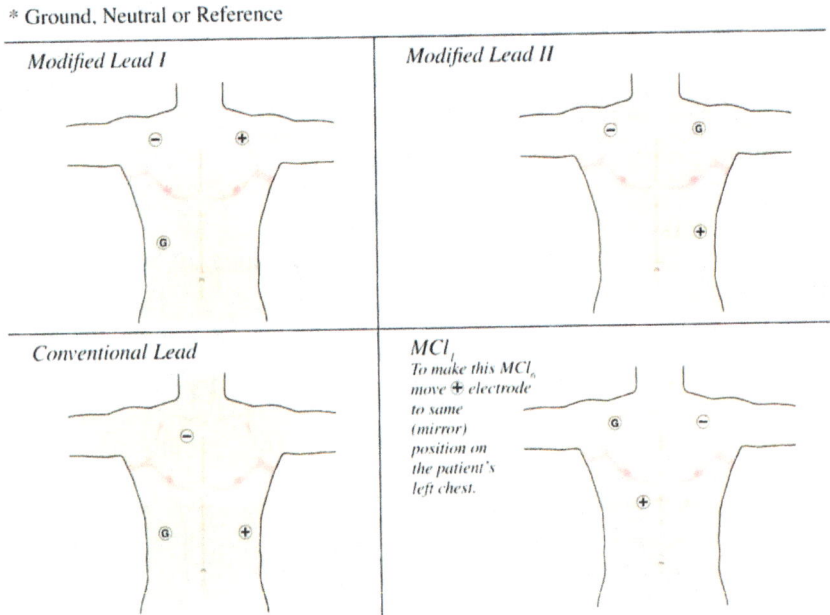

Modified Lead I

Modified Lead II

Conventional Lead

MCl₁
To make this MCl₆ move + electrode to same (mirror) position on the patient's left chest.

EKG Tracings

This section contains EKG tracings (and their interpretation) from various patients. The tracings and interpretations are provided so that you can see how this method of reading EKG's actually works. Try these few examples so that you grow accustomed to this systematic approach. Once you learn how to read an EKG systematically, you will soon become very skilled at routine EKG interpretations.

Patient D.D. is a 29 year old white male known to be a hypochondriac with numerous complaints.

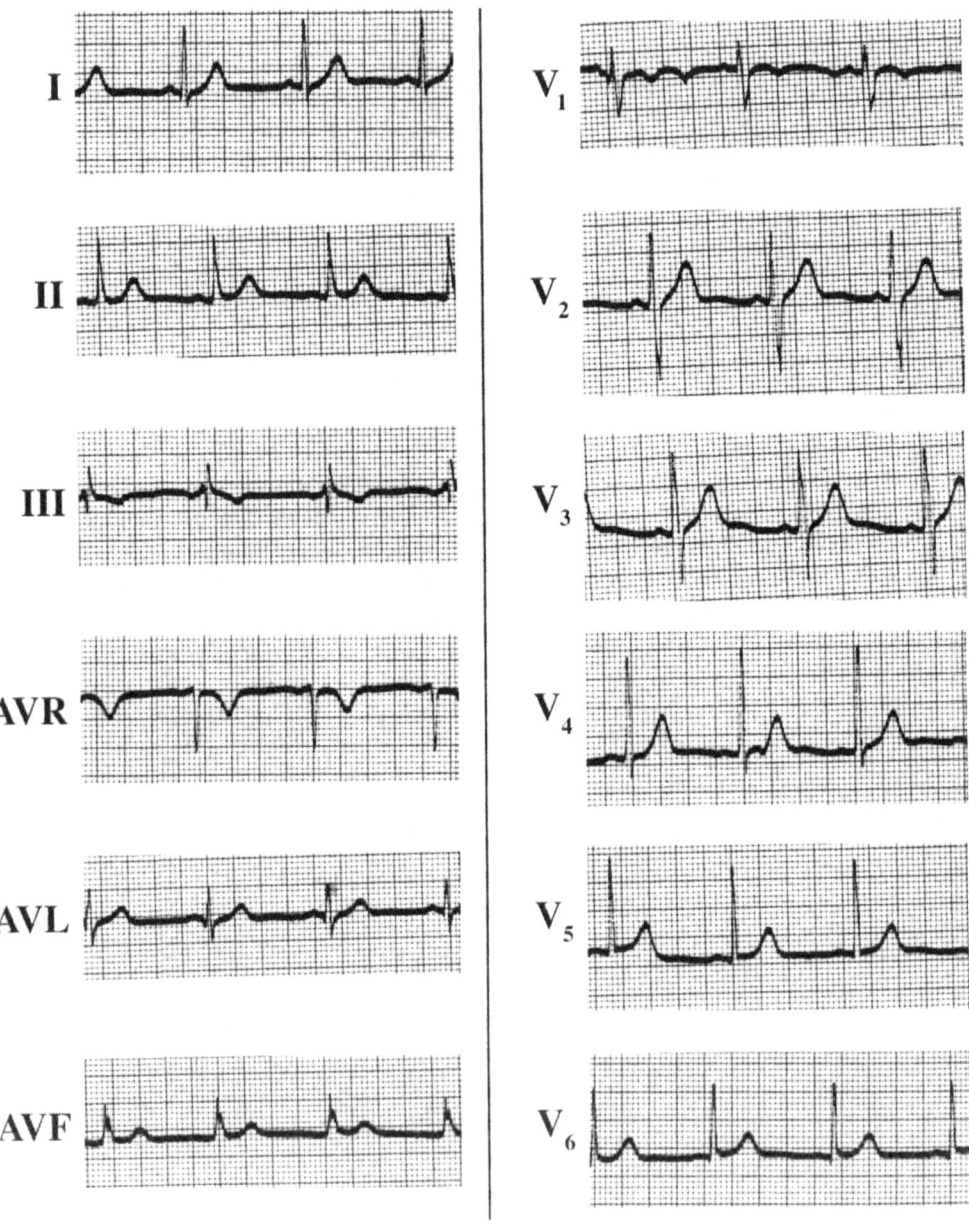

EKG Interpretation

Patient: D.D.

Rate: about 70/minute

Rhythm: Regular Sinus Rhythm
                PR less than .2 sec. (No AV Block).
                QRS less than .12 sec. (No BBB).
                    ...but note the R,R' in III suggesting incomplete
                    Bundle Branch Block.

Axis: Normal Range (about +30°).
                Rightward rotation in the horizontal plane.

Hypertrophy: No atrial hypertrophy.
                No ventricular hypertrophy.

Infarction: No significant *Q waves.*
(coronary   *ST segments*: not elevated, except for V_5 and V_6 where
vascular   ST is elevated 1/2 mm. due to "early repolarization."*
status)   *T waves*: generally upright.

Comment: This is an essentially normal tracing. This is the author's own EKG,
                however he is no longer 29 years old.

---

* Early repolarization is characterized by (minimal) ST elevation in the left chest leads, often with rightward rotation (horizontal plane). It is a normal finding in young athletic males.

This is the followup EKG on patient D.D., 30 years after his last EKG (see previous page.); he has had labile hypertension for the last 25 years. This EKG clearly demonstrates the value of obtaining the patient's prior EKG's for comparison.

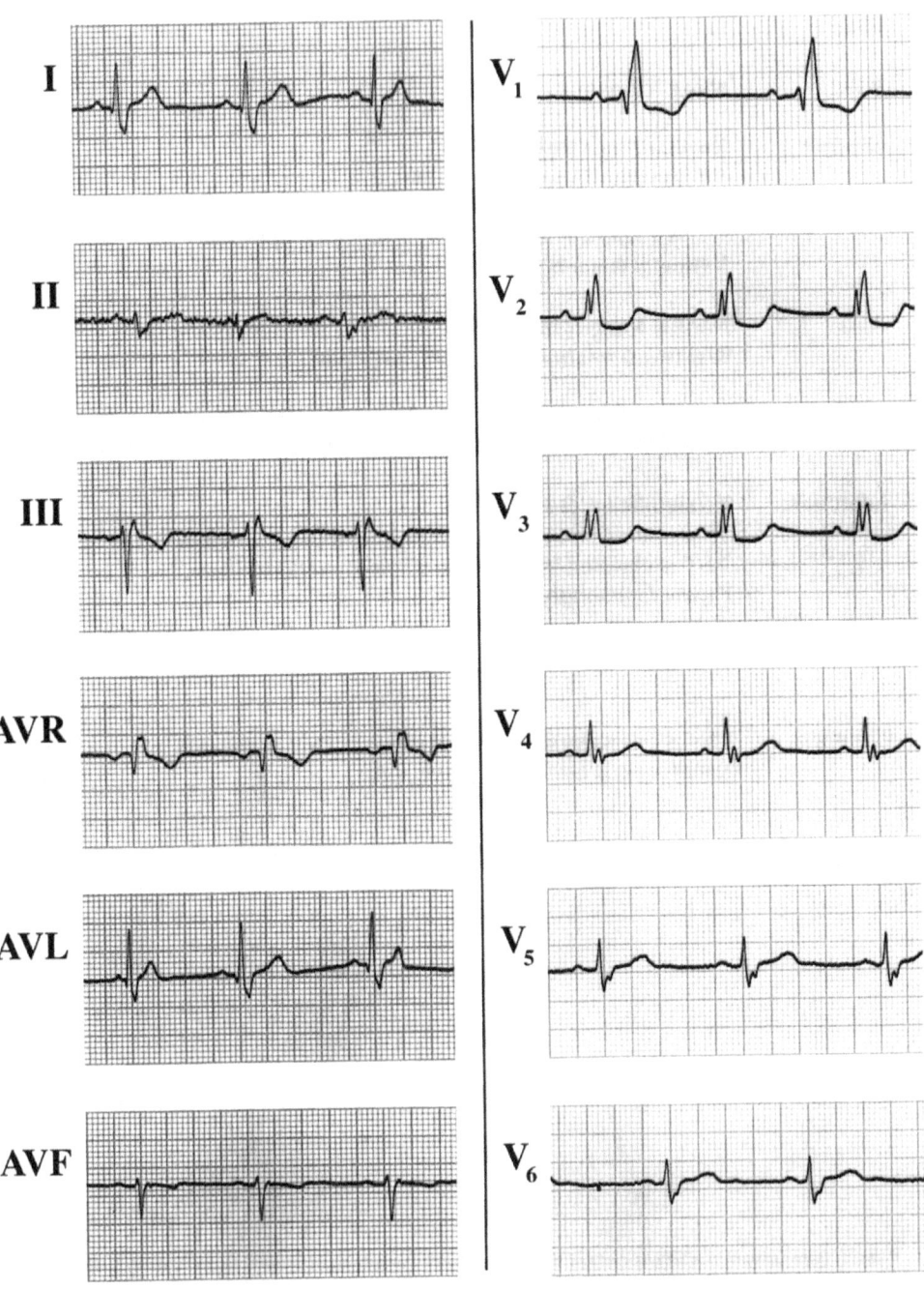

EKG Interpretation

Patient: D.D.

Rate: about 58/minute

Rhythm: Sinus Bradycardia
             PR less than .2 sec. (No AV Block)
             QRS greater than .12 sec. reveals Bundle Branch Block.
                Leads V_1 and V_2 show R,R' complexes typical of Right Bundle
                Branch Block.

Axis: Left Axis Deviation of about -25° (in lead I, R wave greater
                than S wave) and $Q_1 S_3$ indicate probable Anterior Hemiblock.
             Axis rotation in the horizontal plane difficult to assess due to RBBB.

Hypertrophy: Left atrial enlargement.
             Left ventricular hypertrophy verified by other tests
                (difficult to assess on EKG with RBBB present).

Infarction: No significant *Q waves.*
             ST segments: depressed in V_1 and V_2 as related to RBBB
(coronary   *T waves*: generally upright; some T inversion in inferior leads,
vascular   possibly distorted by RBBB.
status)

Comment: Compared to his previous, normal EKG (see page 348), this patient
             has developed significant changes. There is a sinus bradycardia. The
             new Right Bundle Branch Block (previously incomplete) and Anterior
             Hemiblock have occurred in the absense of infarction. After 25 years
             of poorly compensated hypertension, the patient has developed left
             ventricular hypertrophy. The associated left atrial enlargement may
             stretch irritable atrial foci in the ostia of the pulmonary veins, initiating
             atrial fibrillation. A few days later, the patient's rhythm strip of lead I
             (below), shows just that. All EKG's are, unfortunately, authentic.

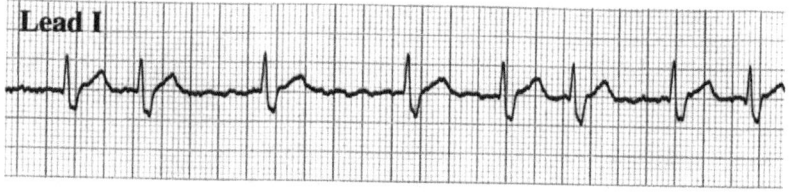

Patient R.C. is a 45 year old black male with a history of coronary vascular disease. Blood pressure was 210/100 on admission.

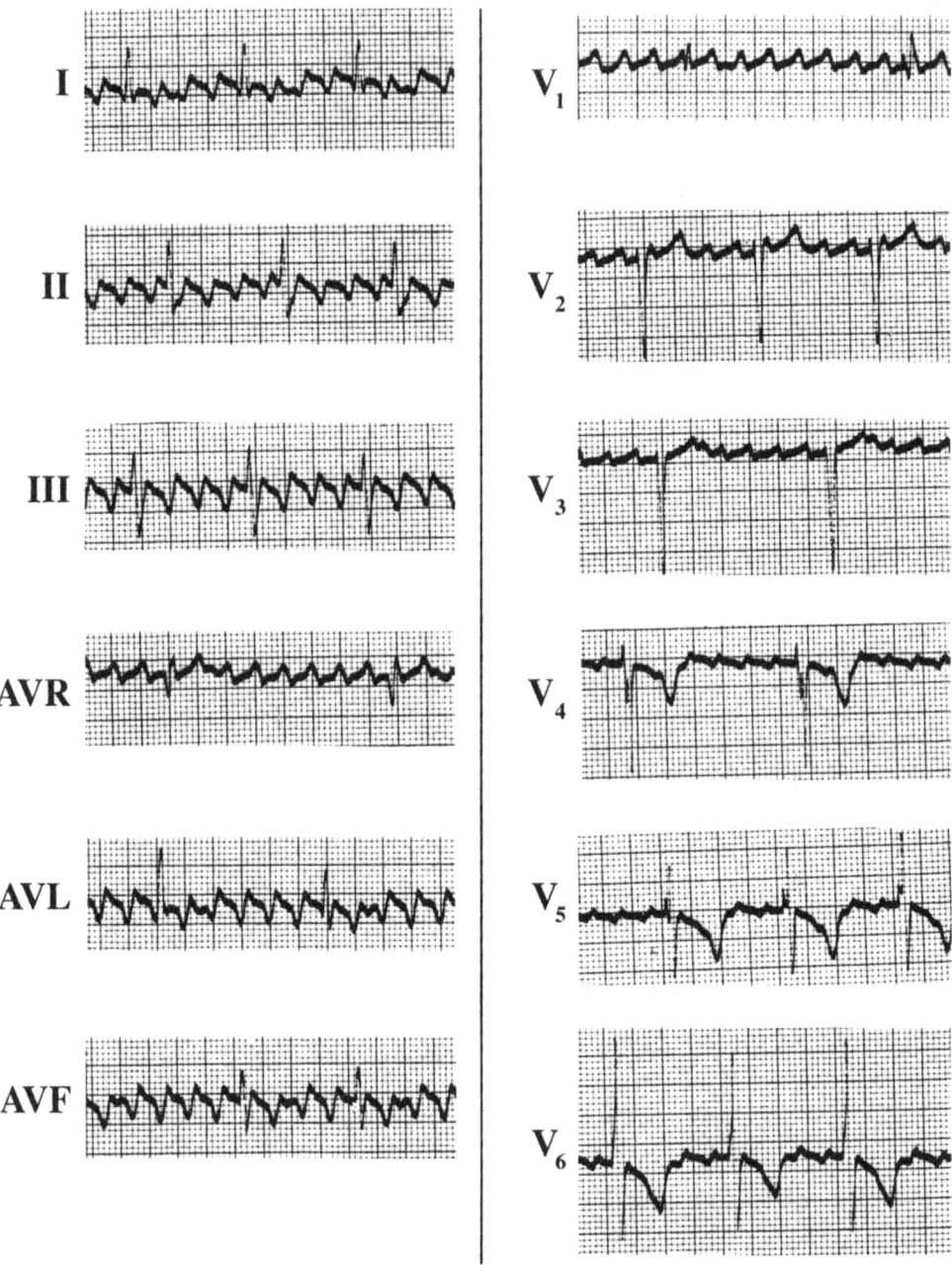

EKG Interpretation

Patient: R.C.

Rate: Atrial rate of 300/minute
                 Ventricular rate generally 60/min. but occasionally slower.

Rhythm: Atrial Flutter (with inconsistent ventricular response, i.e.,
                 no fixed AV ratio).
                 PR is variable.
                 QRS is less than .12 sec. (No BBB).

Axis: Left Axis Deviation (-30°).
                 Leftward rotation in the horizontal plane.

Hypertrophy: Atrial hypertrophy difficult to determine.
                 No ventricular hypertrophy.

Infarction: *Q waves*: Q in lead I (also note large S in Lead III).
(coronary
vascular
status)   *ST segments* are generally isoelectric.
                 T waves are inverted in I and AVL (look closely)
                 and the mid-to-left chest leads.

Comment: The most obvious problem is Atrial Flutter with an atrial rate of
                 300/min. and a variable irregular ventricular rate (average 60/min.)
caused by the variable AV conduction ratio between 3:1 and 7:1.
An old occlusion of the Left Circumflex Coronary artery is evidenced by
the old lateral infarction. New involvement of the Anterior Descending
Coronary artery is suggested by anterior ischemia (T wave inversion in
V_4, V_5, V_6), as well as by the probable Anterior Hemiblock (shift to Left
Axis Deviation with Q_1S_3 configuration; previously R.A.D. with his old
lateral M.I.). Note that if one scrutinizes the T wave regions (somewhat
obscured by flutter waves) in the limb leads, the flutter waves dip lower
(suggestive of negative T waves) rather than higher (if superimposed
on upright T waves) in all but AVR, indicating a generalized cardiac
ischemia, as well as the obvious compromise of both branches of the
Left coronary Artery.

Patient K.T. is a 61 year old obese, black male who was brought into the emergency department by his family. This patient had a sudden episode of severe left chest pain. Blood pressure was 95/65.

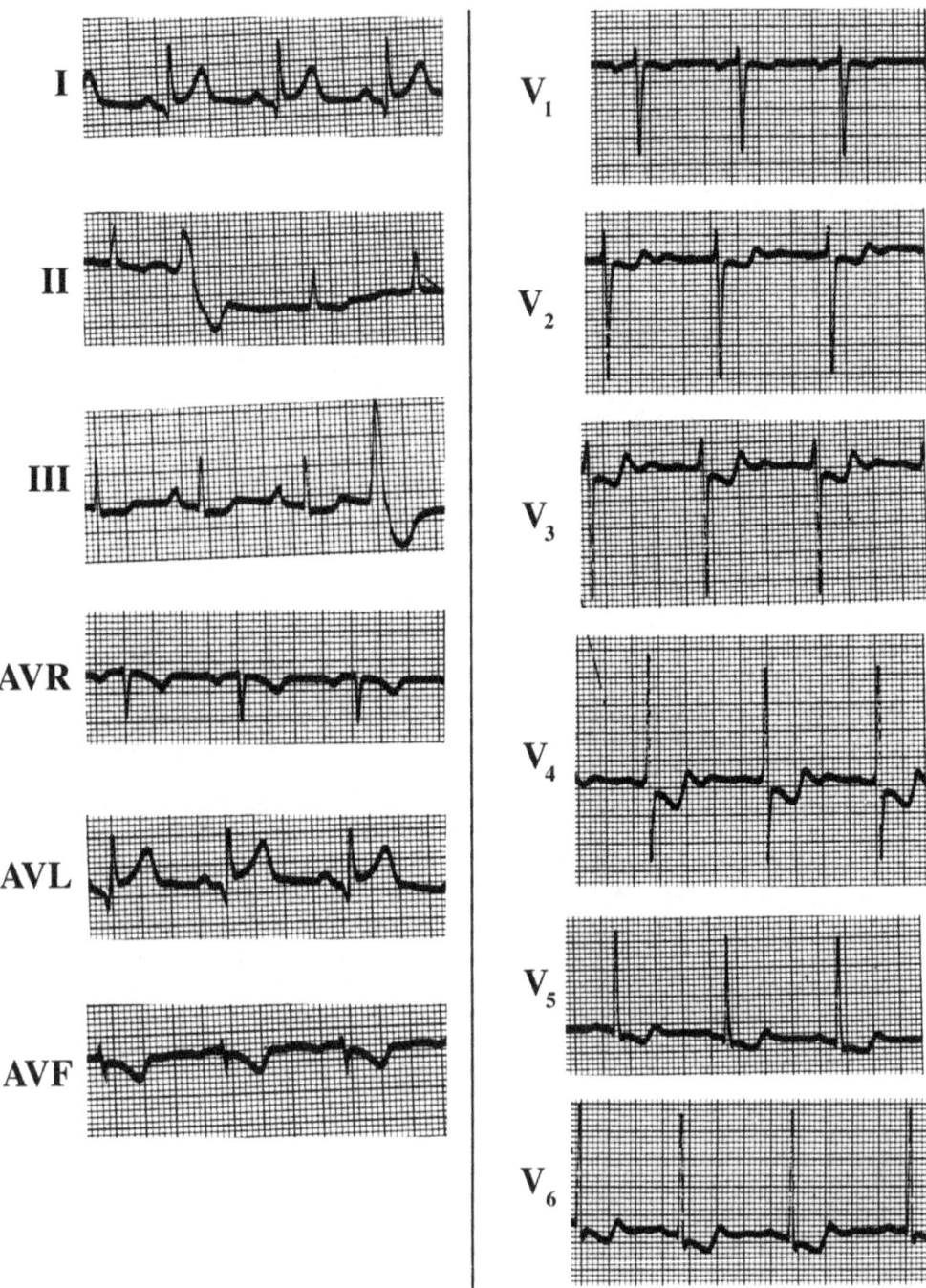

EKG Interpretation

Patient: K.T.

Rate: about 75/minute

Rhythm: Generally regular Sinus Rhythm with occasional PVC's.
                PR is exactly .2 sec. so we will have to say there is a
                    borderline first degree AV Block.
                QRS is less than .12 sec. (No BBB).

Axis: Left Axis Deviation (nearly -90°).
                No rotation in the horizontal plane.

Hypertrophy: Probable left atrial hypertrophy.
                Left ventricular hypertrophy.

Infarction: *Significant Q waves* in I and AVL.
(coronary   *ST segments* are elevated in I and AVL. ST segments
vascular   are depressed in V_1, V_2, V_3, and V_4.
status)   *T waves* are flat or inverted in II, III, and AVF and all chest leads.

Comment: This patient has a classical acute lateral infarction caused by an
                occlusion of the Left Circumflex Coronary Artery. Coincident with this
                is a probable occlusion of the Right Coronary Artery characterized by
                prominent R waves with ST depression in the (V_1 to V_4) chest leads.
                Also, T wave inversion in II, III, and AVF suggests Right Coronary
                compromise. T wave inversion in all chest leads is indicative of ischemia
                of the Anterior Descending Coronary Artery. Note also the tall, peaked
                T waves in I and AVL known as "hyperacute T waves," which,
                although uncommon, characterize a very acute M.I. The Left Axis
                Deviation appeared in this patient's previous EKG's and is most likely
                related to his left ventricular hypertrophy rather than implicating
                Anterior Hemiblock (also, the Bundle Branch System appears to conduct
                normally). Occasional PVC's caused by the ischemia, depending
                on frequency and multiplicity of origin, may forebode more serious
                arrhythmias.

Patient G.G. is a 45 year old Asian male who was doing heavy work when he was overcome by severe, crushing, anterior chest pain. Blood pressure was 110/40 on admission to the hospital.

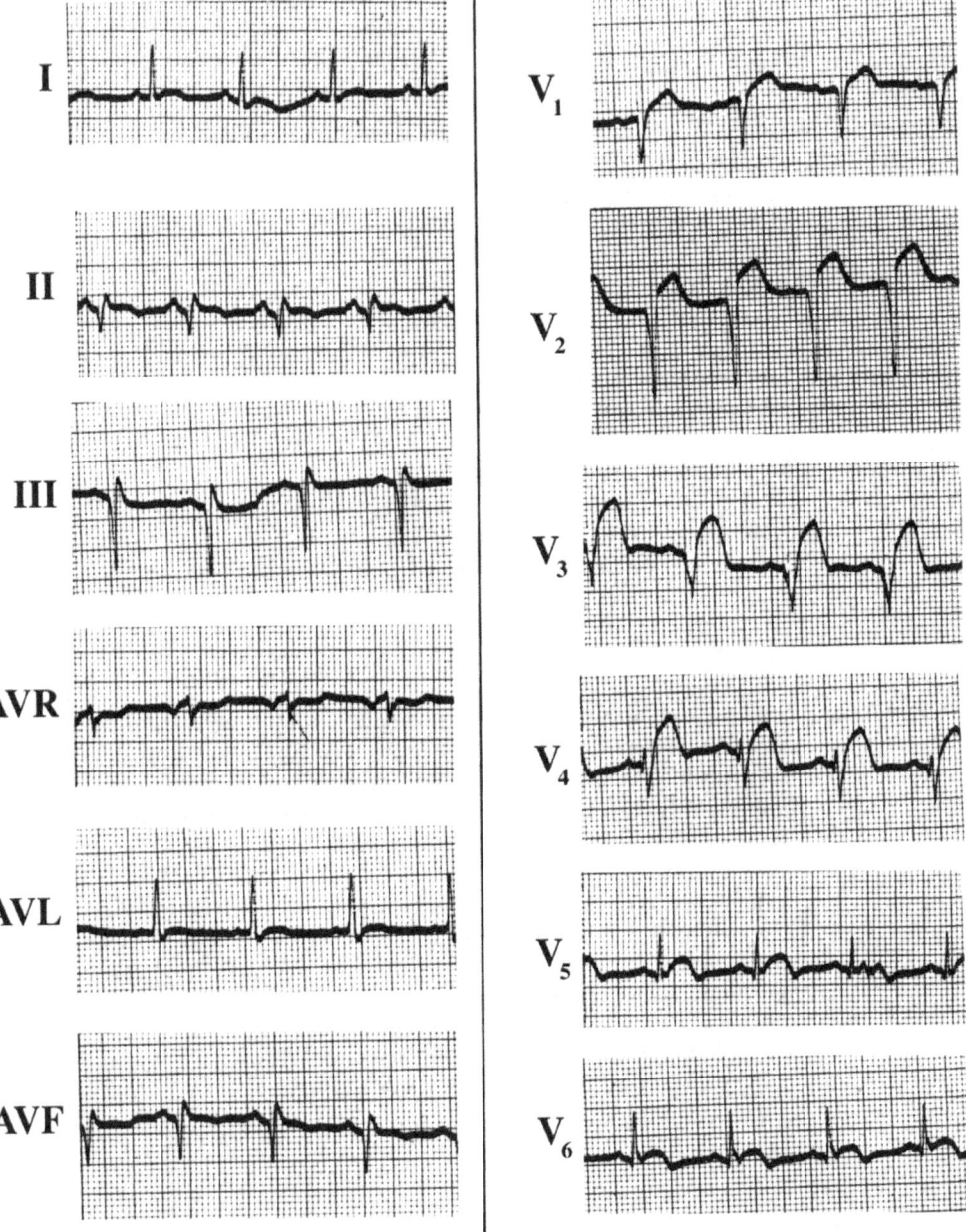

EKG Interpretation

Patient: G.G.

Rate: about 100/minute but variable.

Rhythm: *Sinus* Rhythm, somewhat irregular due to Sinus Arrhythmia.
                   PR less than .2 sec. (No AV Block).
                   QRS less than .12 sec. (No BBB).

Axis: Left Axis Deviation (-30° to -60°).
                   Leftward rotation in the horizontal plane.

Hypertrophy: No atrial hypertrophy.
                   No ventricular hypertrophy.

Infarction: *Significant Q waves* in II, III, and AVF.
(coronary   There are also very large Q waves in V_1, V_2, V_3, and V_4.
vascular   *ST segments* are elevated in V_1, V_2, V_3, and V_4.
status)   *T waves* are difficult to distinguish, but inverted T waves
                      are noted in V_4, V_5, and V_6.

Comment: This patient has an acute antero-septal infarction, probably representing
                   an occlusion of the Anterior Descending branch of the Left Coronary.
                   Generalized ischemia of the myocardium is evident by the flat-to-
                   inverted T waves in nearly every lead. The old inferior infarction
                   demonstrated on this EKG was noted on the patient's previous hospital
                   record and is the documented etiology of his Left Axis Deviation (no
                   Hemiblock). Note that the QRS becomes isoelectric between V_4 and V_5
                   but this is *not* within the normal (V_3, V_4) range; this represents minimal
                   leftward rotation away from the septal infarction. Old EKG's showed
                   no anterior involvement on his previous admission.

Patient E.M. is a 65 year old Hispanic female. She was admitted to the hospital because of constant left chest pain for twelve hours. Blood pressure on admission was 110/75.

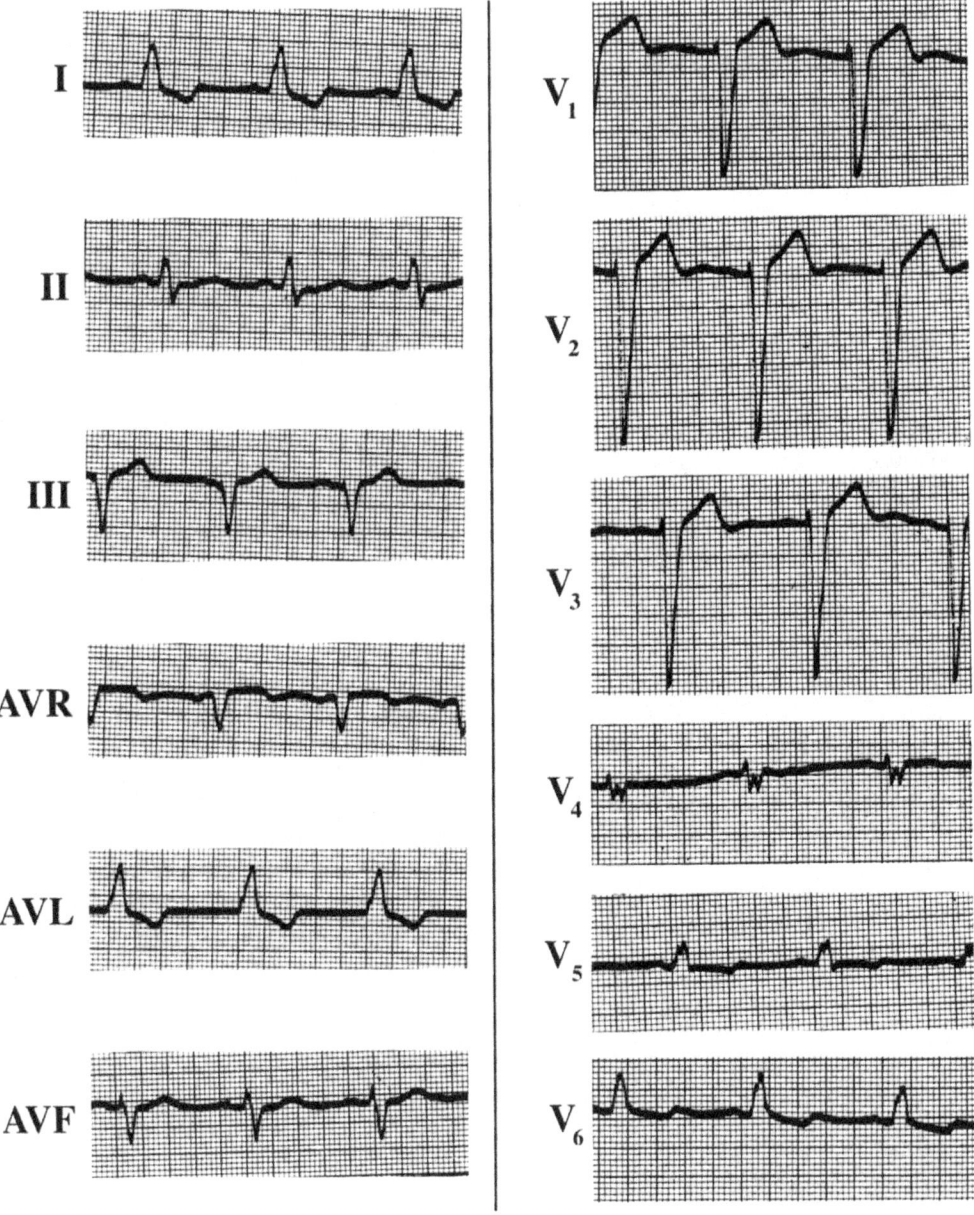

EKG Interpretation

Patient: E.M.

Rate: 60/minute

Rhythm: Sinus Bradycardia
                PR is about .2 sec. so there is probably a
                     first degree AV Block.
                QRS is more than .12 sec. (it is .16 sec. wide). R,R' is present in
                     V_5 and V_6 so there is a Left Bundle Branch Block.

Axis: Suggestive of Left Axis Deviation, but not reliable because of the
                     presence of Bundle Branch Block.

Hypertrophy: No atrial hypertrophy.
                Ventricular hypertrophy is difficult to determine
                     because of Bundle Branch Block.

Infarction: *Q Waves*: not a reliable criterion of infarction in the presence of
(coronary   Left Bundle Branch Block.
vascular   *ST segments*: not reliable in the presence of Left Bundle
status)   Branch Block.
                T Waves are flat in V_4, V_5, and V_6, but not reliable with
                     Left Bundle Branch Block.

Comment: Enzyme studies confirmed a presumptive diagnosis of myocardial
                infarction. The patient's chest pain made us suspicious.

Patient M.A. is a 75 year old black female with a long history of marked hypertension.

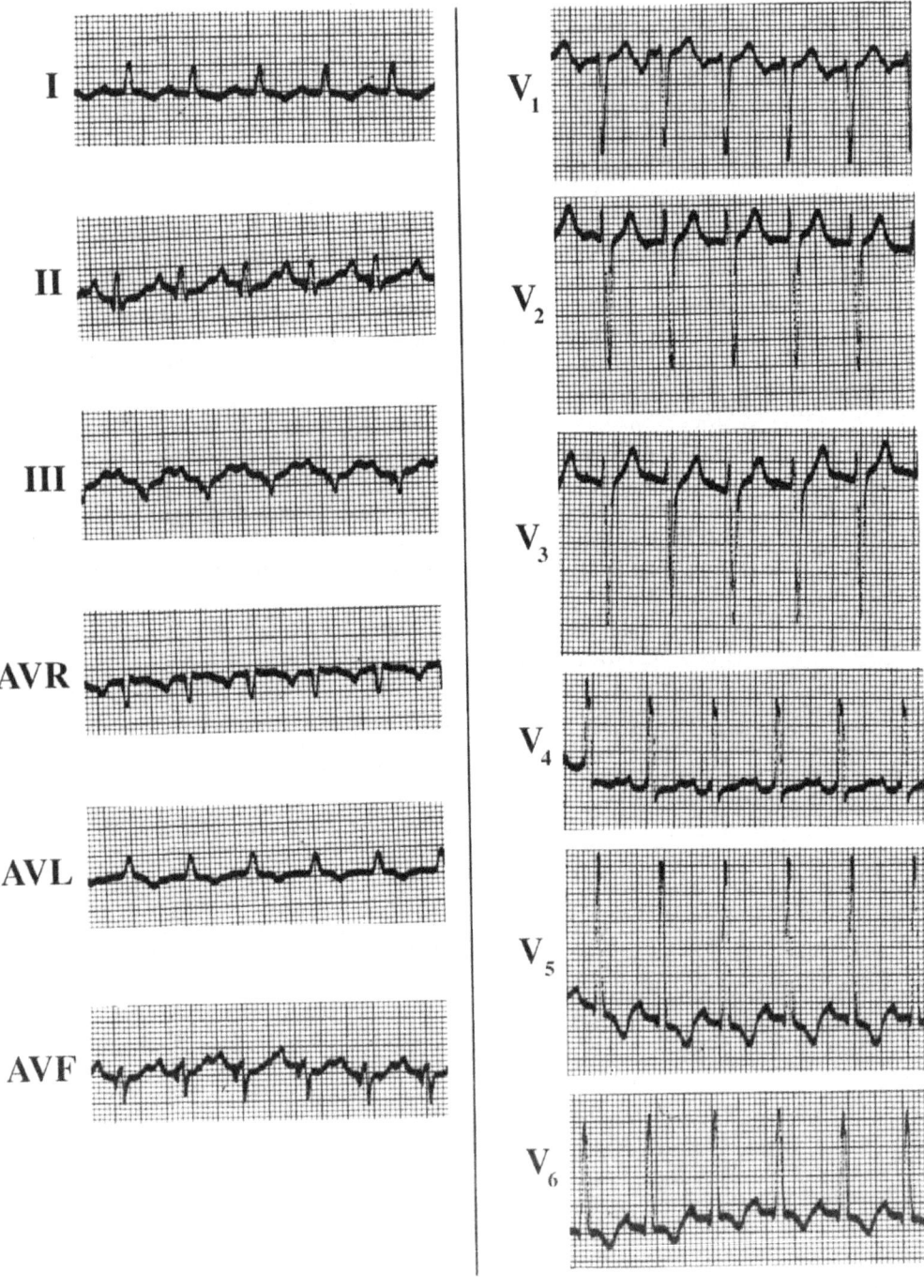

EKG Interpretation

Patient:	M.A.
Rate:	about 125/minute
Rhythm:	Sinus Tachycardia *PR* is less than .2 sec. (No AV Block). *QRS* is less than .12 sec. (No BBB).
Axis:	Left Axis Deviation (minimal amplitude of QRS in limb leads make exact axis determination difficult). No rotation in the horizontal plane.
Hypertrophy:	Left atrial hypertrophy. Left ventricular hypertrophy with strain.
Infarction: (coronary vascular status)	*Q waves* are present in II, III, and AVF. *ST segments*: generally isoelectric (on baseline), but V_5 and V_6 show strain pattern. *T waves* are inverted in I and AVL, and also in V_5, V_6.
Comment:	This patient has hypertrophy of both the left atrium and left ventricle with a left ventricular strain pattern. The patient also had an old inferior infarction. The Left Axis Deviation is caused by the Mean QRS Vector pointing away from the (old) inferior M.I. and toward the thickened left ventricle. It does *not* represent Hemiblock. There is currently (lateral) ischemia in the distribution of the Left Circumflex Coronary Artery.

R.M., an anxious, obese, 57 year old white male whose law practice was failing, complained of "tight, squeezing" pain in his anterior chest. An electrocardiogram was quickly taken by an Emergency Medical Technician.

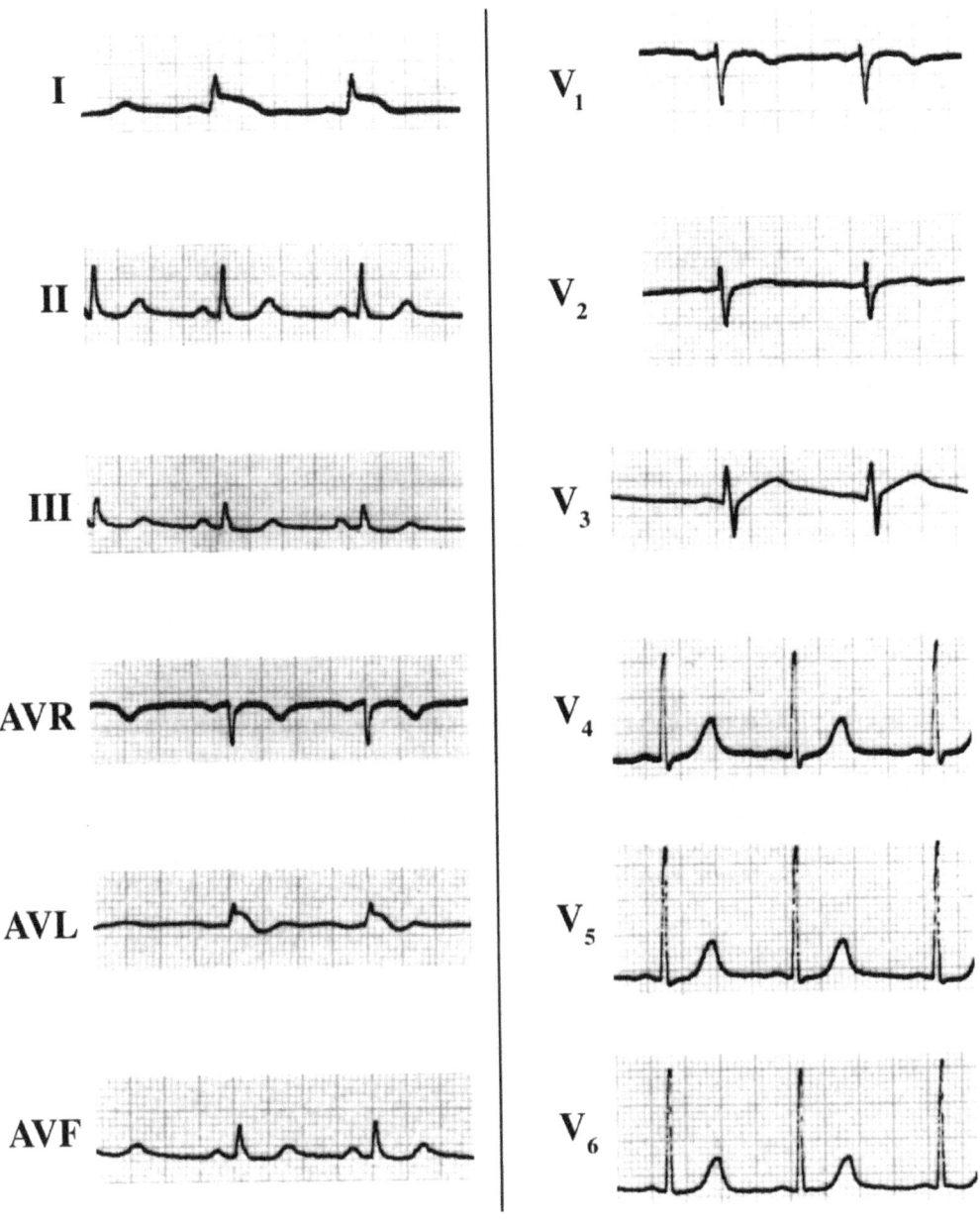

EKG Interpretation

Patient: R.M.

Rate: 75/minute

Rhythm: Sinus Rhythm
                PR .16 sec. (No AV Block).
                QRS .08 sec. (No BBB).

Axis: about +45° (Normal).
                No rotation in the horizontal plane.

Hypertrophy: Possible minimal left atrial hypertrophy.
                No ventricular hypertrophy.

Infarction: *Q waves*: no significant Q waves.
(coronary   *ST segments*: elevated 2+ mm. in I and AVL.
vascular   *T waves*: inverted in I and AVL.
status)

Comment: It is interesting that in this innocuous appearing EKG there is a subtle
                non-Q wave infarction in the lateral left ventricle, which very soon
                developed into a serious lateral infarction. Symptomatology suggestive
                of M.I. always must be investigated and scrutinized.

Index

18874469R00208